CLINICAL PHARMACOLOGY IN PSYCHIATRY
Bridging the Experimental–Therapeutic Gap

Edited by

LARS F.GRAM

Department of Clinical Pharmacology, Odense University, School of Medicine, Odense, Denmark

EARL USDIN

Department of Psychiatry and Human Behavior, University of California at Irvine, Irvine, California, USA

SVEIN G.DAHL

Department of Pharmacology, Institute of Medical Biology, University of Tromsø, Tromsø, Norway

PER KRAGH-SØRENSEN

Department of Psychiatry, Odense University, School of Medicine, Odense, Denmark

FOLKE SJÖQVIST

Department of Clinical Pharmacology, Karolinska Institute, Huddinge University Hospital, Huddinge, Sweden

and

PAOLO L.MORSELLI

L.E.R.S. Synthélabo, Paris, France

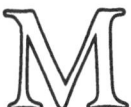

First published 1983 by
The Scientific and Medical Division
MACMILLAN PRESS LTD
London and Basingstoke
Companies and representatives throughout the world

ISBN 978-1-349-06673-5   ISBN 978-1-349-06671-1 (eBook)
DOI 10.1007/978-1-349-06671-1

Designed by Medimedia Ltd, Godalming, Surrey

The members of the Organising Committee for the Third International Meeting on Clinical Pharmacology in Psychiatry held in Odense (Hindsgavl) June 13-16, 1982, were

Lars F. Gram, Odense University
Earl Usdin, University of California at Irvine
Svein G. Dahl, University of Tromsø
Per Kragh-Sørensen, Odense University
Folke Sjöqvist, Karolinska Institute
Paolo L. Morselli, L.E.R.S. Synthélabo

Contents

Participants

AUSTRALIA

Graham D. Burrows
  Department of Psychiatry,
  University of Melbourne,
  Clinical Sciences Block,
  Royal Melbourne Hospital,
  Victoria 3050, Australia

Denis N. Wade
  University of New South Wales,
  School of Physiology and
      Pharmacology,
  St Vincent's Hospital,
  P.O.Box 1,
  Kensington,
  Darlinghurst 2010, Australia

CANADA

Paul A. Mitenko
  Department of Medicine,
  The University of Manitoba,
  Health Sciences Centre - C4,
  7000 William Avenue,
  Winnipeg,
  Manitoba R3E 0Z3, Canada

Edward M. Sellers
  Addiction Research Foundation,
  Clinical Pharmacology Program
      and Clinical Research Unit,
  33 Russell Street,
  Toronto,
  Ontario M5S 2S1, Canada

DENMARK

Lars Andersen
  Ciba-Geigy A/S,
  Lyngbyvej 172,
  DK-2100 København Ø, Denmark

Per Bech
  Department of Psychiatry,
  Frederiksborg County Hospital,
  DK-3400 Hillerød, Denmark

Peder Christensen
  Department of Psychiatry,
  Odense University Hospital,
  J.B. Winsløws Vej 20,
  DK-5000 Odense C, Denmark

Lars F. Gram
  Department of Clinical
      Pharmacology,
  Odense University,
  J.B. Winsløws Vej 19,
  DK-5000 Odense C, Denmark

Lars Bolvig Hansen
  Department B,
  Sct. Hans Hospital,
  DK-4000 Roskilde, Denmark

Axel Jørgensen
  Research Laboratories,
  H. Lundbeck & Co. A/S,
  Ottiliavej 7-9,
  DK-2500 Valby, Denmark

René Klysner
  Department of Pharmacology,
  University of Copenhagen,
  Juliane Mariesvej 20,
  DK-2100 København Ø, Denmark

Per Kragh-Sørensen
  Department of Psychiatry,
  Odense University Hospital,
  J.B. Winsløws Vej 20,
  DK-5000 Odense C, Denmark

Christian Bruun Kristensen
  Department of Clinical
    Pharmacology,
  Odense University,
  J.B. Winsløws Vej 19,
  DK-5000 Odense C, Denmark

Erling T. Mellerup
  Psychochemistry Institute,
  Rigshospitalet,
  DK-2100 Copenhagen Ø, Denmark

Rolf Bang Olsen
  Department of Psychiatry,
  Odense University Hospital,
  J.B. Winsløws Vej 20,
  DK-5000 Odense C, Denmark

Kerstin Fredricson Overø
  Research Laboratories,
  H. Lundbeck & Co. A/S,
  Ottiliavej 7-9,
  DK-2500 Valby, Denmark

Ove L. Pedersen
  Department of Psychiatry,
  Odense University Hospital,
  J.B. Winsløws Vej 20,
  DK-5000 Odense C, Denmark

Mogens Schou
  Psychopharmacology Research
    Unit,
  Aarhus University,
  Psychiatry Hospital,
  DK-8240 Risskov, Denmark

ENGLAND

David G. Grahame-Smith
  MRC Clinical Pharmacology Unit
    and University Dept of
    Clinical Pharmacology,
  Radcliffe Infirmary,
  Woodstock Road,
  Oxford OX2 6HE, England

David Wiles
  MRC Clinical Pharmacology Unit
    and University Dept of
    Clinical Pharmacology,
  Radcliffe Infirmary,
  Woodstock Road,
  Oxford OX2 6HE, England

FRANCE

Guiseppe Bartholini
  L.E.R.S. Synthélabo,
  58 rue de la Glacière,
  F-75013 Paris, France

Jean Paul Brun
  Rhône-Poulenc Santé,
  22 Cours Albert 1er,
  F-75008 Paris, France

Salomon Z. Langer
  L.E.R.S. Synthélabo,
  58 rue de la Glacière,
  F-75013 Paris, France

Paolo L. Morselli
  L.E.R.S. Synthélabo,
  58 rue de la Glacière,
  F-75013 Paris, France

Pierre Simon
  Université Paris IV,
  Département de Pharmacologie,
  Faculté de Médicine
    Pitié-Salpêtriére,
  91 Boulevard de l'Hôpital,
  F-75634 Paris Cédex 13, France

GERMANY

Hendrick M. Emrich
  Max-Planck-Institut für
    Psychiatrie,
  Kraepelinstrasse 10,
  D-8000 München 40, FRG

H.-J. Kuss
  Psychiatrische Klinik und
    Poliklinik,
  Nervenklinik der Universität
    München,
  Nussbaumstrasse 7,
  D-8000 München 2, FRG

THE NETHERLANDS

Robert M. Pigache
  Organon,
  Scientific Development Group,
  The Medical Unit,
  Oss, The Netherlands

Roger M. Pinder
  Organon,
  Scientific Development Group,
  The Medical Unit,
  Oss, The Netherlands

NORTHERN IRELAND

David J. King
  Department of Clinical
    Pharmacology,
  The Queen's University,
  Belfast, N. Ireland

NORWAY

Svein G. Dahl
  Institute of Medical Biology,
  University of Tromsø,
  N-9001 Tromsø, Norway

SPAIN

Dolors Capellà
  Divisió de Farmacologia
    Clínica,
  Unitat Docent de la Facultat
    de Medicina,
  Universitat Autònoma de
    Barcelona,
  Barcelona, España

Joan-Ramon Laporte
  Divisió de Farmacologia
    Clínica,
  Unitat Docent de la Facultat
    de Medicina,
  Universitat Autònoma de
    Barcelona,
  Barcelona, España

SWEDEN

Rolf Axelsson
  Department III,
  Lillhagen Hospital,
  S-422 03 Hisings Backa, Sweden

Ulf Bergman
  Department of Clinical
    Pharmacology,
  Huddinge University Hospital,
  S-141 86 Huddinge, Sweden

Leif Bertilsson
  Department of Clinical
    Pharmacology,
  Huddinge University Hospital,
  S-141 86 Huddinge, Sweden

Gunnar Dahlgren
  Marknadsavdelningen,
  Ciba-Geigy Läkemedel AB,
  Box 605,
  S-421 26 Västra Frölunda,
  Sweden

Gustav Plum Forshell
  Research Division,
  AB Leo, Fack,
  S-251 00 Hälsingborg, Sweden

Margaretha Grind
  Research Division,
  Astra AB,
  S-151 85 Södertälje, Sweden

Håkan Hall
  Research Division,
  Astra AB,
  S-151 85 Södertälje, Sweden

Lothar Herrmann
  Research Division,
  AB Leo, Fack,
  S-251 00 Hälsingborg, Sweden

Folke Sjöqvist
  Department of Clinical
    Pharmacology,
  Huddinge University Hospital,
  S-141 86 Huddinge, Sweden

Kjell Strandberg
  Socialstyrelsens
    Läkemedelsavdelning,
  Box 607,
  S-751 25 Uppsala, Sweden

SWITZERLAND

Luc P. Balant
  Pharmacologie Clinique,
  Zyma SA,
  CH-1260 Nyon, Switzerland

Androniki Balant-Gorgia
  Laboratoire de Monitoring
    Thérapeutique,
  Département de Psychiatrie,
  Centre Médical Universitaire,
  CH-1211 Geneva 4, Switzerland

Pierre Baumann
  Hopital de Cery,
  Clinique Psychiatrique
    Universitaire,
  Canton de Vaud,
  CH-1008 Prilly, Switzerland

USA

Bernard J. Carroll
  The University of Michigan,
  Mental Health Research
    Institute,
  Department of Psychiatry,
  Ann Arbor, MI 48109, USA

Joseph T. Coyle
  Department of Pharmacology,
  Johns Hopkins University,
  School of Medicine,
  725 North Wolfe Street,
  Baltimore, MD 21205, USA

Alexander H. Glassman
  Department of Psychiatry,
  College of Physicians and
    Surgeons,
  Columbia University,
  722 West 168th Street,
  New York, NY 10032, USA

Leo E. Hollister
  Veterans Administration
    Hospital,
  3801 Miranda Avenue,
  Palo Alto, CA 92161, USA

Markku Linnoila
  Clinical Psychobiology Branch,
  National Institute of Mental
    Health,
  9000 Rockville Pike,
  Building 10,
  Bethesda, MD 20205, USA

Steven M. Paul
  Clinical Neuroscience Branch,
  National Institute of Mental
    Health,
  9000 Rockville Pike,
  Building 10,
  Bethesda, MD 20205, USA

Russell E. Poland
  Division of Biological
    Psychiatry,
  Department of Psychiatry,
  Harbor-UCLA Medical Center,
  1000 West Carson Street,
  Torrance, CA 90509, USA

William Z. Potter
  Clinical Psychobiology Branch,
  National Institute of Mental
    Health,
  9000 Rockville Pike,
  Building 10,
  Bethesda, MD 20205, USA

Elliott Richelson
  Departments of Psychiatry and
    Pharmacology,
  Mayo Foundation,
  Rochester, MN 55901, USA

Robert T. Rubin
  Department of Psychiatry,
  Harbor-ULCA Medical Center,
  1000 West Carson Street,
  Torrance, CA 90509, USA

Earl Usdin
  Department of Psychiatry and
    Human Behavior,
  California College of
    Medicine,
  University of California at
    Irvine,
  Irvine, CA 92717, USA

Preface

At the International Meetings on Clinical Pharmacology in Psychiatry (IMCPP), the first held in Chicago 1979, the second in Tromsø 1980 and now the third in Odense (Hindsgavl), experimental pharmacologists, clinical pharmacologists and clinicians have met for in-depth discussion of various fields of psychopharmacology. Particular aims of these meetings have been to increase the mutual understanding of research strategies and methodological problems in these fields, and to bridge the gap between experimental findings and clinical applications of new knowledge.

The 3rd IMCPP, held at Hindsgavl Castle in the western corner of the island Fyn, thus brought together experts from a wide range of fields and from many countries. Nonetheless, a high degree of mutual understanding of principles and problems was achieved, and the 18-20 hours daylight in Denmark in June permitted long and stimulating discussions. The papers presented at the meeting and published in this book illustrate the continuity from experimental research to clinical utilization of psychotropic drugs.

Odense, Irvine, Tromsø, L.F.G.
Huddinge and Paris, E.U.
1982 S.G.D.
P.K.-S.
F.S.
P.L.M.

xv

Acknowledgements

This meeting was supported by international and national institutions as well as a number of European pharmaceutical companies. We gratefully acknowledge support from the following:

International Union of Pharmacology (IUPHAR), Section of
    Clinical Pharmacology
Danish Medical Research Council
Odense University, School of Medicine
A.-L. Pharma, Copenhagen, Denmark
Astra, Södertälje, Sweden
Ciba-Geigy, Copenhagen, Denmark, and Gothenburg, Sweden
Dumex, Copenhagen, Denmark
Essex-Pharma, Copenhagen, Denmark
Ferrosan, Copenhagen, Denmark
Leo, Helsingborg, Sweden
Lundbeck, Copenhagen, Denmark
Organon, Oss, The Netherlands
Rhône-Poulenc, Paris, France
Roche, Copenhagen, Denmark
Synthélabo, Paris, France

In addition we should like to thank Mrs Gitte Halling for excellent technical assistance at all stages of the organizing of the meeting and the editing of the book.

Abbreviations

AAG	α₁-acid glycoprotein (= orosomucoid)	ECS	electroconvulsive shock
ACTH	corticotrophin	ECT	electroconvulsive (shock) therapy
AMP	adenosine monophosphate	ED	equilibrium dialysis
		EEG	electroencephalogram
APS	Adverse Drug Reaction Probability Scale	EPhMRA	European Pharmaceutical Market Research Association
ATC	Anatomical-Therapeutic-Chemical (classification system)	EPS	extrapyramidal side-effects
		GABA	γ-aminobutyric acid
ATP	adenosine triphosphate	GABA-T	GABA transaminase
AUC	area under the curve	GAD	glutamic acid decarboxylase
cAMP	cyclic AMP		
β-CCE	3-carboethoxy-β-carboline	GAS	Global Assessment of Severity
CNS	central nervous system	GFR	glomerular filtration rate
CPRS	Comprehensive Psychiatric Rating Scale	GMP	guanosine monophosphate
c.p.s.	cycles per second	GTP	guanosine triphosphate
CSA	(Northern Ireland) Central Services Agency	HBE	His bundle electrocardiography
CSF	cerebrospinal fluid	HDRS	Hamilton Depression Rating Scale
CVS	cardiovascular system		
DA	dopamine	5-HIAA	5-hydroxyindole acetic acid
DDAVP	desmopressin acetate		
DDD	defined daily dose	5-HT	serotonin
DHA	dihydroalprenolol	5-HTP	5-hydroxytrytophan
DHSS	(UK) Department of Health and Social Services	HVA	homovanillic acid
		ICD	International Classification of Disease (WHO)
dopa	dihydroxyphenylalanine		
DSM-III	Diagnostic and Statistical Manual of Mental Disorders - 3rd edition	ICU	Intensive Care Unit
		i.c.v.	intraventricularly
		IDF	imipramine displacing factor
DST	dexamethasone suppression test	IMCPP	International Meeting on Clinical Pharmacology in Psychiatry
ECG	electrocardiogram		

i.n.	intranasal	PEP	pre-ejection period
Li	lithium (salt)	QNB	quinuclidinyl
LVET	left ventricular		benzilate
	ejection time	REM	rapid eye movement
MAO	monoamine oxidase		(sleep)
MAOI	MAO inhibitor	RIA	radioimmunoassay
5-MeODMT	5-methoxy-N,N-	SADS	Schedule for Affective
	dimethyltryptamine		Disorders and
MHPG	3-methoxy-4-hydroxy-		Schizophrenia
	phenylglycol	SGOT	serum glutamate-
NDA	(US Food and Drug		oxaloacetate
	Administration) New		transaminase
	Drug Application	SLi	serum lithium
NE	norepinephrine	TCA	tricyclic anti-
NHS	(UK) National Health		depressant(s)
	Service	UF	ultrafiltration
PCPA	p-chlorophenylalanine	VMA	vanillylmandelic acid
PDLP	phenylalanine-D-	WHO	World Health
	lysine-phenylalanine		Organization

Section One

Utilization of Psychotropic Drugs: Geographical and Cultural Determinants and Relationship to Morbidity

Utilization of psychotropic drugs in Sweden and the other Nordic countries

Ulf Bergman[1], Ingegerd Agenäs[2] and Monica Dahlström[2]

INTRODUCTION

Marked geographical differences have been found in the utilization of important drugs, e.g. antidiabetics, antihypertensives and psychotropics, both within and between several European countries (Bergman *et al.*, 1975, 1979b; Grimsson *et al.*, 1977; Baksaas, 1978). As there are no data available to suggest correspondingly large differences in the disease patterns between these countries, geographical variations are of great potential interest to public health.

Inappropriate use of drugs is a matter of concern to public health authorities, pharmacologists, doctors and patients (Sjöqvist, 1975). Drug utilization studies are a great help in detecting discrepancies between prescribing practices and acceptable pharmacotherapeutic principles. The studies give additional knowledge that can be used in rational planning and follow-ups of drug information programs. They comprise studies of the use of drugs in different geographical areas, prescribing patterns of physicians and patients' drug-taking behavior.

In agreement with the suggestions made by the WHO Symposium in 1969 (World Health Organization, 1970), statistics on drug utilization have been published regularly in Sweden since the mid-1970s (Svensk Läkemedelsstatistik, 1980-1982). Similarly the Nordic Council on Medicines has decided to publish statistics on medicines regularly. Through these sources, sales figures of psychotropic drugs in the five Nordic countries between 1975 and 1980 have been made available for this paper (Nordic Council on Medicines, 1979, 1982). These data will be discussed in relation to Swedish national prescription data.

---

[1]Department of Clinical Pharmacology, Karolinska Institutet, Huddinge University Hospital, S-141 86 Huddinge, Sweden.
[2]National Corporation of Swedish Pharmacies, S-105 14 Stockholm, Sweden.

In a cross-national interview study of the use of certain psychotropic drugs, differences in use were found between a number of European countries (Balter *et al.*, 1974). This finding and the fact that there are no strict guidelines for the prescribing of many psychotropic drugs make it important to study their utilization and to follow its development with time.

MATERIALS AND METHODS

Type of Data Available

Denmark, Finland, Iceland, Norway and Sweden constitute the five Nordic countries with 22 million inhabitants, ranging from 0.225 million in Iceland to 8.3 million in Sweden.

Drug utilization can be studied using wholesale statistics available from drug manufacturers or national drug control agencies and data available through prescriptions retrieved from pharmacies inside and outside health institutions.

Drug utilization at the patient level can be studied by interviews, recording of the drug purchases of the individual patient and monitoring of drug concentrations.

If not otherwise stated, wholesale data, which are available in all Nordic countries, are used in this paper. These data should not be regarded as synonymous with the real intake of drugs in the populations studied, but they reflect fairly well the attitude among physicians to the use of psychotropic drugs.

Data on drug use in hospitals are available only in Sweden.

A continuous Swedish nationwide prescription survey gives information about, for example, the age and sex of the patient and the number of prescribed daily doses for each drug. The survey is a 1-in-288 representative sample of all prescriptions filled at Swedish pharmacies (Kristoferson and Wessling, 1977).

Since 1978 the Diagnosis and Therapy Survey (Agenäs *et al.*, 1980) has given information about the diagnoses behind drug prescribing (International Classification of Disease: World Health Organization, 1965). The information is obtained from a running random sample of physicians participating for one week each.

Unit of Comparison

In 1981, four companies furnished the Swedish drug market with about 70 diazepam preparations: oral, rectal and parenteral dosage forms in various strengths and pack sizes and at different prices. The difficulty of getting an accurate estimate of the overall utilization of diazepam is thus obvious. It is even more complicated to compare the utilization of similar drugs, e.g. diazepam versus oxazepam or nitrazepam.

To permit convenient comparisons of the utilization of similar drugs, so-called defined daily doses (DDD) were established
for each drug (Baksaas-Aasen *et al*., 1975; Lunde *et al*., 1979).
The DDD was chosen according to what was recommended to be the
average maintenance dose of the particular drug on its assumed
major indication. The DDD shall be regarded as a technical unit
of measurement and comparison.

In Sweden the overall utilization of diazepam (DDD = 10 mg)
was 32 million DDDs in 1981. The corresponding number for nitrazepam (DDD = 5 mg) was 74 million DDDs. The number of DDDs per 1000
inhabitants per day should give a rough estimate of the number of
subjects who might have used the drug in a certain area, e.g. 10.5
DDDs of diazepam per 1000 inhabitants per day compared to 24.3
DDDs of nitrazepam (Svensk Läkemedelsstatistik, 1982).

The sum of all drugs within a therapeutic group represents an
estimate of the 'therapeutic intensity' in the population (e.g.
45.9 DDDs of benzodiazepines per 1000 inhabitants per day in
Sweden in 1981).

For drugs used in various doses for different purposes (e.g.
neuroleptics) and for drugs used in short-term treatment (e.g.
antibiotics, minor analgesics), there is no relevance in morbidity
calculations of the DDD per 1000 inhabitants per day estimate.
Furthermore, the estimate does not take into account differences
in the frequency of combination therapy.

Classification

A prerequisite for comparisons of drug utilization between geographical areas and over time is a common classification of drugs.
The comparisons of wholesale data between the five Nordic
countries were based on the Anatomical-Therapeutic-Chemical
Classification system (ATC code) - a five-level code which is a
development of the three-level EPhMRA/IPMRG code (Nordic Council
on Medicines, 1979). On its fifth level, the ATC code identifies
single chemical substances. (As an example, all plain diazepam
preparations are given the code N 05 B A 01.)

RESULTS AND DISCUSSION

The pattern and extent of psychotropic drug use were different in
the five Nordic countries in the period 1975 through 1980 (figure
1). The publication of the data initially available in four
countries (Denmark excluded) has obviously also had some impact on
the overall sales in the preceding years (Grimsson *et al*., 1977).
Hypnotics, sedatives (N 05 C) and *tranquilizers* (N 05 B) dominated
the sales in all countries but the trends in use were quite different (figure 1). In Denmark, with the highest use of hypnotics

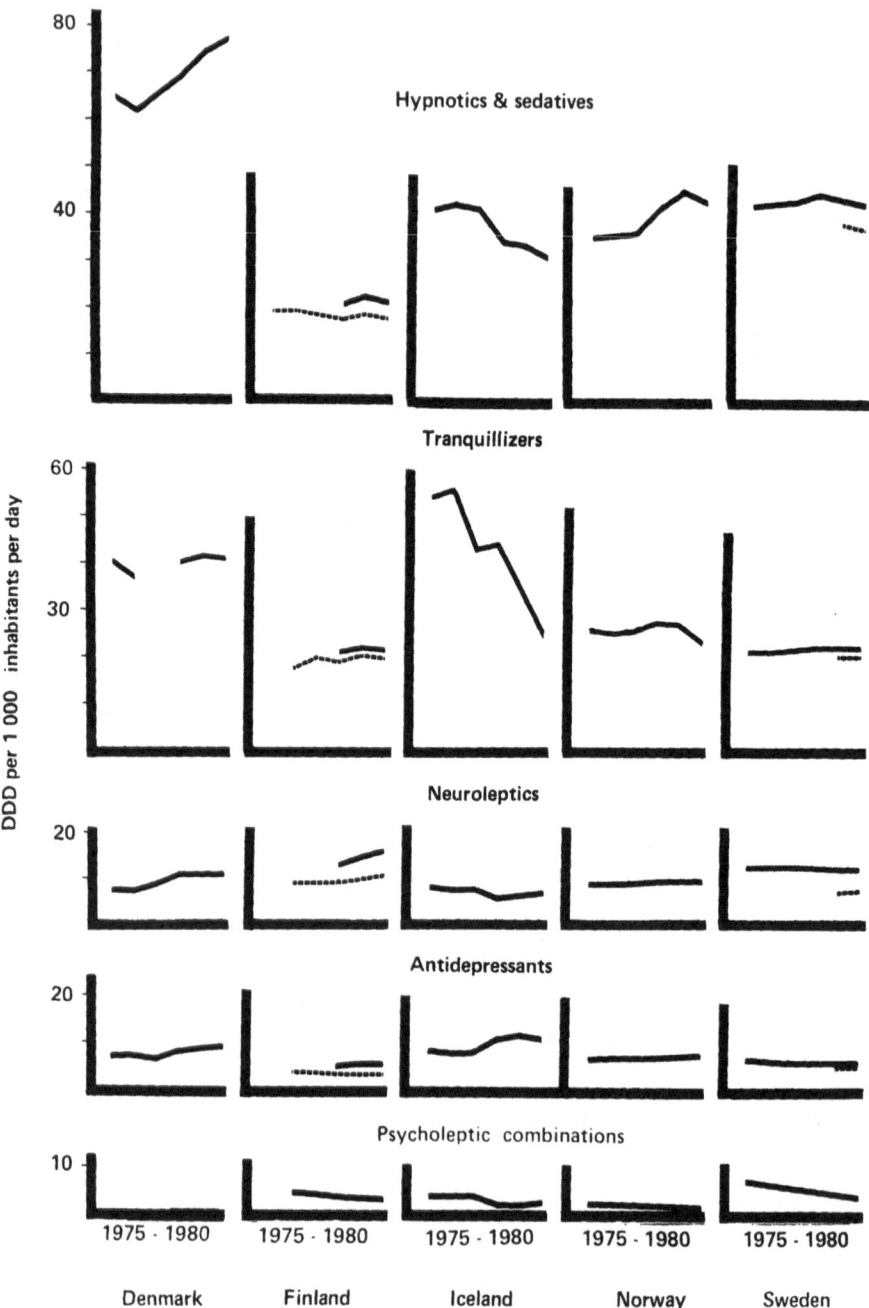

Figure 1.   Trends in sales of psychotropic drugs in the Nordic
            countries.   From the top: hypnotics and sedatives

(N 05 C), tranquilizers (N 05 B), neuroleptics (N 05 A), antidepressants (N 06 A + C) and psycholeptic combinations (A 03 C) (see text). Amitriptyline combined with chlordiazepoxide or perfenazine (N 06 C) were only available in Finland, where it made up 31% of the total outpatient antidepressant use in 1980 and was included here in the figure for antidepressants. Psychostimulants (N 06 B), below 1 DDD per 1000 inhabitants per day in all countries, are not included. The area between the dotted and solid lines indicates hospital sales in Finland (estimates) and in Sweden (Nordic Council on Medicines, 1979, 1982).

and sedatives in 1975, a gradual increase was seen during the study period, whereas the use of these drugs and of tranquilizers decreased in Iceland.

In Iceland, a 20% reduction in the use of hypnotics, sedatives and tranquilizers was found between 1976 and 1978, partly depending on the removal of the 10 mg tablets of diazepam from the market and partly as an effect of feedback to doctors about their prescribing habits (Olafsson *et al.*, 1980), an effect that seems to have persisted through 1980.

In Norway the use of tranquilizers during 1975 through 1977 was 25% higher than that in Finland and Sweden. In 1980 the use was almost at the same level in all three countries due to a new regulation allowing prescriptions for tranquilizers to be dispensed only once and by removing some drugs from the Norwegian market, e.g. most of the barbiturates and methaqualone (Halvorsen and Jøldal, 1981).

In Finland and Sweden, the use of hypnotics, sedatives and tranquilizers was very stable in this six-year period. The sales of hypnotics and sedatives, however, were much lower in Finland than in any other Nordic country. The use of benzodiazepines (N 05 BA and N 05 CD) (figure 2) varied between 73% in Denmark and Sweden and almost 100% in Iceland of the total use of hypnotics/sedatives and tranquilizers in 1980. Diazepam and nitrazepam dominated the use in all five countries in that year.

Barbiturates were still in use in four countries (not in Iceland) with a general downward trend. The use in Denmark (about 22 DDD per 1000 inhabitants per day) was threefold that in Sweden. In 1980 Finland and Norway had the lowest use of barbiturates, 4 and 1 DDD per 1000 inhabitants per day, respectively.

Neuroleptics (N 05 A) are a group of drugs creating special problems in the interpretation of results obtained by the DDD methodology. Neuroleptic drugs are used for several indications besides psychosis and, therefore, in different dosages and modes of administration and in combination with other drugs. The DDDs for neuroleptics are based on the treatment of psychosis (the assumed major indication). A much lower dose is given for minor

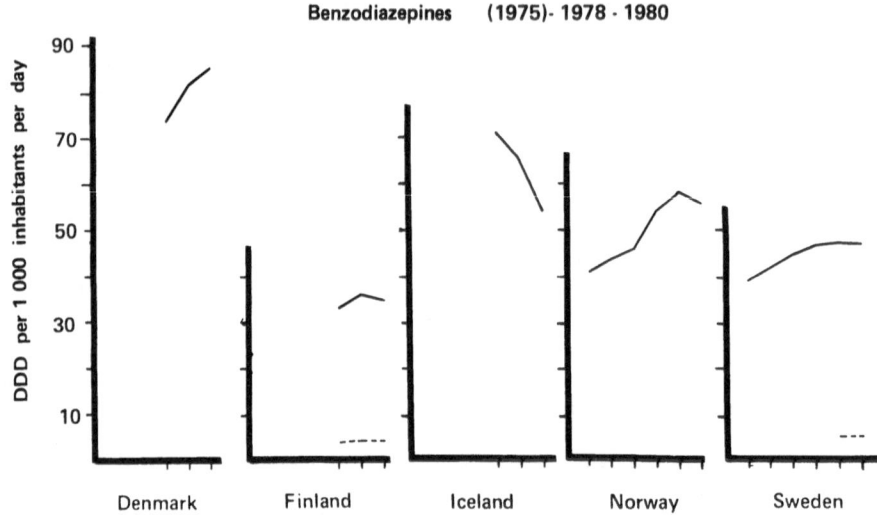

Figure 2. Trends in sales of benzodiazepines (N 05 BA, N 05 CD) in the Nordic countries: Denmark, Finland, Iceland, Norway and Sweden in (1975)–1978–1980. The area between the dotted and base lines indicates hospital sales (Nordic Council on Medicines, 1979, 1982).

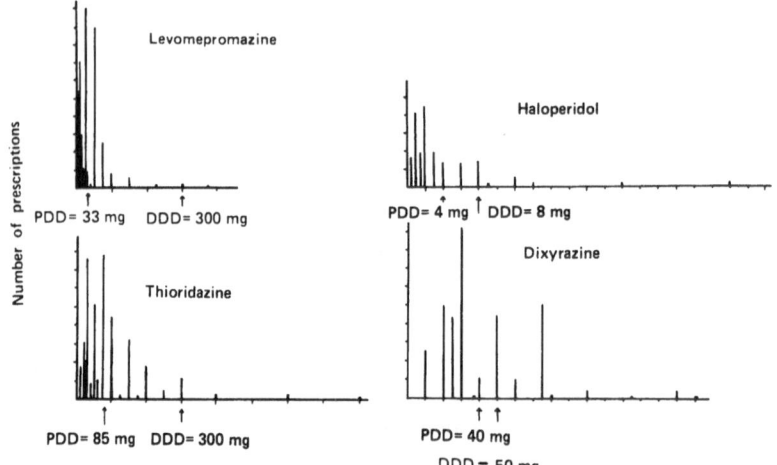

Figure 3. Variability in the prescribed daily doses of certain neuroleptic drugs (N 05 A) in Sweden in 1980 – data from the nationwide prescription survey. As indicated by arrows the average prescribed daily dose (PDD) is lower than the defined daily dose (DDD). For levomepromazine PDD/DDD = 0.11, for thioridazine 0.28, for haloperidol 0.50, and for dixyrazine 0.80.

psychiatric disturbances (figure 3). In Sweden, these drugs have also been recommended to be used as hypnotics and minor tranquilizers (Edgren and Roos, 1970).

At the time of publication of the *Nordic Statistics on Medicines*, no national data on the indications for drug prescribing were available in Sweden or in the other Nordic countries. In a study at a multi-doctor district health center in Sweden, minor psychiatric symptoms, such as sleep disturbances, were found to be common reasons for the prescribing of neuroleptics (Bergman *et al.*, 1979a). The Diagnosis and Therapy Survey (Agenäs *et al.*, 1980) shows that minor psychiatric symptoms were also common reasons for the prescribing of neuroleptics to outpatients in the period 1978 through 1981 (tables 1 and 2). This finding would explain the high use of neuroleptics in Sweden compared with the other Nordic countries with the exception of Finland (see below). Interestingly, hospital consumption represented as much as about 40% of the total use of neuroleptics, a fact which suggests that psychosis may still be the major indication for the overall use of neuroleptics as assumed when establishing DDDs for neuroleptics.

In the first Nordic publication, Finnish hospital data were missing (Nordic Council on Medicines, 1979). In 1978 through 1980 estimated hospital data indicate that Finland had the highest utilization of neuroleptic drugs compared with all the other Nordic countries. No information on indications for drug prescribing in Finland is officially available. However, if neuroleptic drugs were commonly prescribed in minor psychiatric disorders in Finland as well, it could explain the relatively low sales of other psychotropics there compared to other Nordic countries (figure 1).

There was a wide variation in the use of *lithium* (N 05 AX, DDD = 24 mmol) between the five Nordic countries in the period 1978 through 1980 (Nordic Council on Medicines, 1982; Bergman, 1981). Denmark and Sweden were the highest users, their consumption being about five times that of Iceland, which was the lowest user (about 1.3 and 0.3 DDD per 1000 inhabitants per day, respectively). Norway and Finland had an intermediate use of lithium (0.5-0.6 DDD per 1000 inhabitants per day). Since 1976-1977 there has been a decline in the use of lithium in Sweden, possibly related to a report suggesting chronic renal lesions following long-term treatment with lithium (Hestbech *et al.*, 1977). Interestingly, the pattern of use in individual counties in Sweden varied greatly. In a few counties a low and stable level of about the same height as in Finland and Norway was seen during the period 1975 through 1980. In one county there was a steep increase above the Swedish mean. The three counties with the highest use in the period 1975 through 1977 showed marked decrease in the period 1978 through 1980. Recently, a group of experts from the Nordic countries recommended general principles for long-term lithium therapy (Amdisen *et al.*, 1980). It will thus be of great interest

Table 1. Most commonly stated indications for prescribing psychotropic drugs in Sweden (data from the Diagnosis and Therapy Survey in 1978-1981 (Agenäs *et al.*, 1980)).

Neuroleptics (N 05 A) (n = 2057)		Tranquilizers (N 05 B) (n = 4529)	
Psychoneurosis	41%	Psychoneurosis	60%
Psychosis	22%	Disturbance of sleep	18%
Disturbance of sleep	11%	Depression	4%
Alcoholism	5%	Psychosis	2%
Depression	5%	Other indications	16%
Other indications	16%		

Hypnotics and sedatives (N 05 C) (n = 3489)		Antidepressants (N 06 A) (n = 1288)	
Disturbance of sleep	73%	Depression	49%
Psychoneurosis	9%	Psychoneurosis	24%
Depression	2%	Psychosis	13%
Psychosis	2%	Disturbance of sleep	4%
Other indications	14%	Other indications	10%

Table 2. Most commonly stated indications for prescribing certain neuroleptic drugs (N 05 A) in Sweden (data from the Diagnosis and Therapy Survey in 1978-1981 (Agenäs *et al.*, 1980)).

Thioridazine (n = 275)		Levomepromazine (n = 296)	
Psychoneurosis	46%	Disturbance of sleep	46%
Psychosis	27%	Psychoneurosis	19%
Depression	6%	Psychosis	16%
Disturbance of sleep	5%	Alcoholism	3%
Alcoholism	1%	Depression	2%
Other indications	15%	Other indications	14%

Dixyrazine (n = 339)		Haloperidol (n = 137)	
Psychoneurosis	57%	Psychosis	51%
Alcoholism	14%	Psychoneurosis	30%
Disturbance of sleep	11%	Disturbance of sleep	2%
Depression	3%	Depression	2%
Psychosis	2%	Other indications	15%
Other indications	13%		

to follow the future trends in the use of lithium in the Nordic countries, and also to relate the use to the frequency of adverse reactions (Bergman *et al.*, 1978).

Antidepressants (N 06 A + C) also showed differences in the pattern and extent of use between the five countries (figure 1). Amitriptyline was the most common antidepressant drug in all the Nordic countries. Coinciding with the decrease in the use of hypnotics, sedatives and tranquilizers in Iceland, there was an increase of almost 40% in the use of antidepressants, which became twofold that in Finland. A gradual increase in the use of anti-depressants is also seen in Denmark and Norway. Sulpiride, classi-fied as a neuroleptic, is available only in Finland and only for the indication of depression. If this drug is added to the anti-depressant group, the Finnish use of antidepressants approaches the same level as that in Sweden (Nordic Council on Medicines, 1982).

In 1973, a study at a district health center in Sweden showed that the non-specific psychiatric diagnoses *depressio mentis* and psychoneurosis were the principal indications for the prescribing of antidepressants (Bergman *et al.*, 1979a). Manic-depressive psychosis made up about 5% of the total number of antidepressants prescribed. Thus, as earlier shown in the Australian general practice morbidity and prescribing survey (Royal Australian College of General Practitioners, 1976) and now also by national Swedish data (table 1), antidepressants were used for rather non-specific and less well documented psychiatric disturbances.

Controlled clinical trials have shown that the mean effective dose of amitriptyline and nortriptyline in depressed hospitalized patients is around 150 mg per day (50 mg t.i.d.) (Sjöqvist, 1975), which is the dose used in comparisons with new antidepressant drugs. In 1980 the mean dosages prescribed in Sweden for ami-triptyline and nortriptyline were 61 mg and 62 mg, respectively. The dosages corresponded to those found in two earlier Swedish studies (Boethius and Sjöqvist, 1978; Bergman *et al.*, 1979a) - all far below the effective dose (150 mg) suggested for treatment of depressive disorders (Asberg, 1976) and in agreement with earlier English data from general practice (Johnson, 1974). In newly depressed patients receiving tricyclic antidepressants, he found that only one-fourth of the patients were prescribed more than 75 mg per day, and the prescribed daily dose was even lower at sub-sequent consultations. Out of the 73 general practitioners ques-tioned about what maximum dose of tricyclic drugs they would use, only 21 replied 100 mg or more as daily dose in general practice. The almost universal reason given for not using higher doses was the problem of side-effects.

Gastrointestinal antispasmodics and anticholinergics in combination with psychoactive substances (psycholeptic combi-nations) (A 03 C) were included in the section of psychotropic drugs in the first issue of *Nordic Statistics on Medicines* because it had been claimed that considerable use of so-called hidden psychotropics existed (Hemminki, 1974). The sales of psycholeptic combinations were small and decreasing in all the Nordic countries (figure 1). Data on analgesic compounds with psycholeptics were, however, not included in the first issue. In 1980, these compounds made up a low proportion of total analgesics. The lowest sales were found in Finland with most compounds on the market (Nordic Council on Medicines, 1982).

In contrast to many other countries, hidden psychotropics were widely used in Spain in 1980 (Laporte *et al.*, 1981). Nowadays, such use does not seem to be a major problem in the Nordic countries. The need for having these compounds on the market can, however, be questioned, particularly as some countries, e.g. Iceland and Norway, do not have them.

The Pattern of Age and Sex Distribution

A uniform finding in studies of drug consumption is that the use of drugs increases with age and that women are prescribed more drugs than men in almost all age groups. These facts are most pronounced in the groups hypnotics, sedatives and tranquilizers (Westerholm *et al.*, 1978). Thus, differences in age and sex distribution between populations have to be taken into account in comparisons of drug consumption.

The proportion of elderly in Sweden is higher than that in any other Nordic country. However, age and sex distribution alone does not explain the differences in drug use between the Nordic countries.

Indications for Prescribing Psychotropic Drugs

Psychoneurosis and sleep disturbances were the most common reasons for the prescribing of psychotropic drugs in Sweden (figure 4). There was a considerable overlapping in the types of drugs prescribed for the various indications (figure 4) and consequently these drugs are prescribed for a variety of reasons (table 1). Within the therapeutic subgroups the individual drugs also have their diagnostic profiles. The major reason for prescribing the neuroleptic drug levomepromazine was sleep disturbances, while psychoneurosis was the main indication stated for the prescribing of thioridazine and dixyrazine, and psychosis the main one for the prescribing of haloperidol (table 2). National characteristics in the diagnostic profiles of psychotropic drug prescribing may be a major explanation for the striking differences between the Nordic countries.

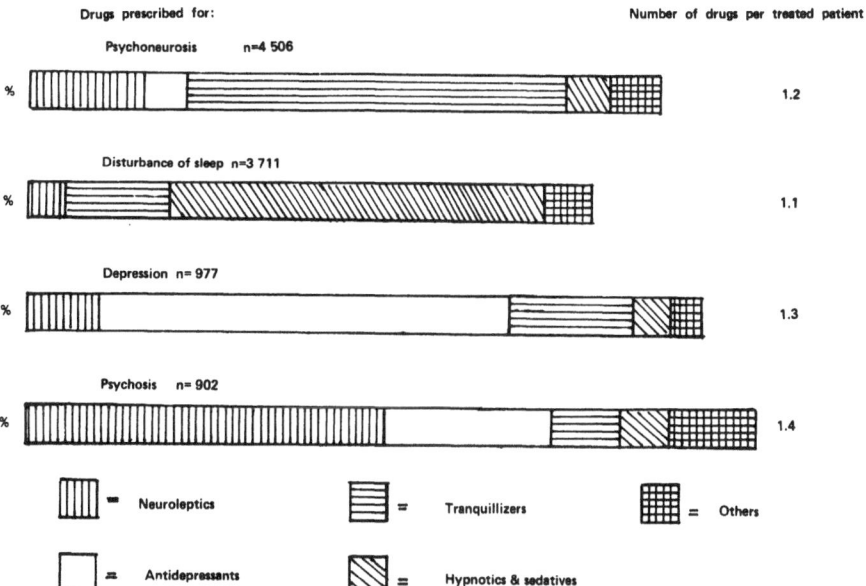

Figure 4. Drugs prescribed for the main psychiatric disorders in outpatients in Sweden from 1978 through 1981 according to the Diagnosis and Therapy Survey (Agenäs *et al.*, 1980). As more than one drug was prescribed on average, the sum is above 100%.

Hospital Drug Utilization

By using a uniform methodology in studies of drug utilization in hospitals, marked differences in the use of hypnotics, sedatives and tranquilizers were found between similar hospital wards in Czechoslovakia, Norway, Spain and Sweden (Stika *et al.*, 1981; Bjørndal, 1982; Laporte *et al.*, 1981; Westerholm, 1974; Bergman *et al.*, 1980). Deliveries of drugs were calculated in number of DDDs per bed–day (Westerholm, 1974; Bergman *et al.*, 1980). This estimate, validated in Sweden and Norway, provides a clinically relevant measure of drug utilization in hospitals (Bergman *et al.*, 1980; Bjørndal, 1982).

The Norwegian study revealed a close correlation ($r = 0.93$) between general and hospital utilization of psychotropic drugs in different parts of Norway (Bjørndal, 1982). Withdrawal of benzodiazepines in normal doses is a clinical problem (Petursson and Lader, 1981). These facts are in agreement with the findings in a Swedish study showing that long-term sleeping medication was most commonly introduced during stays in general medical wards (Bolander *et al.*, 1982).

CONCLUDING REMARKS

In the light of the large geographical variations in psychotropic drug use demonstrated here, problems related to long-term treatment with these drugs may differ between the Nordic countries. An example of such a problem is the balance between the risks of dependence on certain hypnotics, sedatives and tranquilizers and the risk of tardive dyskinesia when using low doses of neuroleptics in minor psychiatric disorders (table 2, figure 3). With available data on drug utilization, such evaluations can be specifically directed to certain geographical areas with vastly different patterns of drug use.

In view of the extensive use of psychotropic drugs reported in many countries (Balter *et al.*, 1974), it is obvious that these drugs are an important part of medical practice. Their use, like the use of alcohol, is related to cultural, social, educational, economic and political conditions. Despite the great socio-economic similarities between the Nordic countries and the close contacts between them, we were able to demonstrate marked differences in the overall use of psychotropic drugs. It is important to study the reasons for the differences, particularly the attitude among physicians to these drugs.

Drug utilization data constitute a valuable feedback instrument in the planning and evaluation of drug information programs, in detecting and identifying areas requiring further investigations and in post-marketing drug evaluations. The DDD methodology, once introduced, is an inexpensive indicator of drug utilization and a suitable basis for therapeutic audit.

Acknowledgement

We thank Mrs Ingrid Nordenstam for her help in preparing this paper.

REFERENCES

Agenäs, I., Jacobsson, M. and Kristoferson, K. (1980). Diagnos – Receptundersökningen. Svensk Farm. Tidskrift., 84, 321-33 (English summary).

Amdisen, A., Bucht, H., Dencker, S.J., Hansen, H.-E., Helgason, T., Lindstedt, G., Nagy, A., Nilsson, G., Rapp, W., Robak, O. and Sjöström, R. (1980). Do you envisage long-term treatment with lithium? Läkartidningen, 77, 35-8 (English summary).

Asberg, M. (1976). Treatment of depression with tricyclic drugs – pharmacokinetic and pharmacodynamic aspects. Pharmacopsychiatry, 9, 18-26.

Baksaas, I. (1978). Antihypertensive drugs. Adv. Pharmacol. Ther., 6, 133-40.

Baksaas-Aasen, I., Lunde, P.K.M., Halse, M., Halvorsen, I. K.,
Skobba, T.J. and Strømnes, B. (1975). Drug Dose Statistics:
List of Defined Daily Doses for Drugs Registered in Norway,
Norsk Medisinal Depot, Oslo.

Balter, M.B., Levine, J. and Manheimer, D.I. (1974). Cross-
national study of the extent of anti-anxiety/sedative drug
use. New Engl. J. Med., 290, 769–74.

Bergman, U. (1981). Studies on patterns and prevalence of
psychotropic drug use – data from the Nordic countries. In
Epidemiological Impact of Psychotropic Drugs (eds G. Tognoni,
C. Bellantuono and M. Lader), Elsevier/North-Holland Biomedical Press, Amsterdam, pp. 183–7.

Bergman, U., Boman, G. and Wiholm, B.E. (1978). Epidemiology of
adverse drug reactions to phenformin and metformin. Br. Med.
J., 2, 464–6.

Bergman, U., Christenson, I., Jansson, B. and Wiholm, B.-E.
(1980). Auditing hospital drug utilization by means of
defined daily doses per bed-day. A methodological study.
Eur. J. Clin. Pharmacol., 17, 183–7.

Bergman, U., Dahlström, M., Gunnarson, C. and Westerholm, B.
(1979a). Why are psychotropic drugs prescribed to outpatients? A methodological study. Eur. J. Clin. Pharmacol.,
15, 249–56.

Bergman, U., Elmes, P., Halse, M., Lunde, P.K.M., Sjöqvist, F.,
Wade, O. and Westerholm, B. (1975). The measurement of drug
consumption. Drugs for diabetes in Northern Ireland, Norway
and Sweden. Eur. J. Clin. Pharmacol., 8, 83–9.

Bergman, U., Grimsson, A., Wahba, A.H.W. and Westerholm, B. (eds)
(1979b). Studies in Drug Utilization – Methods and Applications, Regional Publications European Series no. 8, World
Health Organization, Copenhagen.

Bjørndal, A. (1982). Forbruk av Psykofarmaka i Norge, Institutt
for Almenmedisin, Universitetet i Oslo.

Boethius, G. and Sjöqvist, F. (1978). Doses and dosage intervals
of drugs – clinical practice versus pharmacokinetic principles. Clin. Pharmacol. Ther., 24, 255–63.

Bolander, G., Bolander, P., Edgren, B., Rydin, B. and Ohrvall, M.
(1982). Intervjuundersökning om kroniskt sömnmedelsbruk.
Läkartidningen, 79, 2533–4.

Edgren, B. and Roos, B.-E. (1970). Sedativa, Hypnotika,
Socialstyrelsen kommitté för läkemedelsinformation, 3.

Grimsson, A., Idänpään-Heikkilä, J., Lunde, P.K.M., Olafsson, O.
and Westerholm, B. (1977). Förbrukningen av psykofarmaka i
Finland, Island, Norge och Sverige. Nord. Med., 92, 49–54.

Halvorsen, I.K. and Jøldal, B. (1981). The Health Service of
Norway: Sales statistics in the control of narcotic drugs in
Norway, Paper presented at WHO Drug Utilization Research
Group Meeting, Korcula, Yugoslavia, April 1981.

Hemminki, E. (1974). General practitioners' indications for
psychotropic drugs. Scand. J. Soc. Med., 2, 79–85.

Hestbech, J., Hanse, H.E., Amdisen, A. and Olsen, S. (1977). Chronic renal lesions following long-term treatment with lithium. Kidney Int., 12, 205-13.

Johnson, D.A.W. (1974). A study of the use of antidepressant medication in general practice. Br. J. Psychiat., 125, 186-92.

Kristoferson, K. and Wessling, A. (1977). Tre års receptundersökningar. Svensk Farm. Tidskrift., 81, 309-16.

Laporte, J.-R., Capella, D., Gisbert, R., Porta, M., Frati, M.E., Santemases, M.P.G. and Inesta, A.G. (1981). The utilization of sedative-hypnotic drugs in Spain. In Epidemiological Impact of Psychotropic Drugs (eds G. Tognoni, C. Bellantuono and M. Lader), Elsevier/North-Holland Biomedical Press, Amsterdam, pp. 137-49.

Lunde, P.K.M., Baksaas, I., Halse, M., Halvorsen, T., Strømnes, B. and Øydvin, K. (1979). The methodology of drug utilization studies. In Studies in Drug Utilization - Methods and Applications (eds U. Bergman, A. Grimsson, A.H.W. Wahba and B. Westerholm), Regional Publications European Series no. 8, World Health Organization, Copenhagen, pp. 17-28.

Nordic Council on Medicines (1979, 1982). Nordic Statistics on Medicines 1975-1977, parts I, II (1979), 1978-1980, parts I-III (1982), Statistical Reports of the Nordic Countries, Nordic Council on Medicines, Helsinki and Oslo.

Olafsson, O., Sigfusson, S. and Grimsson, A. (1980). Control of addictive drugs in Iceland 1976-78. J. Epidemiol. Community Health, 34, 305-8.

Petursson, H. and Lader, M.H. (1981). Withdrawal from long-term benzodiazepine treatment. Br. Med. J., 2, 643-5.

Royal Australian College of General Practitioners (1976). The Australian general practice morbidity and prescribing survey 1969 to 1974. Med. J. Austr. Spec. Suppl., 2, 5-28.

Sjöqvist, F. (1975). Drug utilization. Proc. 6th Int. Congr. of Pharmacology, vol. 5, Clinical Pharmacology (eds J. Tuomisto and M.K. Paasonen), Finnish Pharmacological Society, pp. 39-50.

Stika, L., Kubát, K., Elis, J. and Vinař, O. (1981). Studies on patterns and prevalence of psychotropic drug use - data from Czechoslovakia. In Epidemiological Impact of Psychotropic Drugs (eds G. Tognoni, C. Bellantuono and M. Lader), Elsevier/North-Holland Biomedical Press, Amsterdam, pp. 151-69.

Svensk Läkemedelsstatistik (1980, 1981, 1982). Statistiska Sammanställningar 1976-1982, Apoteksbolaget (National Corporation of Swedish Pharmacies).

Westerholm, B. (1974). Patterns of drug utilization. Sources of information on drug usage in Sweden. Clin. Pharmacol. Ther., 19, 644-50.

Westerholm, B., Kristensen, F., Schaffalitzky de Muckadell, H.U., Idänpään-Heikkilä, J., Lahti, T., Grimsson, A., Olaffson, O., McMeekin, C., Lunde, P.K.M. and Øydvin, K. (1978). Drug utilization - geographical differences and clinical implications - psychotropic drugs. Proc. 7th Int. Congr. of Pharmacology, vol. Clinical Pharmacology, Paris, pp. 113-21.

World Health Organization (1965). International Classification of Disease, 8th edn.

World Health Organization (1970). Consumption of Drugs: Report on a Symposium, Oslo, 1969, Regional Office for Europe, World Health Organization, Copenhagen (Euro 3102).

Patterns of use of psychotropic drugs in Spain in an international perspective

Joan-Ramon Laporte[1], Dolors Capellà[1], Miquel Porta[1] and
María Elisa Frati[1]

INTRODUCTION

The increase in the consumption of psychotherapeutic drugs, and
particularly of sedatives and hypnotics, has led to increasing
concern about the overprescribing and abuse of these drugs by the
public. The study of drug consumption, and eventually the identification of particular areas of misuse, soon leads to a search for
medical, social or cultural factors which can influence drug
utilization. Drug utilization has been defined by the World
Health Organization (1977) as 'the marketing, distribution, prescription and use of drugs in a society, with special emphasis on
the resulting medical, social and economic consequences'. Five
questions arise when the utilization of sedatives and hypnotics is
to be studied: (1) which are the characteristics of the milieu
which may have some influence on the consumption of these drugs;
(2) which are the characteristics of the supply of these drugs;
(3) which are the most consumed drugs; (4) how are these drugs
prescribed, dispensed and consumed; and (5) which (if any) are the
effects of the consumption of these drugs.

THE MILIEU

It is well known that the characteristics of the health system
have a relevant influence on the consumption of pharmaceuticals.
The Spanish Social Security System covers 31 million inhabitants,
out of a total population of 37 million inhabitants. National
health costs amounted to around $4800 million in 1980, of which
$1008 million (21%) were spent in pharmaceuticals. In 1980 the

[1]Division of Clinical Pharmacology, Universitat Autònoma de Barcelona, Ciutat
Sanitària de la Vall d'Hebron, P. Vall d'Hebron, s.n., Barcelona - 32/35, Spain.

Social Security System expenditure on drugs accounted for 83% of
total drug expenditure in Spain. The organization of outpatient
services of medical assistance has a decisive influence on drug
abuse and misuse. A recent survey made in Barcelona (Gabinet
d'Assessoria i Promoció de la Salut, 1979) indicated that more
than 30% of the users of general medical services go to the outpatient clinic only to obtain prescriptions. The same survey
showed that 78% of these people get a prescription (mean of 1.35
prescriptions per person). According to general practitioners,
only 31% of their total prescriptions have a clear therapeutic
indication.

Frequently, national drug consumptions are compared in terms
of US dollars per head, but it is not the same thing to spend,
say, $25 per head each year in West Germany as it is in Spain;
gross national products per capita income are very different in
these two countries. If drug consumption is expressed in terms of
per capita income, this results in more valid comparisons
(Laporte, 1981). As table 1 shows, Nordic countries tend to spend
less on drugs than the other European countries included in this
analysis ($p < 0.01$).

Table 1. Per capita drug expenditure related to per capita income
in some European countries (1977).

	(1) Per capita drug expenditure ($, 1977)*	(2) Income per capita ($, 1977)†	(1) as a percentage of (2)
Denmark	42.4	8295	0.51
Finland	52.6	5652	0.93
Norway	49.7	7179	0.69
Sweden	52.6	8266	0.63
France	62.1	6304	0.99
Greece	34.1	2795	1.22
Italy	37.9	2730§	1.39
West Germany	65.7	7328	0.90
Spain	33.2	2925	1.14

*Data from the Nordic Council on Medicines (1979) and Gisbert
 (1981).
†Data from *Statistical Yearbook* (Department of International
 Economic and Social Affairs Statistical Office, 1979).
§1976.

THE SUPPLY OF PHARMACEUTICALS, AND PARTICULARLY OF PSYCHOTROPIC DRUGS

During the last 10-15 years, various groups of health professionals, health authorities in some countries and the WHO have been increasingly concerned with the fact that drugs are not used to their full potential in terms of efficacy, safety or economy (Lunde, 1980a). There are wide geographical variations in overall drug therapy profiles (for review, see Baksaas and Lunde, 1981). While the Nordic countries have a supply of drugs ranging from 2000 to 3000 marketed pharmaceutical specialities, in countries like West Germany, France, Italy and Spain the number of marketed products ranges from 10 000 to 30 000. These variations from one country to another (see table 2) also add to the complex question - what is really rational and optimal drug therapy? As Lunde (1980b) has pointed out, it has never been proven that an infinite number of drugs provides any greater benefits for public health than a more reasonable product offering. On the contrary, a large number of drugs may result in confusion at all levels of the therapeutic chain, and represent a waste of manpower and money.

In Spain 2477 active drugs are marketed; there are 8003 trade names (pharmaceutical specialities) and 17 778 pharmaceutical forms. One distinctive characteristic between the pharmaceutical markets in Nordic and other European countries is that while in the former there is a limited number of fixed-dose combinations, in the latter fixed-dose combinations make up a high proportion of the overall supply. In Spain this proportion is 55.7%, in France it is 58.8%, in Italy 59.2%, in the USA 45.9%, and in the UK 43.1% (Laporte, 1975). Of all these countries, at least in Spain a high percentage of marketed products do not fulfill generally accepted criteria of efficacy and safety (Erill *et al.*, 1973).

With respect to psychotherapeutic drugs, in Spain there are 61 active drugs marketed and classified as 'psycholeptics' (group N 05 in the so-called anatomical classification of the European Pharmaceutical Market Research Association, EPhMRA). The Spanish official drug catalog includes 410 pharmaceutical specialities in the group N 05; however, 346 additional pharmaceutical specialities containing sedative and hypnotic drugs are classified in other groups. This is due to the high proportion of fixed-dose combinations, which are classified according to their main therapeutic indication.

In a previous paper (Laporte *et al.*, 1981) we have described the marketing and consumption of sedatives and hypnotics in Spain: 15 barbiturates, 20 benzodiazepines, 10 sedatives and hypnotics of other classes, 8 tricyclic antidepressants, 2 tetracyclic antidepressants, 5 MAOI antidepressants, 4 antidepressants of other classes, 15 phenothiazines, and 8 antipsychotic drugs of other classes are on the market in our country. All these drugs are marketed in the form of more than 800 pharmaceutical specialities.

Table 2. Consumption of nine groups of medicines in five European countries (percentages of total drug budget) in 1973 *

Group	West Germany	France	Italy	Spain	United Kingdom
Analgesics	5.0	5.5	4.4	3.3	5.1
Antibiotics and chemotherapeutic agents	4.1	8.5	10.8	27.3	13.5
Anti-inflammatory drugs	6.3	4.0	4.0	3.7	7.5
Cardiovascular drugs	18.2	14.6	8.1	5.2	11.0
Dermatological products	5.9	4.6	4.7	4.3	1.5
Hormones	2.9	4.4	8.4	4.3	7.2
Psychopharmacological agents	5.0	7.0	1.9	4.5	7.9
Respiratory system drugs	6.7	7.2	6.2	4.1	6.4
Vitamins	3.4	3.0	5.1	5.4	2.2
Total	57.5	58.8	53.6	62.1	62.3

*Data from Gisbert (1981).

While in Spain there are 20 benzodiazepines on the market, the number of these drugs marketed in other countries is smaller: 16 in Italy (1979); 11 in Germany (1978); 9 in Switzerland (1978); 8 in the UK (1978); 7 in Finland (1976), in the USA (1978) and in Norway (1976); 5 in Sweden (1979); and 3 in Israel (1976) (Bellantuono *et al.*, 1980). The regulations which allow the marketing of this high number of active drugs have been reviewed by Erill (1974). The last modification of the law regulating the requirements for marketing drugs in Spain, made in March 1970 (Ministerio de la Gobernación, 1970), required, for the first time, pharmacokinetic data (although it is not clearly stated that they should be obtained in human studies) and reports from clinical trials in the applications submitted for the marketing of new drugs. It is not surprising, therefore, that the need for more complete and updated marketing regulations is felt strongly.

THE CONSUMPTION OF PSYCHOTROPIC DRUGS

It has been suggested that the consumption of psychotropic drugs in Spain is much lower than in other European or American countries (Bellantuono *et al.*, 1980; Balter *et al.*, 1974). The outcome of any survey on psychotherapeutic drug use obviously depends on which drugs are included. Differences in drug classification can lead to very different conclusions about the character, extent and appropriateness of drug prescribing and use. A classification scheme based on chemical structure or pharmacological action tends to group drugs with very different clinical uses and with little relation to clinical practice; however, it can be useful as a consumption denominator when adverse effects of drugs are evaluated, or when public health decisions have to be taken. On the other hand, a classification based on clinical applications in medicine would be most appropriate when the use of psychotherapeutic drugs in the treatment of psychic symptoms associated with anxiety and depression is to be investigated. Table 3 shows the distribution of pharmaceutical specialities containing sedatives and hypnotics, according to their sales figures in 1980. As this table shows, 20 out of 33 pharmaceutical specialities with sales figures higher than half-a-million units are not classified as tranquilizers, hypnotics or sedatives in classifications frequently used to compare consumption of drugs from one country to another. It is clear from these figures that very different results can be obtained depending on the criteria used to include or exclude the pharmaceutical specialities marketed in one country.

Comparisons of drug consumption from one country to another or from one period to another in the same country can be done in terms of expenditure per capita. Although these data can be useful in the investigation of the health budget of a group of countries (see table 2), the drug bill does not permit comparisons

Table 3. Hidden sedatives and hypnotics – pharmaceutical specialities containing sedative and hypnotic drugs, according to their sales volumes and to their classification.*

Units sold in 1980	Number of pharmaceutical specialities		
	Classified in group N 05	Classified in other groups	Total
More than 1 million	4	8	12
500 000-999 999	9	12	21
100 000-499 999	52	44	96
50 000-99 999	33	30	63
10 000-49 999	90	68	158
5000-9999	7	6	13
Less than 1000	188	154	342
Total	410	346	756

*Catálogo de Especialidades Farmacéuticas, 1981(Consejo General de Colegios Oficiales de Farmacéuticos, 1981).

of drug utilization between different countries or within one country in different periods of time. A more suitable unit of comparison has been defined by the Drug Utilization Research Group (Lunde *et al.*, 1979). This unit is the 'defined daily dose' (DDD), which is the mean daily dose used for the main indication of each drug. The DDD is an amount of an active substance. The number of DDDs consumed is usually given per 1000 inhabitants per day, and this provides a gross estimation of the number of patients being treated with each drug (Bergman *et al.*, 1983). Table 4 lists the DDDs of the most consumed psychotropic drugs marketed in Spain. In order to define the consumption of sedatives and hypnotics in our country better, and in order not to overlook hidden sedatives and hypnotics (see table 3), active substances, whether as single drugs or fixed-dose combinations, have been taken into account to make up the final figures of DDDs consumed.

Figure 1 shows the consumption of barbiturates, benzodiazepines and other sedatives and hypnotics in 1980 in Spain. The total consumption of tranquilizers, sedatives and hypnotics in Spain is not very different from that in other European countries (Laporte *et al.*, 1981), as other authors had suggested (Bellantuono *et al.*, 1980; Balter *et al.*, 1974). However, the consumption of benzodiazepines is lower in Spain (Laporte *et al.*, 1981) than in Northern Ireland (King *et al.*, 1980), and in the majority of Nordic countries (Grimsson *et al.*, 1979).

In Spain, among single drugs, barbiturates account only for 9.8% of total consumption. As a whole, two-thirds of the total consumption of sedative/hypnotic drugs is made up of medicines which are fixed-dose combinations of two or more drugs. For most

Table 4. Some of the principal psychotropic drugs and
their defined daily doses (mg)

Barbiturates	DDD	Benzodiazepines	DDD
Allobarbital	100	Chlordiazepoxide	30^a-50^b
Amobarbital	100	Clonazepam	8^a-2^b
Aprobarbital	100	Clorazepate potass.	20
Butalbital	250	Cloxazolam	8
Heptabarbital	200	Diazepam	10
Hexobarbital	250	Flunitrazepam	2
Phenobarbital	100	Flurazepam	30
Secobarbital	100	Lorazepam	2.5
		Medazepam	20
		Nitrazepam	5
		Oxazepam	50
		Oxazolam	50

Antidepressants	DDD	Antipsychotics	DDD
Tricyclic		Phenothiazines	
Amitriptyline	75	Acepromazine	100^a-50^b
Clomipramine	100	Chlorpromazine	300^a-100^b
Doxepin	100	Fluphenazine	10^a-1^b
Imipramine	100	Levomepromazine	300^a-100^b
Nortriptyline	75^a-30^b	Perphenazine	30^a-10^b
Trimipramine	150	Perphenazine enant.	7^b
		Pipotiazine	5
		Propericiazine	50^a-20^b
Tetracyclic		Thioproperazine	75^a-20^b
Maprotiline	100	Thioridazine	300
		Trifluoperazine	20^a-8^b
		Others	
MAOI		Haloperidol	8
Nialamide	100	Trifluperidol	2
Tranylcypromine	10	Tiotixene	30
		Lithium carbonate	2400

[a] Oral route.
[b] Parenteral route.

of these drugs the main indication is not anxiety, insomnia or
nervousness, but pain, and less frequently digestive symptoms,
cardiovascular conditions and non-specific problems of old age. A
high consumption of these hidden sedatives and hypnotics has also
been noted in other countries, where barbiturates are marketed in

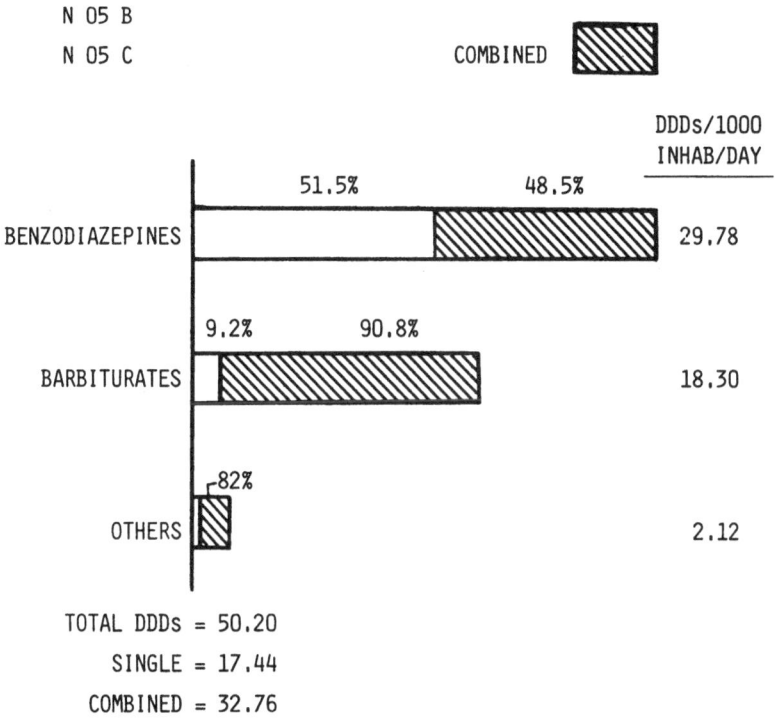

Figure 1. Consumption of tranquilizers, hypnotics and sedatives in 1980 in Spain.

fixed-dose combinations with analgesics-antipyretics. Thus, in Czechoslovakia 16.9 DDDs per 1000 inhabitants per day of single-sedative hypnotics were consumed in 1977, while 22.3 DDDs per 1000 inhabitants per day of combinations containing barbiturates were consumed in the same period (Stika and Vinař, 1980). On the other hand, in Northern Ireland the consumption of fixed-dose combinations containing barbiturates only amounted to 12% of total barbiturate consumption in 1979 (King *et al*., 1980). In Finland 110.4 DDDs per 1000 inhabitants per day of the 10 most sold psychotropic substances were consumed in 1977, of which 36.6 DDDs per 1000 inhabitants per day (33%) were hidden psychotropic drugs. In Norway these figures were respectively 121.0 DDDs per 1000 inhabitants per day and 11.3 DDDs per 1000 inhabitants per day (9%). In Sweden the proportion of hidden psychotropic drugs among the 10 most sold of these products was 16% (Hemminki, 1981). Attitudes of doctors, pharmacists and the public in relation to the consumption of drugs are influenced by drug regulations, and this may explain, at least partly, the striking differences in the consumption of hidden sedative-hypnotics from one country to another. As table 5 shows, fixed-dose combinations account for 91% of the barbiturate consumption. In particular, a pharmaceutical speciality containing propyphenazone, caffeine and 50 mg of butalbital (Optalidon®) is most popular in Spain. Almost 17 tons of butalbital were sold in 1980 in the form of Optalidon®.

Table 5. Consumption of barbiturates in Spain (1980)* (defined daily doses per 1000 inhabitants per day).

Barbiturate	Single	Combined	Total
Butalbital	–	6.3	6.3
Phenobarbital	1.3	4.7	6.0
Amobarbital	0.2	2.5	2.7
Allobarbital	–	2.1	2.1
Others	0.2	1.0	1.2
Total	1.7	16.6	18.3
(%)	(9.3)	(90.7)	(100)

*Data from Laporte *et al.* (1981).

HOW PSYCHOTROPIC DRUGS ARE PRESCRIBED, DISPENSED AND CONSUMED

A survey made in Barcelona in 1980 showed that 8% of all prescriptions written by doctors in the outpatient clinics of the Social Security System are of medicines which contain some psychotropic drug. No differences in the prevalence of prescriptions of psychotherapeutic drugs were found among elderly people, as compared to younger people (Mas *et al.*, in press). Another survey, in which 395 elderly people were interviewed at home, showed that 21.3% of them were taking some psychotropic drug regularly, the prevalence of use of these drugs being higher in women than in men (Mas *et al.*, in press). Another survey, in which 232 people over 55 years old and living in the community were interviewed, yielded similar results about the prevalence of use of psychotropic drugs. More interestingly, many people (22 out of 232) were taking additive doses of the same drug contained in different marketed pharmaceutical specialities. The most frequently repeated drugs were phenylbutazone, barbiturates, corticosteroids, diazepam and codeine, most of them known as common or serious causes of adverse reactions in the elderly (Mas *et al.*, 1981).
     A recent survey in which the prescription of sedative/hypnotic drugs in all the hospitals of the Spanish Social Security System was studied (Laporte *et al.*, 1981), showed that the consumption of these drugs amounted to 287 DDDs per 1000 bed-days, and that the pattern of use of the different groups of these drugs

in hospitals was approximately the same as in the community: benzodiazepines accounted for 53% of total consumption, and barbiturates accounted for 43%.

With the aim of determining which were the drugs most frequently found at home (regularly consumed or merely hoarded), a survey was made in 538 randomly chosen homes in five different socio-geographical areas of Catalonia (Martín *et al.*, 1980). The mean number of medicines found was 21.7 ± 9.7. Medicines containing tranquilizers were found in 78% of visited homes; in their majority they were not regularly consumed by people living in these homes, but they had been merely hoarded. Optalidon®, one of the most popular fixed-dose combinations used as analgesic (containing 50 mg of butalbital per tablet), was found in 60% of visited homes, and it was consumed as an analgesic with varying frequencies.

We feel that these data are relevant when the prevention of acute drug overdoses is considered (see below). Optalidon® is the most frequent offending drug among cases of acute drug overdoses admitted to the Hospital de Sant Pau in Barcelona (Camí et al., 1980). As butalbital is an intermediate-acting barbiturate, overdosage by this drug is potentially more serious than overdosage by long-acting preparations (Harvey, 1980; Berman *et al.*, 1956). In Spain Optalidon® is not included in the official list of over-the-counter medicines (Ministerio de Trabajo, Sanidad y Seguridad Social, 1981). However, a recent survey shows that it can be readily obtained in pharmacies without a medical prescription (see table 6), as compared to Luminal®.

Table 6. Results of a survey on the dispensation of two medicines containing barbiturates in 60 pharmacies in Barcelona (1982)

	Number of pharmacies visited	Dispensed without any prescription	Prescription required
Luminal® was asked for	30	0	30
Optalidon® was asked for	30	30	0

LOOKING FOR CLINICAL AND EPIDEMIOLOGICAL END-POINTS OF BARBITURATE MISUSE: SEVERE ACUTE OVERDOSE IN A UNIVERSITY HOSPITAL

In order to know the severity, in terms of morbidity and mortality, of acute overdoses caused by different drugs, an analysis was made of all the 91 cases admitted to the Intensive Care Unit (ICU) of the Hospital de Sant Pau in Barcelona between 1974 and

1980 (Frati, 1982). As during this period only two patients with an acute overdose died in this hospital before their admission to the ICU (one before admission to the emergency room and the other in the emergency room), this sample can be considered as representative of the more severe cases of acute overdoses. Optalidon® was the most commonly implicated medicine in this series (see table 7).

The barbiturates with short half-life and high lipid solubility are more toxic than the more polar, long-acting compounds, such as phenobarbital, and poisoning with the short-acting agents is more dangerous. Among 39 deaths by barbiturate poisoning reported by Poklis and Gantner (1981), only three were related to phenobarbital and two to barbital, the rest being related to amobarbital, butalbital, pentobarbital, secobarbital and other short-acting barbiturates. In our series, out of 25 cases of acute overdose by butalbital, 19 presented with deep coma on admission, and six with superficial coma, whereas among the six cases related to phenobarbital, only two presented with deep coma ($p < 0.05$). Respiratory complications were also more common among patients with butalbital intoxication: nine suffered bronchoaspiration and pneumonitis while admitted to the ICU, whereas only one case of pneumonitis was recorded among patients with a phenobarbital overdose. Out of the 91 patients with acute drug overdose admitted to the ICU, five died; in two of these cases the implicated drug was butalbital.

Table 7. Medicines most commonly implicated in acute overdoses among 91 patients with acute overdose admitted to the Intensive Care Unit of the Hospital de Sant Pau (Barcelona) during the period 1974–1980

Medicine	n
Optalidon® (butalbital + propyphenazone + caffeine)	25
Nobitrol® (amitriptyline + medazepam)	7
Luminal® (phenobarbital)	6
Meleril® (thioridazine)	6
Valium® (diazepam)	4
Tranxilium® (dipotassium clorazepate)	4
Tofranil® (imipramine)	3
Dormodor® (flurazepam)	3

SUMMARY AND CONCLUSIONS

Drug utilization statistics provide one of the tools needed for the understanding of the role that drugs, prescribed or unprescribed, play in a society, and for adjusting that to the real needs of the society. In recent years, some astonishing differences have arisen between drug markets in different countries, largely as a result of variations in drug regulation policy. The use of psychotropic drugs, and particularly that of sedatives and hypnotics, shows wide geographical variations. The high number of drugs and the high proportion of fixed-dose combinations marketed in many countries make comparisons of drug use more difficult, and confuse the real indications for the use of drugs at all the levels of the therapeutic chain (prescriber, dispenser and user). Some scientifically unsound cultural attitudes tend to appear when the number of drugs is not restricted to an optimal level. As an example, the ease of obtaining intermediate-acting barbiturates, sold for indications other than the treatment of psychic symptoms, is illustrated in this paper with figures of consumption and by some medical consequences in the field of drug overdosage and poisoning.

Acknowledgements

This work has been supported partly by a Grant from the Instituto de Estudios de Sanidad y Seguridad Social (Ministerio de Trabajo, Sanidad y Seguridad Social, Madrid).

REFERENCES

Baksaas, I. and Lunde, P.K.M. (1981). Drug utilization: pharmacokinetics in the community. Trends in Pharmacol. Sci., 2(2), V-VII.

Balter, M.B., Levine, J. and Manheimer, D.I. (1974). Cross-national study of the extent of anti-anxiety/sedative drug use. New Engl. J. Med., 290, 769-74.

Bellantuono, C., Reggi, V., Tognoni, G. and Garattini, S. (1980). Benzodiazepines: clinical pharmacology and therapeutic use. Drugs, 19, 195-219.

Bergman, U., Agenäs, I. and Dahlström, M. (1983). Utilization of psychotropic drugs in Sweden and the other Nordic countries. This volume, pp. 3-17.

Berman, L.B., Jeghers, H., Schreiner, G.E. and Pallotta, A.J. (1956). Hemodialysis, an effective therapy for acute barbiturate poisoning. J. Am. Med. Assoc., 161, 820-7.

Camí, J., Frati, M.E. and Martín, M.L. (1980). Intoxicación aguda en Barcelona. Epidemiología y consideraciones sobre su terapéutica. Med. Clin. (Barcelona), 75, 287-91.

Consejo General de Colegios Oficiales de Farmacéuticos (1981). Catálogo de Especialidades Farmacéuticas 1981, CGCOF, Madrid.

Department of International Economic and Social Affairs Statistical Office (1979). Statistical Yearbook 1978, United Nations, New York.

Erill, S. (1974). Clinical pharmacology in Spain. <u>Clin. Pharma-col. Ther.</u>, 16, 597-604.

Erill, S., García Sevilla, J.A. and Laporte, J.R. (1973). Las especialidades farmacéuticas en España: un análisis del Vademecum Daimon 1971. <u>Anales de Medicina</u>, 54, 215-20.

Frati, M.E. (1982). Intervención farmacológico-clínica en el tratamiento de las intoxicaciones agudas en la UCI. <u>Tesis doctoral</u>, Universitat Autònoma de Barcelona, Barcelona.

Gabinet d'Assessoria i Promoció de la Salut (1979). <u>L'Assistència Externa de la Seguretat Social a Barcelona</u>, Col.legi Oficial de Metges, Barcelona.

Gisbert, R. (1981). La demanda y el consumo de medicamentos en España durante el período 1970-1979. In <u>Primeres Jornades Sobre Economia de la Salut</u>, Col.legi d'Economistes de Catalunya, Barcelona, pp. 65-79.

Grimsson, A., Idänpään-Heikkilä, J., Lunde, P.K.M., Olafsson, O. and Westerholm, B. (1979). The utilization of psychotropic drugs in Finland, Iceland, Norway and Sweden. In <u>Studies in Drug Utilization</u> (eds U. Bergman, A. Grimsson, A.H.W. Wahba and B. Westerholm), WHO Regional Office for Europe, Copenhagen, pp. 163-73.

Harvey, S.C. (1980). Hypnotics and sedatives. In <u>The Pharmaco-logical Basis of Therapeutics</u>, 6th edn (eds A. Goodman Gilman, L.S. Goodman and A. Gilman), Macmillan, New York, p. 359.

Hemminki, E. (1981). <u>Sales of Psychotropic Drugs in Finland, Norway, and Sweden in the 1960s and 1970s: Descriptive Material</u>, Publications of the University of Kuopio, Kuopio.

King, D.J., Griffiths, K., Hall, C.E., Cooper, N.C. and Morrison, D.J. (1980). Effect of the CURB campaign on barbiturate prescribing in Northern Ireland. <u>J. R. Coll. Gen. Pract.</u>, 30, 614-8.

Laporte, J. (1975). El abuso de medicamentos. In <u>Avances en Terapéutica</u>, vol. 6 (eds J. Laporte and J.A. Salvà), Salvat, Barcelona, pp. 1-25.

Laporte, J.R. (1981). Drug consumption in Spain. <u>Lancet</u>, i, 103-4.

Laporte, J.R., Capellà, D., Gisbert, R., Porta, M., Frati, M.E., García Santesmases, M.P. and García Iñesta, A. (1981). The utilization of sedative-hypnotic drugs in Spain. In <u>Epidemi-ological Impact of Psychotropic Drugs</u> (eds G. Tognoni, C. Bellantuono and M. Lader), Elsevier/North-Holland, Amsterdam, pp. 137-49.

Lunde, P.K.M. (1980a). The World Health Organization essential drug concept - three years afterwards. In <u>Clinical Pharma-cology and Therapeutics: Proc. of Plenary Lectures, Symposia and Therapeutic Sessions of the First World Conf. on Clinical Pharmacology and Therapeutics</u> (ed P. Turner), Macmillan, London, pp. 529-35.

Lunde, P.K.M. (1980b). Drug and product selection - an essential part of the therapeutic benefit/risk ratio strategy? In Drug-Induced Sufferings: Proc. of the Kyoto Int. Conf. Against Drug-Induced Sufferings (ed T. Soda), Elsevier/North-Holland, Amsterdam, pp. 129-36.

Lunde, P.K.M., Baksaas, I., Halse, M., Halvorsen, I.K., Strømmes, B. and Øydvin, K. (1979). The methodology of drug utilization studies. In Studies in Drug Utilization (eds U. Bergman, A. Grimsson, A.H.W. Wahba and B. Westerholm), WHO Regional Office for Europe, Copenhagen, pp. 17-28.

Martín, M.L., Busquet, L., Arnau, J.M., Arboix, M., Frati, M.E. and Casas, M. (1980). Medicines at home and attitudes of public towards medicines. In World Conf. on Clinical Pharmacology and Therapeutics (eds P. Turner and C. Padgham), Macmillan, London, Abstracts, no. 0749.

Mas, X., Laporte, J.R., Frati, M.E., Busquet, L., Arnau, J.M., Ibañez, L., Séculi, E., Capellà, D. and Arbonés, G. (in press). Drug prescribing and drug use among elderly people in Spain. Drug. Intell. Clin. Pharm.

Mas, X., Laporte, J.R. and Martín, M.L. (1981). Drugs and the elderly. Br. Med. J., 282, 824.

Ministerio de la Gobernación (1970). Decreto 849/1970 de 21 de marzo, por el que se actualizan algunas disposiciones vigentes en materia de registro, comercialización y publicidad de especialidades farmacéuticas. Boletín Oficial del Estado, 310-82, 5370-1.

Ministerio de Trabajo, Sanidad y Seguridad Social (1981). Real Decreto 2730/1981 de 19 de octubre, sobre registro de especialidades farmacéuticas publicitarias. Boletín Oficial del Estado de 25 de noviembre de 1981.

Nordic Council on Medicines (1979). Nordic Statistics on Medicines 1975-1977, part 1, Statistical Reports of the Nordic Countries, 35, Nordic Council on Medicines, Helsinki.

Poklis, A. and Gantner, G.E. (1981). Drug deaths in St. Louis City and County: a brief survey, 1977-1979. Clin. Toxicol., 18, 141-7.

Stika, L. and Vinař, O. (1980). Utilization of psychotropic drugs. An international comparison. Activ. Nerv. Sup. (Praha), 22, 221-4.

World Health Organization Expert Committee (1977). The Selection of Essential Drugs, WHO Technical Report Series, 615, WHO, Geneva.

Heavy drug use among the elderly: prescription surveys in Manitoba

P.A.Mitenko[1], D.S.Sitar[1] and F.Y.Aoki[1]

INTRODUCTION

Infirmity and disease have always been identified with old age, but it is only within the last generation that some relief from the discomforts and disabilities of aging has really been possible. Appropriate drug therapy can bring substantial benefits to older patients, but benefits must be carefully weighed against risks. The hazards of adverse drug effects are markedly increased with aging. This is in part due to changes in drug disposition and drug effect with age, but is more likely related to the number of drugs used by the elderly, drugs which are often prescribed simultaneously and chronically.

Thus, drug use in itself must be considered as an important risk factor. The elderly use more drugs than the young (Boethius, 1977; Skoll *et al.*, 1979), and the number of drugs prescribed increases with the variety of illnesses being treated. Polypharmacy is a real danger for the elderly, and each drug prescribed adds measurably to the risk of adverse drug effects. Hurwitz (1969) demonstrated this for hospitalized patients, and more recently, Williamson and Chopin (1980) found that the prevalence of adverse reactions increased markedly with the number of drugs prescribed for a series of geriatric patients requiring admission to hospital.

Studies on changes in disposition and drug effect must be undertaken to identify drugs of risk to older patients, but patients at risk must also be identified, namely those elderly patients who receive multiple prescription drugs for long periods with the attendant danger of adverse reactions. There is a need for information concerning the number and type of drugs used by heavy drug users among the elderly, and it was the purpose of these studies to provide such observations.

[1]Geriatric Clinical Pharmacology Unit, Departments of Medicine and Pharmacology, University of Manitoba, Winnipeg, Manitoba R3E 0Z3, Canada.

METHODS

Manitoba's Pharmacare plan offers partial reimbursement to individuals or families whose annual prescription drug costs are more than $50.00. Each application for Pharmacare benefits provides specific information as to the type, amount and cost of all prescribed drugs, as well as the route of administration and duration of therapy. These variables were related to the age and sex of the claimants by examining random samples of applications for the years 1975 and 1978.

The sample for 1975 consisted of 429 applications from claimants aged 65 and older whose individual drug costs were more than $50.00 in that year. In addition, the applications of 387 claimants aged 50 to 64 were reviewed as a control sample to determine age-related differences in prescription frequencies. Although the numbers of claims reviewed in 1975 and 1978 were approximately equal (Aoki *et al.*, 1982), the application of a correcting factor for inflation reduced the number of 1978 applications surveyed for the purposes of this study to 365 for those aged 65 and older and 380 for those aged 50 to 64. Since the mean cost per Pharmacare claimant rose from $132.39 to $171.34 between 1975 and 1978, only these individuals who spent more than $64.70 on prescription drugs in 1978 are included in the comparisons made in this publication.

The data were analyzed to relate the number and types of drugs to the age and sex of the claimants. Differences between means were tested by analysis of variance, and differences between frequencies by chi-square analysis. Values $p < 0.05$ were taken to indicate statistically significant differences for a two-tailed test.

RESULTS

The population of Manitoba is just over a million, and in 1978 there were 117 000 Manitobans older than 65 years of age. In that year, 24% of this population spent more than $64.70 on prescription drugs, and are characterized as heavy drug users for this study.

Sample Characteristics

The two samples are compared in table 1. In both years, more women than men were represented, especially among claimants aged 50 to 64. More drugs were prescribed for women than men in both samples, but the difference was not statistically significant for the older claimants in either year. There was no difference in the number of drugs prescribed between younger and older claimants.

Table 1. Sample characteristics *

| | 50 to 64 years | | 65 years and older | |
	Men	Women	Men	Women
1975				
Number in group	160	227	201	228
Number of drugs/year	8.5 ± 0.4	10.3 ± 0.4	8.6 ± 0.4	9.8 ± 0.4
Cost in dollars/year	209 ± 13	221 ± 10	188 ± 8	170 ± 6
Number of doctors/year	2.3 ± 0.1	2.6 ± 0.1	2.1 ± 0.1	2.2 ± 0.1
1978				
Number in group	163	217	163	202
Number of drugs/year	7.1 ± 0.4	8.7 ± 0.4	8.2 ± 0.4	8.9 ± 0.4
Cost in dollars/year	199 ± 10	200 ± 15	183 ± 11	187 ± 9
Number of doctors/year	2.1 ± 0.1	2.3 ± 0.1	2.0 ± 0.1	2.0 ± 0.1

*Mean and standard error (S.E.M.) are shown for each group.

The proportion of drugs prescribed as combination products was quite constant over all groups in both years, and ranged from 38% to 45% of the annual total. Similarly, the proportion of drugs prescribed chronically, that is, for more than 120 days annually, was also consistent, ranging from 36% to 41% of the number of drugs prescribed. Women tended to receive more drugs chronically and more drugs as combination products, but no statistically significant differences were found.

Prescription Frequencies

Drugs prescribed for claimants were classified into categories containing one or more drugs with similar pharmacological properties. The most commonly prescribed categories for claimants aged 65 or older are shown in table 2, which ranks the percentage of older claimants receiving prescriptions for drugs in these categories in 1975 and 1978. There were relatively few differences in prescription frequency apparent over the interval, but the substantial decline in the use of phenobarbital and of barbiturates other than phenobarbital should be noted.

Psychotherapeutic agents were very commonly prescribed in both years, and occupied seven of the first 25 places in our survey out of a total of 154 categories. For these older Manitobans, benzodiazepines were second only to thiazide-type diuretics in prescription frequency.

In 1975, the five categories most commonly prescribed chronically for older claimants were thiazide-type diuretics, benzodiazepines, digoxin, α-methyldopa and barbiturates other than phenobarbital. By 1978, salicylates had displaced other barbiturates from this ranking.

Table 2. Most commonly prescribed drug categories for claimants
aged 65 years and older*

	1975 (n = 429)		1978 (n = 365)	
1	Thiazide-type diuretics	55.9	Thiazide-type diuretics	53.2
2	Benzodiazepines	47.1	Benzodiazepines	41.9
3	Salicylates	31.2	Salicylates	28.5
4	Sympathomimetics	25.9	Sympathomimetics	24.7
5	Other barbiturates†	25.6	Digoxin	24.1
6	Codeine	24.9	Codeine	22.7
7	Digoxin	24.2	Furosemide	17.5
8	Tetracyclines	20.5	Tetracyclines	17.3
9	Phenobarbital†	20.0	α-Methyldopa	17.3
10	Anticholinergics†	19.8	β-Blocking drugs	14.8
11	Sulfonamides†	17.7	Phenobarbital	14.0
12	Furosemide	15.6	Other barbiturates	13.7
13	Theophylline	15.4	Anticholinergics	13.7
14	α-Methyldopa	14.5	Tricyclic antidepressants	13.7
15	Profen-type drugs	14.5	Theophylline	13.2
16	Tricyclic antidepressants	13.8	Potassium supplements	12.9
17	Ampicillin	13.5	Ampicillin	12.6
18	Potassium supplements	13.5	Triamterene	12.3
19	Phenylbutazone†	13.3	Profen-type drugs	10.7
20	Systemic corticosteroids†	13.1	Indomethacin	10.4
21	β-Blocking drugs	12.1	Phenothiazines	9.9
22	Phenothiazines	12.1	Co-trimoxazole	9.3
23	Propoxyphene	10.0	Sulfonamides	8.5
24	Triamterene	9.8	Systemic corticosteroids	8.2
25	Indomethacin	8.9	Phenylbutazone	7.7

*Percentage of claimants aged 65 and older who received prescriptions for drugs from these categories in 1975 and 1978.
†Designates significant difference in prescription frequency between 1975 and 1978 ($p < 0.05$).

Prescription of Psychotherapeutic Drugs

In table 3 the prescription of the major psychotherapeutic drug categories is detailed. Other drugs may alter neurological or psychological function in the elderly, but the drug categories listed in table 3 clearly have their major effects on the central nervous system and are prescribed for these effects. It is in this context that these agents are grouped together as psychotherapeutic drugs.

Sedative-hypnotic drugs were prescribed for many heavy drug users. The benzodiazepines were frequently prescribed, and more than half the prescriptions in both years were considered chronic

Table 3. Most commonly prescribed psychotherapeutic categories*

		50 to 64 years		65 years and older	
		Men	Women	Men	Women
Benzodiazepines	1975†	49.4 (31.3)	64.8 (46.3)	39.3 (25.4)	53.9 (35.1)
	1978	34.4 (19.0)	55.3 (31.8)	37.4 (16.6)	45.5 (25.7)
Phenobarbital	1975	18.1 (9.4)	18.9 (7.5)	17.9 (10.4)	21.9 (10.5)
	1978	11.0 (4.9)	12.4 (4.1)	10.4 (4.9)	16.8 (6.4)
Other barbiturates	1975	18.1 (9.4)	25.6 (15.0)	22.4 (14.4)	28.5 (17.1)
	1978	6.7 (3.1)	13.8 (7.8)	10.4 (4.9)	16.3 (10.9)
Codeine	1975	23.8 (4.4)	33.5 (8.4)	26.4 (3.0)	23.7 (3.9)
	1978	21.5 (4.3)	25.8 (6.9)	20.8 (1.8)	24.3 (8.4)
Propoxyphene	1975	7.5 (1.3)	16.3 (5.3)	7.0 (2.0)	12.7 (3.9)
	1978	1.2 (0.0)	5.5 (2.3)	5.5 (1.2)	7.4 (2.5)
Tricyclic antidepressants	1975†§	17.5 (6.3)	24.2 (15.9)	9.5 (7.0)	17.5 (13.6)
	1978	11.7 (8.6)	15.2 (9.7)	11.7 (8.0)	15.3 (10.4)
Phenothiazines	1975†§	8.1 (4.4)	23.8 (16.7)	10.4 (6.5)	13.6 (8.8)
	1978	7.4 (4.3)	13.8 (8.8)	4.9 (1.8)	13.9 (7.4)

*Open figures indicate the percentage of claimants in each group who received prescriptions for drugs from these categories, and figures in parentheses indicate the percentage in each group who received prescriptions for more than 120 days.

†Designates differences related to age at $p < 0.05$ (50 to 64 yr vs. 65 yr and older).

§Designates differences related to sex at $p < 0.05$ (all men vs. all women).

because the drug was prescribed for more than 120 days during the year. More women than men used benzodiazepines in 1978, but the age-related difference observed for the 1975 survey was not apparent in 1978.

Phenobarbital is included in a variety of combination products in Canada, usually with anticholinergic drugs, and this accounts for most of the use recorded in our surveys. There were no differences in prescription frequency related to age or sex in either year, and prescriptions for phenobarbital decreased between 1975 and 1978 for all groups.

The other barbiturates marketed in Canada are available only as single drugs or barbiturate combinations and are prescribed solely as sedative-hypnotics. More women than men received prescriptions for these drugs in both years, but there were no age-related differences. Use of sedative-hypnotic barbiturates fell

for all groups over the three-year interval, and indeed decreased
more than phenobarbital use.

Several salicylate-codeine combination products are popular
in Canada, and prescriptions for these agents accounted for most
of the codeine given to these heavy drug users. Similarly, most
of the propoxyphene prescribed was contained in various salicy-
late-propoxyphene combinations. As well, the only minor sedative-
hypnotic to be prescribed to any extent, meprobamate, was used as
a salicylate-codeine-meprobamate combination. (It was prescribed
for 4.7% of older claimants in 1975 and 3.8% in 1978.) The prescription of codeine was high and not different between groups in
both years, and although the use of propoxyphene declined between
1975 and 1978, the decrease was statistically significant only for
the younger claimants.

Tricyclic antidepressants were prescribed for many claimants
in both 1975 and 1978, as were the phenothiazines, and the prescription frequencies for these categories did not change over the
interval. More of both these categories were prescribed for
younger claimants than for older in 1975, and more for women than
for men. Only the sex-related difference in phenothiazine prescription held in 1978.

Multiple Psychotherapeutic Prescriptions

Many of these heavy drug users received more than one drug with
major effects on the central nervous system. As table 4 indicates,
over 65% of the claimants aged 65 and older received at least one
such psychotherapeutic drug in either year, and over 40% were
given such drugs chronically.

Concurrent use of psychotherapeutic drugs was considered
probable if two or more such drugs were prescribed chronically.
In 1975, 48% of the women and 33% of the men over the age of 65
met this criterion, and in 1978, 34% of the older women and 18% of
the older men had concurrent psychotherapeutic prescriptions.
Similar patterns were observed for the younger claimants, and both
the sex-related difference in concurrent prescriptions and the
decrease over the interval were statistically significant for
older and younger claimants.

DISCUSSION

Several studies have examined the use of prescription drugs by the
elderly and the World Health Organization (1981) estimates that,
where the proportion of elderly in the population approaches 20%,
they account for over 50% of the total drug consumption. In
Canada, a study in our neighboring province found that the 11% of
Saskatchewan's population aged 65 and older received 28% of all
prescriptions written in 1976 (Skoll *et al.*, 1979). In that year,

Table 4. Multiple psychotherapeutic prescriptions*

Number of prescriptions		50 to 64 years		65 years and older	
		Men	Women	Men	Women
One	1975	23.8 (15.6)	22.9 (13.7)	33.3 (19.9)	25.0 (12.7)
	1978	25.8 (13.5)	34.6 (17.1)	39.3 (18.4)	26.7 (14.9)
Two	1975	23.8 (17.5)	25.1 (17.2)	19.9 (13.4)	25.4 (19.3)
	1978	14.1 (11.7)	17.1 (10.1)	13.5 (9.2)	22.3 (16.3)
Three	1975	11.9 (10.6)	12.8 (11.0)	11.9 (11.4)	20.6 (17.1)
	1978	8.0 (6.7)	11.5 (8.8)	9.8 (4.9)	14.4 (9.9)
Four	1975	5.0 (5.0)	11.0 (11.0)	7.0 (5.0)	7.9 (7.5)
	1978	4.3 (2.5)	9.2 (6.9)	4.9 (3.7)	5.0 (4.0)
Five	1975	7.9 (6.6)	7.9 (6.6)	2.5 (2.0)	3.9 (3.1)
	1978	1.2 (1.2)	1.8 (1.8)	0.6 (0.0)	3.0 (2.5)
Six or more	1975	4.4 (3.8)	7.0 (7.0)	1.0 (1.0)	0.9 (0.9)
	1978	1.2 (1.2)	2.8 (2.8)	0.6 (0.6)	1.5 (1.5)

*Open figures indicate the percentage of claimants in each group who received that number of psychotherapeutic drugs, and figures in parentheses indicate the percentage in each group who received that number for more than 120 days.
A prescription for a psychotherapeutic drug specified a drug from one of the following categories: phenothiazines, other major tranquilizers, tricyclic antidepressants, MAO inhibitors, lithium, benzodiazepines, chloral hydrate and other minor sedative-hypnotics, levodopa, codeine, other narcotic analgesics, propoxyphene, phenobarbital, other barbiturates, hydantoins, and other anticonvulsants.

77% of those over 65 received at least one prescription drug, and the average number prescribed for the elderly in that province was 4.1.

Our surveys in 1975 and 1978 have attempted to define the drugs prescribed for that portion of the older population that could be characterized as heavy drug users. Although a $50 annual expenditure for prescription drugs provides a rather arbitrary limit, we feel that it reasonably encompasses all the heavy drug users in Manitoba. This study indicates that 24% of all Manitobans aged 65 or older in 1978 met this criterion, and actually had a mean expenditure of $185 for an average 8.6 prescription drugs that year. It should be noted that these surveys did not include hospitalized or institutionalized elderly who might be predicted to be heavy drug users.

Although there were more women than men represented in the random samples from both years, it was only for the claimants aged 50 to 64 that this sex-related difference was statistically significant. For the claimants aged 65 and older, the female:male distribution approximated the female:male distribution of Manitoba's over 65 population (1.24:1 in 1978). Similarly, women received more drugs than men in both 1975 and 1978, but the difference was statistically significant only for the younger groups.

This study has focused on the use of psychotherapeutic drugs by older heavy drug users, and the widespread prescription of these drugs to the elderly was predictable. A study in Boston found that 20% of all patients admitted to general medical and surgical wards there had used psychotropic agents in the three months prior to hospitalization, and that 'use of these drugs was higher in middle and older-aged groups, and higher in women than among men' (Greenblatt *et al.*, 1975). Similarly, a study of American adults showed differences in psychotherapeutic drug use related to sex and age, such that 28% of the men and 35% of the women over 60 years of age had used such drugs in the preceding year (Parry *et al.*, 1973).

As might be expected, the prescription of psychotherapeutic drugs was much higher in our surveys of heavy drug users. Approximately two-thirds of the claimants aged 65 and older had been given psychotherapeutic agents in both 1975 and 1978. Although the percentage of men and women who had received at least one such prescription was not different in either year, there were more women than men who got more than one of these drugs, and more women who used psychotherapeutic drugs chronically.

It was not unexpected that prescriptions for benzodiazepines made up the bulk of this drug use, but the amount of sedative-hypnotic barbiturate prescribed for this population is surprising. By 1975, barbiturates were well recognized as being obsolete and potentially dangerous drugs, especially for the elderly (Koch-Weser and Greenblatt, 1974). Thus, although their prescription frequency decreased for 1975 to 1978, it is difficult to understand why these barbiturates were still being used by a substantial proportion of elderly Manitobans. If new prescriptions were not being written, it is likely that this use represents a continuation of prescriptions originally given to these heavy drug users some years earlier. In this way aging patients, possibly assisted by aging physicians, may tend to accumulate drugs.

Our surveys indicate that antidepressants and antipsychotic agents were often given to these heavy drug users and, in most instances, prescribed chronically. There may be more justification for the prescription of these drugs for the elderly than for the prescription of barbiturates. However, what Fries (1980) refers to as 'the loss of the ability to maintain homeostasis' makes these medications more hazardous for the elderly because of their prominent cardiovascular and anticholinergic effects.

It is not clear why the age-related differences in prescription frequency of the tricyclic antidepressants and phenothiazines recorded in 1975 were not present in 1978. Indeed, there were no age-related differences in prescription frequency for any of the major psychotherapeutic categories in 1978, suggesting further

that the patterns of psychotherapeutic drug use shown by these
Manitobans had actually been established before they reached old
age.

Codeine was widely prescribed for these elderly Manitobans
and its use is emphasized because the prescription of codeine and
other narcotic analgesics adds to the burden of drugs borne by
geriatric patients. The demonstration in our study of the substantial number of older heavy drug users who receive multiple and
concurrent psychotherapeutic drugs is particularly worrisome.
Deterioration of intellectual and emotional function are the major
adverse effects associated with the use of these agents in the
elderly, and the study of Williamson and Chopin (1980) demonstrates that drugs acting on the central nervous system are the
most likely to result in adverse effects leading to hospital
admission for geriatric patients.

These surveys provide a database by which we can examine the
magnitude of this problem in Canada, and through which we may
confirm that elderly patients at risk may be identified by the
amount and type of drugs prescribed for them.

SUMMARY AND CONCLUSIONS

Claims submitted under Manitoba's Pharmacare plan are being
sampled at three-year intervals to provide information on elderly
Manitobans who spend more than $50 annually on prescription drugs.
In 1975 and 1978, the claims of individuals aged 65 and older were
compared with those of claimants aged 50 to 64. In both years,
there were more younger women than men who spent more than $50 on
drugs, and the younger women received more drugs than the younger
men. In contrast, the sex distribution of older claimants approximated that of the province's over-65 population (55% females), and
the difference in number of drugs received was not statistically
significant. The most frequently prescribed drug categories for
the elderly claimants were thiazide-type diuretics, benzodiazepines, salicylates, sympathomimetics, digoxin and codeine.

Benzodiazepines, codeine, phenobarbital, other barbiturates,
tricyclic antidepressants and phenothiazines were the most commonly prescribed psychotherapeutic categories for the elderly
claimants. There were few differences in prescription frequency
between 1975 and 1978, but there were substantial decreases in the
prescription of phenobarbital and other barbiturates. More women
than men aged 65 and older received prescriptions for benzodiazepines, phenothiazines and barbiturates other than phenobarbital in
both years. Over two-thirds of the elderly claimants received
prescriptions for at least one psychotherapeutic drug in both
years, and concurrent prescriptions of these agents was relatively
common.

Drugs prescribed for the elderly tend to accumulate like the maladies for which they are prescribed, and each drug adds to the risk of adverse drug effects. Psychotherapeutic drugs are no exception to this rule and, indeed, are often associated with the most devastating consequences.

These surveys have demonstrated that a substantial proportion of Manitoba's elderly population are heavy drug users, and that much of that drug use consists of psychotherapeutic agents. Our information on the hazards posed by this use is incomplete, but enough is known to make us promote the appropriate and considerate prescription of psychotherapeutic drugs as an essential goal for those who care for the elderly.

Acknowledgements

The generous support of Dr J.A. MacDonell is gratefully acknowledged, as is the expert assistance of Mr Gary Scott. The Manitoba Health Services Commission continues to be most accommodating in allowing access to the Pharmacare records.

REFERENCES

Aoki, F.Y., Hildahl, V.K., Large, G.W., Mitenko, P.A. and Sitar, D.S. (1982). Aging and heavy drug use: a prescription survey in Manitoba. J. Chronic Dis., in press.

Boethius, G. (1977). Recording of drug prescriptions in the county of Jamtland, Sweden. Acta Med. Scand., 202, 241–51.

Fries, J.F. (1980). Aging, natural death and the compression of morbidity. New Engl. J. Med., 303, 130–5.

Greenblatt, D.J., Shader, R.I. and Koch-Weser, (1975). Psychotropic drug use in the Boston area. Arch. Gen. Psychiatry, 32, 518–21.

Hurwitz, N. (1969). Predisposing reactions in adverse reactions to drugs. Br. Med. J., 1, 536–9.

Koch-Weser, J. and Greenblatt, D.J. (1974). The archaic barbiturate hypnotics (Editorial). New Engl. J. Med., 291, 790.

Parry, H.J., Balter, M.B., Mellinger, G.D., Cisin, I.M. and Manheimer, D.I. (1973). National patterns of psychotherapeutic drug use. Arch. Gen. Psychiatry, 28, 769–83.

Skoll, S.L., August, R.J. and Johnson, G.E., (1979). Drug prescribing for the elderly in Saskatchewan in 1976. Can. Med. Assoc. J., 121, 1074–81.

Williamson, J. and Chopin, J.M. (1980). Adverse reactions to prescribed drugs in the elderly: a multicentre investigation. Age Ageing, 9, 73–80.

World Health Organization (1981). Health care in the elderly: report of the technical group on the use of medicaments by the elderly. Drugs, 22, 279–94.

To what extent are inter- and intra-regional differences in psychotropic drug use explained by demographic and socio-economic factors?

David J. King[1] and Kathryn Griffiths[2]

INTRODUCTION

Geographical comparisons made between psychotropic drug usage levels in different countries (Grimsson *et al.*, 1979) or particular regions (Westerholm, 1979; Elmes *et al.*, 1976a) have not usually taken into consideration the varying proportions of inhabitants that constitute the 'at risk' population, or any differences in their living conditions, and without reference to these characteristics of the people receiving drug treatment it is difficult to judge the clinical relevance of any disparities found. Furthermore, since comparable and reliable psychiatric morbidity data are particularly difficult to obtain, regional differences in psychotropic drug prescribing are probably more usefully related to objective demographic and socio-economic measures in the first instance. A Central Mental Health Records Scheme, based on returns from all psychiatric hospitals and units in Northern Ireland, has been in operation since 1960. Although these data are incomplete in some respects, it is hoped to make some comparisons with the drug utilization data in a subsequent study.

Drug prescribing studies in Northern Ireland benefit from a number of advantages, which are as follows. (i) Data on general practice prescribing can be supplied by the Northern Ireland Central Services Agency (CSA) which has been processing over 95% of the National Health Service (NHS) prescriptions in the province through a computerized pricing system since 1966. (ii) There is no hospital prescribing for outpatients, and tentative estimates

---
[1] Department of Therapeutics and Pharmacology, The Queen's University of Belfast, and Consultant Psychiatrist, Holywell Hospital, Antrim, N.Ireland.

[2] Department of Therapeutics and Pharmacology, The Queen's University of Belfast, N.Ireland.

of hospital prescribing for inpatients indicate that this only accounts for between 5 and 10% of total NHS psychotropic prescribing, and therefore the CSA data represent virtually all the psychotropic drugs prescribed in the province. (iii) With the exception of the Belfast area, the Department of Health and Social Services (DHSS) districts in Northern Ireland correspond to groups of district council areas for which census and more recent housing condition data are available. The DHSS districts can also be related to the travel to work areas or aggregations of employment service office areas for unemployment statistics. (iv) Our department has collaborated for a number of years in the WHO 'Drug Utilization Research Group', which has coordinated the work of a number of European countries which have agreed on a common system of drug classification and quantification. The classification system adopted is the so-called anatomical classification of the European Pharmaceutical Market Research Association (EPhMRA) and the unit of measurement, the defined daily dose (DDD), is used as a technical unit of measurement and of comparison, which can be applied to drug data from any source (Lunde *et al.*, 1979).

METHODS

General practice prescribing data were obtained from the Northern Ireland CSA for all practices for a one-month period (October) of each year until 1970 but thereafter a three-month sample (April to June) was provided. This was then collated and converted to a measure of drug consumption per 1000 of the population per day using DDDs provided by the Nordic Council on Medicines (1979b), and expressed as DDD per 1000 inhabitants per day for each drug, as described previously (Elmes *et al.*, 1976b; McDevitt and McMeekin, 1979). The term 'tranquilizer' includes all benzodiazepines (excluding clonazepam) normally prescribed for daytime use, together with meprobamate, hydroxyzine and benzoctamine. 'Hypnotic' is synonymous with 'hypnotics and sedatives' in the EPhMRA classification. Barbiturate and non-barbiturate hypnotics are considered separately. Antidepressants include all tricyclics and monoamine oxidase inhibitors; L-tryptophan, viloxazine, mianserin and tofenacin were included from 1977 onwards and nomifensine from 1978. The term 'major tranquilizer' has been avoided and 'neuroleptic' used instead to avoid confusion. The European data were provided from sales figures, but since the Northern Ireland prescribing data cover 90-95% of all NHS psychotropic drug use in the province, the two sets of data were considered to be comparable.

The general practice psychotropic drug prescribing data for each of Northern Ireland's 17 health districts were then analyzed in detail for the year 1978. The drug usage level 'dependent' variables were mapped and their degree of association with 11 'independent' socio-economic variables examined. These demographic or socio-economic measures were chosen on the basis of factors which had previously been linked with high drug utiliz-ation or psychiatric morbidity, social indicators related to these reported factors, and variables suggested by the geographical pattern of Northern Ireland psychotropic drug utilization as being suitable for investigation. Details of these variables and their sources have been published elsewhere (King *et al.*, 1982). The district council areas for which these data were available corre-sponded closely to the DHSS health districts except for Belfast, which was treated as one area for some of the official statistics. The city data could not be subdivided according to the three health districts which were therefore treated as tied ranks for some of the socio-economic variables.

The degree of association between psychotropic drug utiliz-ation and each socio-economic variable for the 17 districts was found by calculating zero-order Spearman rank correlation coef-ficients. A multivariate analysis was performed on the psycho-tropic drug 'dependent' variables of tranquilizers, hypnotics, neuroleptics, antidepressants and psychostimulants with respect to six demographic and social indicators - the five that appear to be most highly correlated with drug utilization at the zero order, plus list size per doctor to standardize workload. Fifth-order Spearman partial correlation coefficients were calculated between the prescribing levels and each of the 'independent' variables in turn (population density, overcrowding, the proportion of females aged 45-59 in the population, the percentage of people over the age of 65, the unemployment rate, and list size per doctor) by keeping the effects of the remaining five socio-economic variables constant. The utilization figures were then transformed into logarithms and subjected to multiple regression analyses against population density, overcrowding, females aged 45-59, persons aged over 65 years, and list size per doctor. This procedure was repeated using unemployment rather than overcrowding as the fifth 'independent' socio-economic variable.

RESULTS

The overall pattern of psychotropic drug prescribing in Northern Ireland from 1966 to 1980, and the comparisons with Great Britain and other European countries, have been reported in detail else-where (King *et al.*, 1982). Total psychotropic drug consumption reached a peak of 88 DDD per 1000 inhabitants per day, i.e. ap-proximately 8.8% of the total population, or 12.5% of the adult population (over 15 years), in 1975. The subsequent decline has been due to the changing pattern of benzodiazepine use since this has represented an increasingly large proportion of the total psychotropic drugs prescribed, so that in 1980 they constituted 98% of all tranquilizer, 78% of all hypnotic and 75% of all psy-chotropic drugs prescribed. Thus both total tranquilizer and

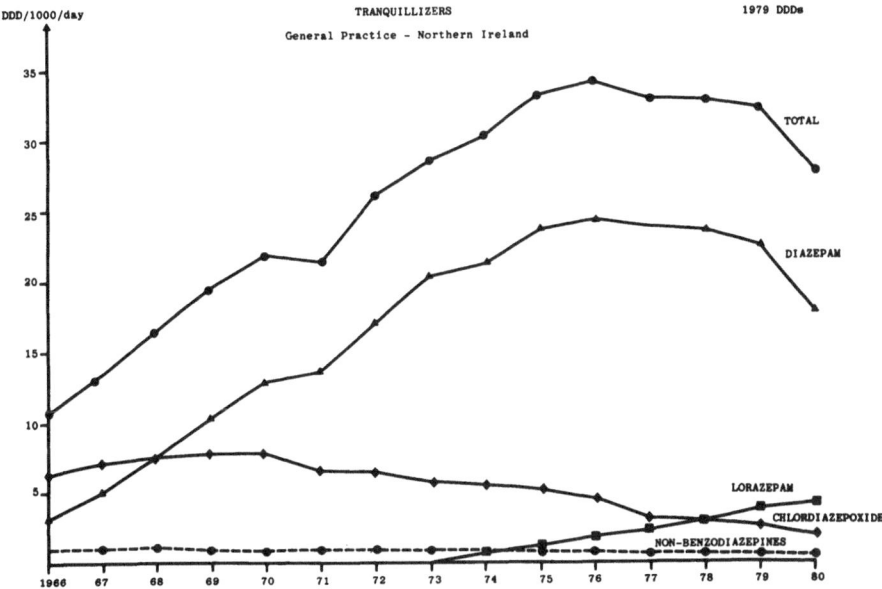

Figure 1. Psychotropic drug prescribing levels in Northern Ireland 1966-80. Defined daily doses per 1000 per day for diazepam, lorazepam, chlordiazepozide, non-benzodiazepines and total tranquilizers.

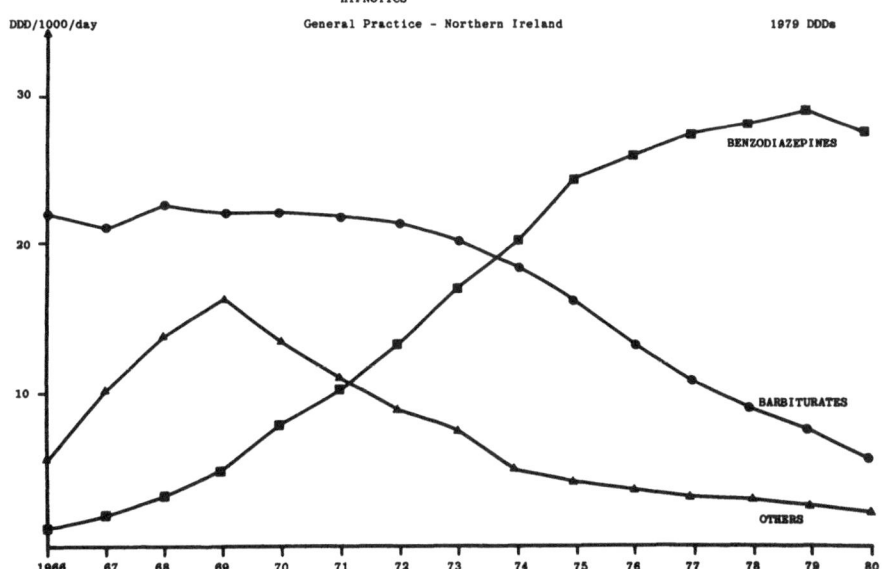

Figure 2. Psychotropic drug prescribing levels in Northern Ireland 1966-80. Defined daily doses per 1000 per day for barbiturate and benzodiazepine hypnotics.

diazepam prescribing showed a similar pattern to the total psychotropic drug use, reaching a peak a year later (1976) and after a three-year plateau began to decline after 1979 (figure 1). Earlier decreases were evident in psychostimulant and barbiturate hypnotic use. The latter has been falling steadily since 1968 (figure 2). The main effect of the 1975-77 CURB campaign on this trend was to accelerate the decline in the quantity of barbiturates prescribed but not in the number of barbiturate prescriptions written (King *et al.*, 1980). The successful reduction in barbiturate prescribing has probably been due to the ready availability of alternative hypnotics, for although non-barbiturate exceeded barbiturate hypnotic prescribing in 1972, and benzodiazepine exceeded barbiturate hypnotics two years later (figure 2), total hypnotic drug use did not show any reduction until 1979.

The remaining drug groups have continued to show steady but more gradual increases over the period of study. Antidepressant prescribing doubled between 1966 and 1975 (King *et al.*, 1977) and neuroleptic use also almost doubled from 1.5 to 2.9 DDD per 1000 per day between 1966 and 1980 (figure 3). It is evident that

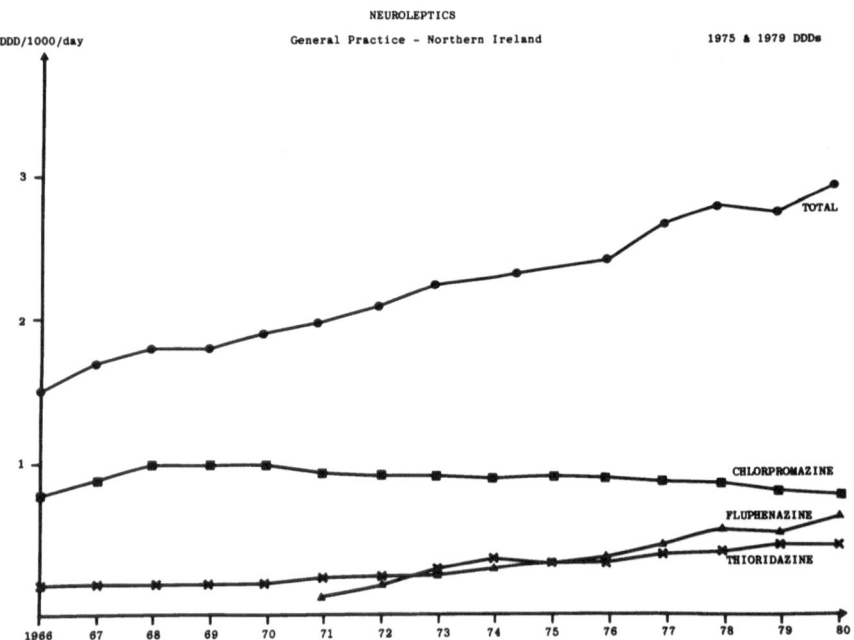

Figure 3. Psychotropic drug prescribing levels in Northern
Ireland 1966-80. Defined daily doses per 1000 per day
for chlorpromazine, thioridazine, fluphenazine and
total neuroleptics.

general practitioners have been making increasing use of depot neuroleptic preparations while chlorpromazine prescribing has remained remarkably static.

The inter-regional comparisons of the use of the largest psychotropic drug group, benzodiazepine tranquilizers, are shown in figure 4. Clearly for the decade after 1966 the rise in tranquilizer use in Northern Ireland was more rapid than elsewhere, but the decline since 1976 means that the utilization here is now less than in Iceland and Denmark but still higher than in Norway, Sweden, Finland and Czechoslovakia. Although it has been speculated that various local factors such as the introduction of a monitoring scheme for benzodiazepines in Finland (Idänpään-Heikkilä, 1977), or the widening of the advertised indications for tranquilizer use (Hemminki *et al.*, 1981) may account for the fluctuations in consumption, the wide differences between Iceland on the one hand and Czechoslovakia on the other are difficult to

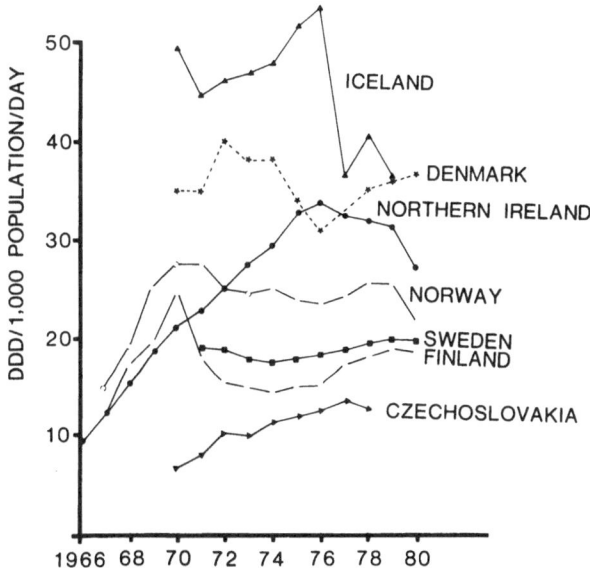

Figure 4. Benzodiazepine tranquilizer use in Czechoslovakia, Finland, Iceland, Norway, Sweden, Denmark and Northern Ireland for 1966-80, in defined daily doses per 1000 per day. (Figures for Iceland for 1976 and 1977 estimated from total benzodiazepines (Olafsson *et al.*, 1980) and tranquilizers (Nordic Council on Medicines, 1979a.) From King *et al.* (1982). Psychotropic drug use in Northern Ireland 1966-80. *Psychol. Med.* (in press). Reproduced by permission of Cambridge University Press.

explain. Differences in clinical indications for using these
drugs seem to be unlikely since they have been predominantly
prescribed for women and for persons in the 45-59 year old age
range in all regions studied (Balter *et al.*, 1974; Skegg *et al.*,
1977; Böethius and Westerholm, 1977; Anderson, 1980; Grímsson and
Olafsson, 1981). Our inter-regional analysis was designed to see
to what extent differences in demographic structure or socio-
economic circumstances explained variations in psychotropic drug
use.

When the psychotropic drug utilization rates were mapped out
for 1978, high tranquilizer and hypnotic prescribing appeared to
be associated with predominantly urban districts whereas neuroleptic and antidepressant use seemed to be greater in the rural
areas. The striking contrast between these two patterns of prescribing is shown for tranquilizers and neuroleptics in figures 5
and 6. The eastern border area of Newry and Mourne ranked highly
in each type of psychotropic drug usage but other country areas
adjacent to the Republic of Ireland tended to have low tranquil-

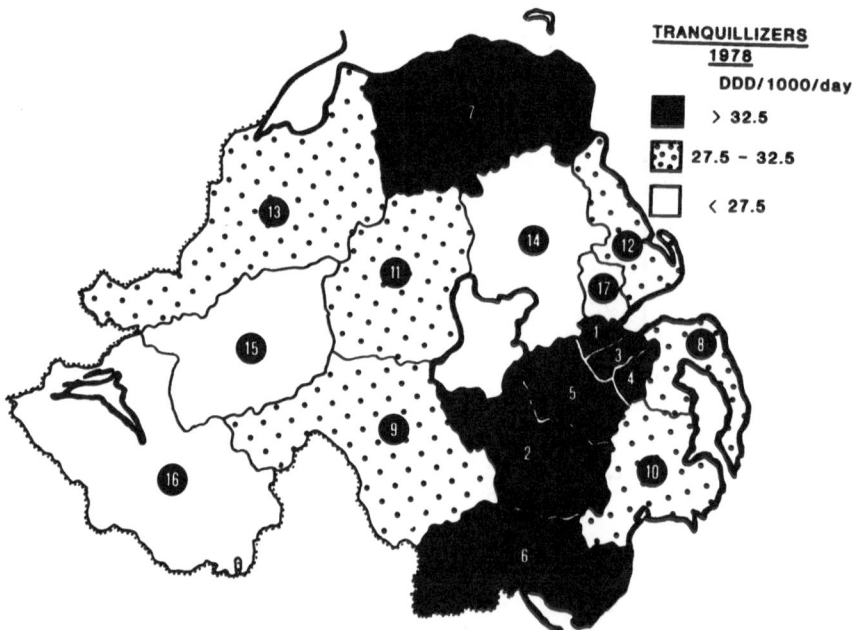

Figure 5.   Seventeen health districts in Northern Ireland ranked
according to high, intermediate and low prescribing of
tranquilizers in 1978. From King *et al.* (1982).
Psychotropic drug use in Northern Ireland 1966-80.
Psychol. Med. (in press). Reproduced by permission of
Cambridge University Press.

izer, hypnotic and psychostimulant utilization rates with slightly higher antidepressant prescribing and above-average neuroleptic use.

The zero-order Spearman rank correlation coefficients showed that antidepressant and neuroleptic utilization rates were significantly inter-related although neither correlated well with the other types of psychotropic drug usage. High antidepressant prescribing was associated with a low benzodiazepine proportion of tranquilizer and hypnotic use ($r_s = -0.52$) and a high barbiturate proportion of hypnotic prescribing tended to be linked with high psychostimulant and antidepressant utilization ($r_s = 0.51$). Some of the 'independent' socio-economic variables were also strongly inter-related, the most striking association being between unemployment and overcrowding ($r_s = 0.87$). Both poor housing conditions, measured in terms of overcrowding (the proportion of people living at more than 1.5 persons per room), and high unemployment existed in rural areas with low population density ($r_s = 0.68$ and $r_s = 0.69$ respectively).

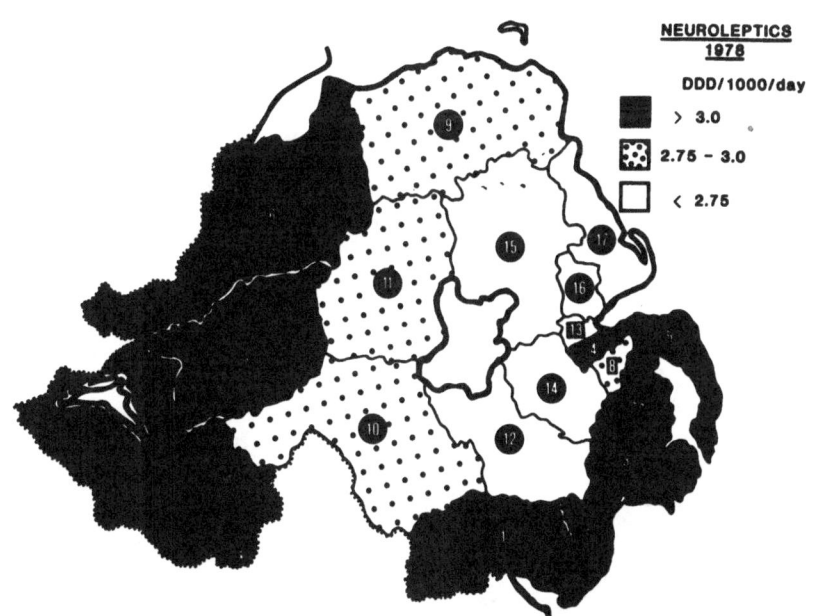

Figure 6. Seventeen health districts in Northern Ireland ranked according to high, intermediate and low prescribing of neuroleptics in 1978. From King *et al.* (1982). Psychotropic drug use in Northern Ireland 1966-80. *Psychol. Med.* (in press). Reproduced by permission of Cambridge University Press.

The main psychotropic drug group and socio-economic variable
zero-order correlation coefficients are shown in table 1. These
indicated a significant correlation between population density and
tranquilizer but not neuroleptic prescribing. Neuroleptic prescribing correlated most highly with overcrowding and unemployment, whereas hypnotic prescribing was most significantly correlated with females aged 45-59 and persons over 65 years. The
fifth-order multivariate analyses are shown in table 2. These led
to the loss of significance for a number of the zero-order correlations but the emergence of population density as significantly
correlated with neuroleptic prescribing. Age above 65 years was
significantly correlated with both hypnotic and neuroleptic prescribing. The exclusion of overcrowding or unemployment did not
account for the 'disappearance' of their significance and the
emergence of population density as the most relevant variable in
neuroleptic prescribing. There were no significant correlations
between list size per doctor and any of the psychotropic drug
prescribing levels, nor between estimated population movement and
psychotropic drug prescribing.

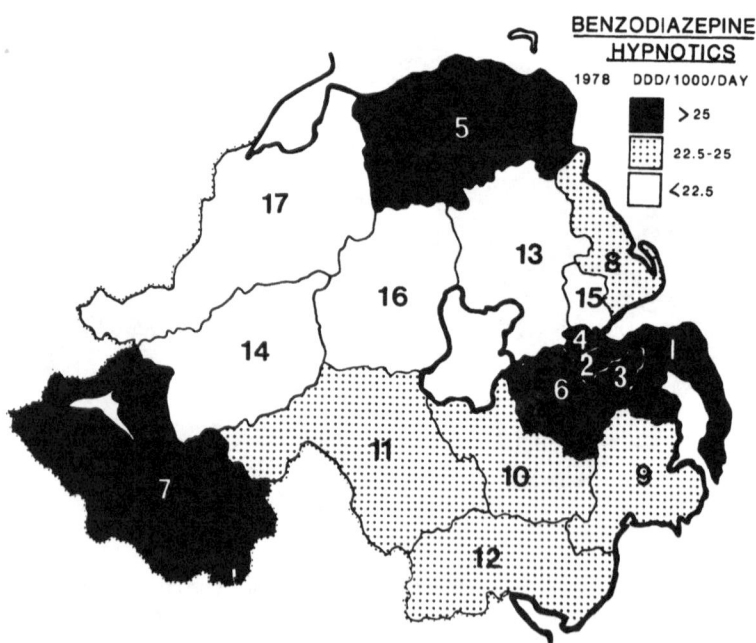

Figure 7.   Seventeen health districts in Northern Ireland ranked
according to high, intermediate and low prescribing of
benzodiazepine hypnotics in 1978.

Table 1. Zero-order Spearman correlation coefficients*

Prescribing level	Population density	Overcrowding	Females aged 45-59	Persons aged 65+	Unemployment	List size per doctor
1 Tranquilizers	0.56†	- 0.14	0.47	0.43	- 0.19	- 0.10
2 Benzodiazepine hypnotics	0.50	- 0.49§	0.74†	0.85†	- 0.44	0.10
3 Barbiturate hypnotics	0.33	- 0.08	0.29	0.44	- 0.13	- 0.10
4 Hypnotics	0.48§	- 0.28	0.57†	0.73†	- 0.25	- 0.03
5 Neuroleptics	- 0.25	0.60†	- 0.41	0.25	0.59†	- 0.30
6 Antidepressants	- 0.32	0.37	- 0.29	0.28	0.46	- 0.41
7 Psychostimulants	0.42	- 0.20	0.32	0.32	- 0.14	0.06

* From King et al. (1982). Psychotropic drug use in Northern Ireland 1966-80. Psychol.Med. (in press). Reproduced by permission of Cambridge University Press.
† $p < 0.02$
§ $p < 0.05$

The findings of the multiple regression analyses including unemployment are summarized in table 3. Here it can be seen that although population density is once again the most relevant socio-economic variable associated with tranquilizer prescribing, it only accounted for 31.7% of the variance, and the total variance explained was only 32.5%, which did not reach statistical significance. A significant proportion (75%; $p < 0.01$) of neuroleptic prescribing, however, was accounted for by overcrowding, the proportion of elderly (persons over 65 years), females aged 45-59 years, and population density, in that order. An even greater proportion of hypnotic (82%; $p < 0.01$), particularly benzodiazepine hypnotic (95.1%; $p < 0.01$), but not barbiturate hypnotic (38.8%; n.s.), prescribing was accounted for by the socio-economic variables. For all hypnotic groups the proportion of elderly was the most important explanatory variable. Substituting unemployment for overcrowding did not materially alter the results. The geographical pattern of benzodiazepine hypnotic prescribing is shown in figure 7.

Table 2. Fifth-order partial correlation coefficients*

Prescribing level	Population density	Overcrowding	Females aged 45-59	Persons aged 65+	Unemployment	List size per doctor
1 Tranquilizers	0.42	0.27	0.11	0.21	0.06	- 0.19
2 Benzodiazepine hypnotics	0.08	- 0.13	0.12	0.76†	- 0.04	0.07
3 Barbiturate hypnotics	0.36	0.03	- 0.19	0.40	- 0.10	- 0.20
4 Hypnotics	0.38	- 0.03	- 0.08	0.60§	0.05	- 0.16
5 Neuroleptics	0.60§	- 0.08	- 0.53	0.64§	0.15	- 0.40
6 Antidepressants	0.23	- 0.30	- 0.34	0.49	0.22	- 0.45
7 Psychostimulants	0.44	- 0.18	- 0.24	0.34	0.10	- 0.08

* From King et al. (1982). Psychotropic drug use in Northern Ireland 1966-80. Psychol.Med. (in press). Reproduced by permission of Cambridge University Press.
† $p < 0.02$
§ $p < 0.05$

DISCUSSION

The recent decline in Northern Ireland tranquilizer prescribing may reflect an effect of the 'Systematic review of benzodiaze-pines' in 1980 (Committee on the Review of Medicines, 1980) and the associated media publicity at that time about the dangers of benzodiazepine dependence. It certainly suggests that major campaigns such as was mounted for barbiturates are unnecessary to influence prescribing (King *et al.*, 1980). Clearly the severe rioting from 1969, which peaked in 1972, bears no direct relation-ship to tranquilizer prescribing in the province as a whole, although who can say that those civil disturbances did not have prolonged or delayed effects?

It seems likely that broad trends in psychotropic drug use follow certain world-wide changes in prescribing fashions and patient demands. For instance, in the United States the number of

Table 3. Order of independent variables (in parentheses) in the regression equation*, and the percent cumulative variance explained

	Tranqui-lizers	Benzodiazepine hypnotics	Barbiturate hypnotics	Hypnotics	Neuro-leptics	Anti-depressants	Psycho-stimulants
Population density	(1) 31.7	(3) 92.7	(5) 38.8	(4) 78.7	(4) 75.0	(3) 33.0	(4) 21.9
Overcrowding	(3) 32.3	(4) 94.6	(3) 33.7	(5) 82.0	(1) 42.6	(1) 12.2	(3) 17.6
Females aged 45–59	(4) 32.5	(2) 92.3	(4) 34.0	(2) 76.4	(3) 71.6	(5) 40.3	(1) 14.7
Persons aged 65+	(2) 32.0	(1) 81.9	(1) 28.3	(1) 70.6	(2) 69.8	(2) 21.9	(5) 27.2
List size per doctor	(5) 32.5†	(5) 95.1	(2) 32.0	(3) 78.0	(5) 75.1	(4) 40.0	(2) 16.8
F	1.44	43.04**	1.39	10.00§	6.65§	1.49	0.82
Unemployment	(2) 32.2	(5) 94.4	(3) 35.8	(4) 79.7	(1) 36.9	(1) 11.0	(2) 16.8

* From King et al. (1982). Psychotropic drug use in Northern Ireland 1966-80. Psychol.Med. (in press). Reproduced by permission of Cambridge University Press.
† No more variance accounted for than in 4.
§ $p < 0.01$
** $p < 0.001$

tranquilizer prescriptions reached a peak in 1973, and the total quantity prescribed peaked in 1978 (Rickels, 1981). There remain marked inter- and intra-regional differences, however, which are not easily accounted for and raise the question as to whether some regions are over-treating or others under-treating psychiatric illness.

In our intra-regional study of the 1978 psychotropic drug data, the most striking differences appeared at first sight to be due to the urban/rural divide (see figures 5 and 6). Total psychotropic prescribing in Belfast was approximately 50% higher than in country districts. This may partly reflect less readily available services in rural districts, and, indeed, the district average number of rural practitioner fund units paid to doctors for patients living more than three miles from the surgery was inversely (but non-significantly) correlated with psychotropic drug prescribing. The higher use of tranquilizers and hypnotics in urban areas was expected and was consistent with previous findings in Northern Ireland (Elmes *et al.*, 1976a), Iceland (Olafsson, 1981) and the higher urban 'anxiety' consultation rates reported by the Royal College of General Practitioners (1979) in Great Britain. On the other hand, the higher use of neuroleptics in rural areas had not been predicted.

The statistical comparisons yielded different answers for different drug subgroups. An association between tranquilizer and hypnotic prescribing and population density was confirmed in the zero-order Spearman rank correlation coefficients. However, when the separate effects of the different demographic and socio-economic variables were controlled in the multivariate analysis, it emerged that, while neuroleptic prescribing was significantly correlated with population density, tranquilizer and hypnotic prescribing were not (table 2). Moreover both hypnotic and neuroleptic prescribing were also significantly correlated with the proportion of elderly persons (aged over 65 years). In fact the two most potent explanatory variables identified by the multiple regression analyses were the relative proportions of elderly persons (over 65 years) and females aged 45-59 years, which alone accounted for 92.3% of the variance in benzodiazepine hypnotic prescribing, and also contributed substantially to the variance in use of most of the other psychotropic drug groups. The variables included in the multiple regression analysis accounted for 75.1% of neuroleptic prescribing but only 32.5% of tranquilizer prescribing. Combining the results of these two statistical exercises it must be concluded, therefore, that as far as Northern Ireland is concerned, the prescribing of benzodiazepine hypnotics is a function of the proportion of elderly and women aged 45-59 years; neuroleptic prescribing is largely a function of factors associated with rural areas (overcrowding and unemployment) together with the proportion of elderly in the community; but that neither tranquilizer, antidepressant, barbiturate hypnotic nor psychostimulant prescribing were satisfactorily explained by any of the variables we studied.

Nevertheless, the success of demographic and socio-economic factors in explaining benzodiazepine hypnotic and neuroleptic prescribing suggests that further extensions or refinements of this approach should be able to account for the variations in prescribing in the remaining psychotropic drug groups. Other factors which we were unable to include in this first study, such as marital status and social class, may have been responsible for some of the unexplained variance and should be included in future studies. In addition, data on alcohol consumption and, of course, morbidity should greatly improve the degree of explanation reached for intra-regional psychotropic drug prescribing differences. Some of the differences in psychiatric morbidity data in turn might also be expected to be subjected to demographic and socio-economic determinants (Hollingshead and Redlich, 1958; Langer and Michael, 1963; Shepherd *et al.*, 1966; Factor and Waldron, 1973). Thus these variables must be taken into account before valid conclusions about any inter- or intra-regional differences in either psychotropic drug utilization or psychiatric morbidity data can be drawn, or any inferences made about relative over-treatment or under-treatment of psychiatric illness in particular regions.

SUMMARY

A study of psychotropic drug prescribing derived from the computerized pricing data in Northern Ireland from 1966 showed that the use of these drugs reached a peak in 1975, when about 12.5% of the adult population were estimated to have been receiving them, and declined in the following five years. The rate of increase in benzodiazepine tranquilizer utilization was greater than in other European countries, but the level was generally lower than in Iceland and Denmark. The influence of 11 demographic and socio-economic variables was studied in an intra-regional analysis of the 1978 data for the 17 health districts in the province, using multivariate and multiple regression statistics. In benzodiazepine hypnotic prescribing 92.3% of the variance was accounted for by the proportion of elderly (over 65 years) and women aged 45-59 years; neuroleptic prescribing was largely a function of factors associated with rural areas (overcrowding and unemployment) and the proportion of elderly; but neither tranquilizer, antidepressant, barbiturate hypnotic nor psychostimulant prescribing were satisfactorily explained by these variables.

Acknowledgements

We wish to thank Dr J.D. Merrett for statistical assistance; Dr A.L. Walby and Mr J. Barry of Research and Intelligence, Department of Health and Social Services, Northern Ireland, for providing the district drug analyses; Mr R. McMullan of the Central Services Agency, for supplying additional prescribing statistics; and Mr R. Beckett and Mr J. Birch of Manpower Services and Miss E. Hume of the Registrar General's Office, Northern Ireland, for their help and advice.

Figures 4, 5 and 6 and tables 1, 2 and 3 have been reproduced by the kind permission of the editor of *Psychological Medicine* and the publishers, Cambridge University Press.

We are also indebted to the following for providing their drug information:

Czechoslovakia
Dr J. Elis and Dr L. Stika, Institute of Pharmacology, Academy of Sciences, Prague.

Denmark
Mr H.U. Schaffalitzky de Muckadell, National Board of Health, Copenhagen.

Finland
Dr J. Idänpään-Heikkilä, National Board of Health, Helsinki.

Great Britain
Mrs M.J. Roberts, Statistics and Research Division, Department of Health and Social Services, London.

Iceland
Dr O. Olafsson, Medicinaldirektor, Arnarhvali, Reykjavik.
Mr I. Petersen, Pharmaceutical Division, Ministry of Health and Social Security, Reykjavik.

Norway
Mr B. Jøldal, Pharmaceutical Division, The Health Services of Norway, Oslo.

Sweden
Mrs I. Agenäs, Apoteksbolaget, Stockholm.

REFERENCES

Anderson, R. (1980). Prescribed medicines: who takes what? J. Epidem. Comm. Health, 34, 299–304.
Balter, M.B., Levine, J. and Manheimer, D.I. (1974). Cross-national study of the extent of anti-anxiety/sedative drug use. New Engl. J. Med., 290, 769–74.
Böethius, G. and Westerholm, B. (1977). Purchases of hypnotics, sedatives and minor tranquilizers among 2566 individuals in

the county of Jamtland, Sweden – a 6 years' follow up. _Acta Psych. Scand._, **56**, 147–59.

Committee on the Review of Medicines (1980). Systematic review of benzodiazepines. _Br. Med. J._, **280**, 910–12.

Elmes, P.C., Hood, H., McMeekin, C. and Wade, O.L. (1976a). Prescribing in Northern Ireland: study number 1, sleeping tablets. _Ulster Med. J._, **45**, 166–77.

Elmes, P.C., Hood, H. and Wade, O.L. (1976b). Prescribing in Northern Ireland: methods of analysis. _Ulster Med. J._, **45**, 56–58.

Factor, R.M. and Waldron, I. (1973). Contemporary population densities and human health. _Nature_, 243, 381–4.

Grímsson, A., Idänpään-Heikkilä, J., Lunde, P.K.M., Olafsson, O. and Westerholm, B. (1979). The utilization of psychotropic drugs in Finland, Iceland, Norway and Sweden. In _Studies in Drug Utilization, Methods and Applications_ (eds U. Bergman, A. Grímsson, A.H.W. Wahba and B. Westerholm), Regional Publications European Series no. 8, WHO Regional Office for Europe, Copenhagen, pp. 163–7.

Grímsson, A. and Olafsson, O. (1981). Drug prescriptions in Reykjavik according to age, sex and marital status. In _Drugs in Iceland_ (ed. O. Olafsson), Landlaeknisembaettid, Reykjavik, pp. 65–74.

Hemminki, E., Bruun, K. and Jensen, T.O. (1981). Use of benzodiazepines in the Nordic countries in the 1960s and 1970s. Paper presented at _WHO Drug Utilization Research Group Meeting_, Korcula, 28–30 April.

Hollingshead, A.B. and Redlich, F.C. (1958). _Social Class and Mental Illness: A Community Study_, John Wiley and Sons, New York, p. 210.

Idänpään-Heikkilä, J. (1977). Use of anxiolytics, sedatives, hypnotics, antidepressants and neuroleptics in Finland in 1966–1976. _Suomen Apteekkarilehti_, 1, 20–31.

King, D.J., Griffiths, K., Hall, C.E., Cooper, N.C. and Morrison, D.J. (1980). Effect of the CURB campaign on barbiturate prescribing in Northern Ireland _J. R. Coll. Gen. Pract._, **30**, 614–18.

King, D.J., Griffiths, K., Reilly, P.M. and Merret, J.D. (1982). Psychotropic drug use in Northern Ireland 1966–80: prescribing trends, inter- and intra-regional comparisons and relationship to demographic and socioeconomic variables. _Psychol. Med._, (in press).

King, D.J., McMeekin, C. and Elmes, P.C. (1977). Are we as depressed as we think we are? _Ulster Med. J._, **46**, 105–12.

Langer, T.S. and Michael, S.T. (1963). _Life Stress and Mental Health. The Midtown Manhattan Study_, Thomas A.C. Rennie Series in Social Psychiatry, vol. II, Collier-Macmillan, London.

Lunde, P.K.M., Baksaas, I., Halse, M., Halvorsen, I.K., Strømnes, B. and Øydvin, K. (1979). The methodology of drug utilization studies. In <u>Studies in Drug Utilization, Methods and Applications</u> (eds U. Bergman, A. Grímsson, A.H.W. Wahba and B. Westerholm), Regional Publications European Series no. 8, WHO Regional Office for Europe, Copenhagen, pp. 17-28.

McDevitt, D.G. and McMeekin, C. (1979). Data collection in Northern Ireland. In <u>Studies in Drug Utilization, Methods and Applications</u> (eds U. Bergman, A. Grímsson, A.H.W. Wahba and B. Westerholm), Regional Publications European Series no. 8, WHO Regional Office for Europe, Copenhagen, pp. 103-11.

Nordic Council on Medicines (1979a). <u>Nordic Statistics on Medicines 1975-1977</u>, part I, Nordic Council on Medicines, Helsingfors.

Nordic Council on Medicines (1979b). <u>Nordic Statistics on Medicines 1975-1977</u>, part II, <u>The Anatomical-Therapeutic-Chemical Classification System (ATC) and Defined Daily Doses</u>, Nordic Council on Medicines, Helsingfors.

Olafsson, O. (1981). Prescription habits of G.P. in Reykjavik and rural areas of Iceland on hypnotics and psychotropic drugs. In <u>Drugs in Iceland</u> (ed O. Olafsson), Landlaeknisembaettid, Reykjavik, pp. 33-40.

Olafsson, O., Sigfusson, S. and Grímsson, A. (1980). Control of addictive drugs in Iceland 1976-1978. <u>J. Epidem. Comm. Health.</u>, 34, 305.

Rickels, K. (1981). Are benzodiazepines overused and abused? <u>Br. J. Clin. Pharmacol.</u>, 11, 71S-83S.

Royal College of General Practitioners, Office of Population Censuses and Surveys and Department of Health and Social Security (1979). <u>Morbidity Statistics from General Practice 1971-1972</u>, Second National Study. Studies on Medical and Population Subjects no. 36, HMSO, London, p. 119.

Shepherd, M., Cooper, B., Brown, A.C. and Kalton, G. (1966). <u>Psychiatric Illness in General Practice</u>, Oxford University Press, London, pp. 97-105.

Skegg, D.C.G., Doll, R. and Perry, J. (1977). Use of medicines in general practice. <u>Br. Med. J.</u>, 1, 1561-3.

Westerholm, B. (1979). Data collection in Sweden. In <u>Studies in Drug Utilization, Methods and Applications</u> (eds U. Bergman, A. Grímsson, A.H.W. Wahba and B. Westerholm), Regional Publications European Series no. 8, WHO Regional Office for Europe, Copenhagen, pp. 73-82.

Section Two

Methodology of Clinical Trials in Psychopharmacology

Methodology of clinical trials: current issues

Bernard J.Carroll[1]

INTRODUCTION

One of the most sobering problems in the clinical pharmacology of depression is that, although we have had antidepressant drugs available for the past 25 years, we still do not know who responds specifically to them. As several authors in this volume have observed, the tricyclic antidepressant drugs are widely prescribed, mostly by non-psychiatrist physicians. Much of this widespread prescribing of tricyclic antidepressants is appropriate: hospital first-admission rates are declining and untreated severely depressed patients are rarely seen any more. On the other hand, we must strongly suspect that many simply unhappy or dysphoric patients are given these drugs unnecessarily and with predictable consequences in terms of morbidity from side-effects, mortality from overdosage, economic waste, and irrational, unproductive clinical management.

As the new generation of antidepressant drugs enlarges, the need to document *specificity of drug effect* in particular types of depressed patients grows correspondingly. Even for the tricyclic antidepressants there are no generally accepted criteria to select 'depressed' patients for drug treatment. Roland Kuhn originally emphasized that patients with the syndrome of 'vital depression' were the most likely to respond to imipramine (Kuhn, 1957). This diagnostic category corresponds to the syndrome 'endogenous depression' or 'melancholia' in other European, British and American settings. Yet we all know that in practice the diagnostic distinction between melancholic and non-endogenous depression is regarded as a difficult decision for many individual patients. As a result, many patients are 'given the benefit of the doubt' and receive tricyclic antidepressants on an empirical basis. Such a practice

---

[1]Department of Psychiatry, The University of Michigan, Ann Arbor, Michigan 48109, USA.

is not good medicine, any more than is the indiscriminate prescribing of antibiotics for non-bacterial respiratory infections.
Even in cases where the depression is clearly recognized as non-
endogenous there are no firm guidelines established for the use or
avoidance of antidepressant drugs.

This problem of nosology affects us not only from a public
health perspective and in our clinical practice but also in our
scientific work of identifying effective new drugs and understanding their pharmacokinetics. As one example, it seems likely that
a relationship between plasma imipramine concentration and clinical effect obtains for endogenous but not for non-endogenous
depressed patients (Gram *et al.*, 1977). Good studies of this
question with other antidepressants are difficult to find.

Clearly, our elegant studies of the chemistry, metabolism,
pharmacokinetics and pharmacodynamics of antidepressant drugs need
to be supplemented by equivalent rigor in the design of our clinical trials. Some of the more important aspects of this area are
briefly summarized below.

DESCRIPTION OF THE PATIENTS

No report of a clinical trial is adequate unless the reader can
judge from it the extent to which the results can be generalized.
The *clinical setting* is well known to affect the selection and
referral of depressed patients (Paykel *et al.*, 1970). Some
research units deal mainly with atypical, chronic or refractory
patients but this circumstance is rarely apparent in their published reports.

The group of patients studied needs to be clearly described
in the following ways in addition to the usual demographic features of age and sex:

(a) inpatient or outpatient;
(b) acute or chronic depression;
(c) first episode or recurrent;
(d) untreated or refractory;
(e) delusional or non-delusional;
(f) unipolar or bipolar;
(g) associated physical disorders;
(h) associated psychiatric disorders (e.g. personality
     disorder);
(i) overall level of social and occupational functioning
     (e.g. the Global Assessment of Severity (GAS) rating
     from the Schedule for Affective Disorders and
     Schizophrenia (SADS) (Spitzer *et al.*, 1977));
(j) severity of depressive symptoms, preferably with both
     observer ratings and self-ratings.

DIAGNOSTIC CRITERIA

Explicit, operationally defined diagnostic criteria are required for ease of communication from one clinical group to another. This is the primary purpose of such criteria. At the same time, it must be understood that *all* sets of diagnostic criteria are arbitrary conventions. So far, no one set of criteria is proven superior to others in terms of validity.

For this reason, it is an advantage if patients entered in clinical trials can be characterized simultaneously according to several sets of criteria - ICD, Washington University (St Louis or Feighner criteria), Research Diagnostic Criteria, DSM III, Newcastle Diagnostic Index I and II, and so forth. This will allow the respective performances of the sets of criteria to be compared and partly validated against response to treatment. Such a process can contribute to the eventual selection of some criteria in preference to others.

Misuse of Diagnostic Criteria

Considering the current state of nosologic problems in depression, the selection of patients for a clinical trial is an important task that should be carried out by the most experienced clinicians available. All sets of diagnostic criteria require a thorough knowledge of clinical phenomenology. The most appropriate way to use diagnostic criteria is to confirm that patients selected by the experienced clinicians have the specified number of relevant clinical features as part of the current episode of depression. On the other hand, since many psychiatric symptoms and signs are non-specific, it is *not* appropriate to use a set of diagnostic criteria in stand-alone fashion as a simple checklist (Carpenter *et al.*, 1980; Carroll *et al.*, 1980). The criteria should be regarded as necessary but not in themselves sufficient for the diagnosis, which must first be made by standard clinical assessment. Those patients who also meet the diagnostic criteria can then be entered into the clinical trial.

It is especially deplorable to entrust the diagnostic assessments to research assistants or medical students who are not well trained in clinical psychiatry. In some centers such raters are trained to administer a structured interview from which items on the diagnostic criteria sets are checked off, sometimes by computer programs. However, raters of this kind are not necessarily skilled in identifying complex or subtle phenomenologic features and they lack the experience of interpreting what they see in a clinical context. In particular, they lack the ability to discriminate a syndromal depressive illness from a collection of dysphoric complaints. A related issue is the use of symptomatic volunteers in clinical trials. These subjects are recruited either from newspaper advertisements or from checklist screening in general practice settings. While they might satisfy the nominal diagnostic criteria for depression, few of them would be likely candidates for antidepressant drug treatment when their overall clinical status is considered.

Finally, since most clinical trials now include a 7-10 day placebo washout period, a requirement for entry should be that the patient still meets the *diagnostic criteria at that time*. In many current trials the only requirement is that the patient meet a predetermined severity criterion after the placebo washout period. The problem with that approach is that many non-depressed patients will score significantly on any depression rating scale. Hamilton and others have long cautioned that such scales cannot be used for diagnostic purposes (Hamilton, 1960; Carroll *et al.*, 1973).

DOCUMENTING THE RELIABILITY OF CLINICAL ASSESSMENTS

In our laboratory work we have come to expect that quality control measures, estimates of laboratory error, between-assay variance and so forth will be routinely documented. By now, the same principles can be expected for the clinical measures of diagnosis and severity. Any clinical research unit today should be able to publish estimates of diagnostic reliability such as kappa coefficients. Similarly, for ratings of severity among members of the group the intra-class correlation coefficients and coefficients of variation should be stated. In the author's unit the kappa coefficient for the diagnosis of melancholia among the senior clinicians is 0.80. The intra-class correlation coefficient for Hamilton Rating Scale measures by multiple raters for the same subjects is 0.74, while the coefficient of variation of these ratings is 10%. This last figure is comparable to the coefficient of variation of many laboratory assays.

NEED FOR PLACEBO CONTROL

Despite some opinions to the contrary, there still are cogent reasons for insisting on the inclusion of a placebo control in the evaluation of new antidepressant drugs. These reasons will remain at least until the current problems of identifying specific subtypes of depression that respond to drugs are resolved.

From a statistical point of view the danger of using only an active drug control group is that very large numbers of patients are needed to avoid Type II errors. The new drug may not be statistically inferior to the standard antidepressant drug but at the same time it may not be statistically superior to placebo. Obviously, unless a placebo control group is included this information will never be obtained.

The finding of a new drug to be equivalent in efficacy to a standard drug is especially likely to occur when both drugs are tested in patients with only a broad, non-specific diagnostic entity such as 'major depressive disorder' in DSM III. This category is so heterogeneous that it will accommodate large numbers of depressed patients whom experienced clinicians would never elect to treat with drugs in the first place. Those who object most strongly to the use of a placebo control on ethical grounds are those who use antidepressant drugs selectively in more typical unipolar and bipolar melancholic patients.

In other centers, however, such typical patients are in the minority. Certainly, in the United States pharmaceutical firms target their new products mostly at the large market of milder, ambulatory, non-melancholic dysphoric patients. It is not difficult to see the potential danger of this approach. A new drug may be tested in the population of non-specific depressed patients, compared only with a standard tricyclic drug, found to be not inferior to the standard drug, and then approved for clinical use as an 'antidepressant'. Under these circumstances, there is no guarantee that the new drug will be effective for severely depressed melancholic patients. The ethical responsibility of the investigator extends, in other words, beyond the patients in his particular study to future patients who may be given the drug with the expectation derived from his trial that it will be effective for them. For this reason the Food and Drug Administration in the United States continues to require a placebo control in the testing of new antidepressants.

Another reason for a placebo control is a check on the ability of the investigators. To be qualified as a unit for the testing of new drugs each group of investigators needs to establish their credentials. This means they must be able to show that in their clinical program the referral, selection, diagnostic and treatment practices are adequate to demonstrate the efficacy of a standard drug over placebo.

USE OF LABORATORY MARKERS

Several promising laboratory tests are now receiving widespread evaluation as markers for the diagnosis of subtypes of depression. Some of these tests may also be found to have prognostic utility or to aid in the selection of specific antidepressant drugs. As in the case of clinical diagnostic criteria discussed above, the use of laboratory diagnostic tests requires informed judgement, common sense and knowledge of conditional probability theory on the part of the psychiatrist (Carroll, 1981, 1982a).

The potential contribution of laboratory diagnostic tests to clinical trials of antidepressant drugs is considerable. For example, both the dexamethasone suppression test (DST) and the sleep EEG are abnormal in patients with melancholic depression rather than in those with simple major depressive disorder. As in other areas of medicine, such laboratory tests can provide a degree of objectivity in the diagnosis and selection of patients that is impossible to achieve with clinical features alone.

In a multicenter trial of a new drug, for example, the investigators in different units will agree to use similar selection procedures and standardized clinical diagnostic criteria. At the same time, we are all aware that the standardization of these clinical procedures among units is not always uniform, despite the best efforts of all concerned. Thus, if a group in one center finds an abnormal DST rate of 80% in their patients, while the rate in another center is only 20% - even though both units claim to be using the same clinical diagnostic criteria - then we can tell that the two centers are not studying comparable groups of patients. The laboratory tests can then serve as a measure of the consistency of selection and diagnostic practice among the participating centers in a clinical trial. Further, the treatment results in the overall study can be analyzed by stratifying the total sample according to the laboratory test results and this analysis may provide very useful information.

The ultimate validity of tests like the DST is still being assessed by many clinical research groups. In time, it is likely that new definitions of depressive subtypes will be developed that give weight to the laboratory test results along with the classical clinical features (Carroll, 1982b). Even before this point is reached by consensus in the field, however, the applications of such tests for the purposes described above in clinical trials can already be adopted.

CONCLUSIONS

The need to identify specific drug-responsive types of depressed patients is a serious problem for all concerned with the clinical pharmacology of antidepressant drugs. Diagnostic precision with standardized clinical criteria and new laboratory tests will help to improve the current situation and should lead eventually to a more effective nosology of depression. The generalizability of a clinical trial is of critical importance for other centers to assess and this can only be done if adequate, comprehensive descriptions of the patients are provided, along with documented reliability and consistency estimates for the clinical assessment procedures. For the time being, placebo controls are still necessary in the development of new antidepressant drugs and individual units need to establish that in their own clinical setting a standard drug can be distinguished from a placebo.

REFERENCES

Carpenter, W. T., Strauss, J. S. and Bartko, J. J. (1980). Diagnostic systems and prognostic validity. Arch. Gen. Psychiatry, 37, 228-9.

Carroll, B. J. (1981). Implications of biological research for the diagnosis of depression. In New Advances in the Diagnosis and Treatment of Depressive Illness (ed. J. Mendlewicz), Elsevier, Amsterdam, pp. 85-107.

Carroll, B. J. (1982a). Clinical applications of the dexamethasone suppression test for endogenous depression. Pharmacopsychiatria, 15, 19-24.

Carroll, B. J. (1982b). The dexamethasone suppression test for melancholia. Br. J. Psychiatry, 140, 292-304.

Carroll, B. J., Feinberg, M., Greden, J.F., Haskett, R. F., James, N. McI., Steiner, M. and Tarika, J. (1980). Diagnosis of endogenous depression: comparison of clinical, research and neuroendocrine criteria. J. Affective Disorders, 2, 177-94.

Carroll, B. J., Fielding, J. M. and Blashki, T. G. (1973). Depression rating scales: a critical review. Arch. Gen. Psychiatry, 28, 361-6.

Gram, L. F., Søndergaard, I., Christiansen, J., Petersen, G. O., Bech, P., Reisby, N., Ibsen, I., Ortmann, J., Nagy, A., Dencker, S. J., Jacobsen, O. and Krautwald, O. (1977). Steady-state kinetics of imipramine in patients. Psychopharmacology, 54, 255-61.

Hamilton, M. (1960). A rating scale for depression. J. Neurosurg. Psychiat., 23, 56-62.

Kuhn, R. (1957). Uber die Behandlung depressiver Zustands mit einem iminodibenzyedeviat (G22355). Schweiz Med. Wochenschr., 87, 1135-40N.

Paykel, E. S., Klerman, G. L. and Prusoff, B. A. (1970). Treatment setting and clinical depression. Arch. Gen. Psychiatry., 22, 11-21.

Spitzer, R. L., Endicott, J. and Robins, E. (1977). Research Diagnostic Criteria, New York State Psychiatric Institute, New York.

Practical aspects of the utilization of double-blind trials using adjusted doses of psychotropic drugs

Pierre Simon[1], Laurence Landragin[1], Alain J. Puech[1] and Yves Lecrubier[1]

INTRODUCTION

Controlled clinical trials usually compare a fixed dose of a drug x with either a placebo or a fixed dose of a reference drug. In the first case, the question to be answered is: 'Is x an efficient drug?' In the second case: 'Is x more (or equally, or less) efficient than the reference drug?'

It is clear that bias can interfere in such comparisons, particularly the choice of the dosages. Moreover, the conditions under which the drugs are prescribed differ completely from the usual therapeutic attitude.

Even if these studies are sometimes sufficient to satisfy the drug registering authorities, it remains to answer various practical questions: How should the drug be prescribed to patients? What is the 'ideal' dosage? Is it a collective one or an individual one? And, in the second case, what is the best way to reach it? What are the equi-active dosages of two drugs? Could one compare the therapeutic margins of two drugs? At different dosages, what are the percentages of occurrence of various effects, either positive or negative?

Before looking at the possible solutions to these questions, one could try to define the 'proper dose of a drug'. It has been said to be that amount of drug which is 'enough but not too much', that is enough to produce the optimum therapeutic effect with the smallest possible amount of the drug.

The definition of 'optimum' is difficult, but it clearly refers to the ratio between risks and benefits: where is the limit between an acceptable side-effect and an unacceptable one? 'The least possible amount of the drug' is a very often forgotten concept and its appreciation, necessary from economical and ecologi-

[1]Department of Clinical Pharmacology, Hospital Pitié-Salpêtrière, 47 Boulevard de L'Hôpital, 75634 Paris Cédex 13, France.

cal points of view, is not devoid of ethical problems: when an effective and safe dosage is found for an individual patient, are we allowed to decrease the dosage until the disappearance of the effect?

POSSIBLE ADAPTATIONS OF CLASSICAL CONTROLLED TRIALS

Adjustment of Dosage According to Simple Characteristics of the Subjects

Usually the dosage is predetermined and cannot be changed. In case of unbearable side-effects, the drug is stopped and the result is 'negative'.
Just a few published studies consider adapting the dosage according to weight or to body surface.

Adjustment of Dosage According to the Plasma Level of the Drug

If one has to compare lithium with a new drug expected to be an alternative preventive treatment of bipolar patients, everybody would agree that the dosage of patients receiving lithium has to be adapted according to the plasma level. One could predict that it will be the case for other drugs in the near (?) future.

Adjustment of Dosage According to Biological Criteria

This is supposed to be related to the therapeutic effect, but it is not yet true for psychotropic drugs. The discovery of biological markers sensitive to treatment could change this situation.

Classical Trials Comparing Different Dosages of the Same Drug (or of Two Drugs)

The comparison of two drugs at three different dosages is certainly a minimum to define the dose-effect relationship of the two drugs. The number of patients necessary to undertake such a comparison is generally unachievable. Some intensive designs with multiple crossover in the same patients have been proposed but necessitate both very stable disease and short-acting drugs.

Trials with Systematic Variations of Dosage in the Same Patients

For example, the dosage is increased every week or every second day. Of course, it is difficult to increase the dosage if important side-effects occur or if the symptoms (or the disease) disappear.

CLINICAL TRIALS WITH INDIVIDUAL ADJUSTMENT OF DOSAGE DURING THE
TRIAL ACCORDING TO A DECISION TABLE

Difficulties Related to the Decision Table

This decision table could be prepared according to side-effects,
according to efficacy, or according to side-effects and efficacy.
In this last case, a schematic representation is given in table 1.
The decisions to take if the situation corresponds to 1, 2, 6, 7
and 9 are easy and are respectively increase, increase, decrease,
stop and decrease. In fact, this is true only if the activity
increases with the dosage; of course, inverted U shaped curves
(described e.g. with nortriptyline) would necessitate other
decisions.

Table 1.

		Efficacy		
		0	+	++
	0	↑ 1	↑ 2	? 3
Side-effects	+	? 4	? 5	↓ 6
	++	Stop 7	? 8	↓ 9

What to decide if the situation corresponds to 4, 5 and 8
depends on the severity (and risks) of the side-effects and on the
benefit expected with the drug. In position 3, some doctors would
consider it unethical to decrease the dosage and others would
consider it unethical to continue the same dosage. If one accepts
that the proper dose of a drug corresponds to the least possible
quantity of drug, the decision - during a trial - must be to
decrease the dosage.
     The latency of effects - either therapeutic or adverse -
could make the use of the decision table more difficult. For
example, with tricyclic antidepressant drugs, the lack of efficacy
during the first or even the second week must not be taken into
consideration.
     The greatest difficulty is related to the multicenter charac-
ter of these trials: it implies a standardization. Even if all
the psychiatrists or doctors involved agree with the decision
table, it is very improbable that they would always take the same
decision in front of a patient.

Difficulties Related to the Frequency of Evaluations

Have these evaluations to be performed at regular intervals? It
would not be realistic, especially if side-effects occur. Differ-

ent patients do not react in the same way: some will wait for some days to complain (either of a side-effect or of a lack of activity), some will phone immediately to their psychiatrist.

The ideal frequency of evaluations would have to consider the half-lives of the drugs and one could imagine the difficulties in double-blind conditions in comparing two drugs with different half-lives.

Theoretically it would be better if the clinical evaluations were dependent of validated scales: for example, increase dosage if the Hamilton Anxiety Rating Scale did not decrease at least 5 points. Practically, the decisions have to be taken quickly, especially with outpatients and the use of such rating scales is not realistic to adjust dosage from one consultation to another.

Analysis of the Results

When two drugs are compared in these conditions, the only acceptable analysis is the comparison between the percentages of 'good results' with drug *A* and with drug *B*. Of course, it is absolutely necessary to define clearly, *before the study*, what is a 'good result'.

Two possible sources of bias must be avoided:

(1) The non-equivalent unitary dosages of *A* and *B*. Whatever decision table is used, one could think that the habit of the prescribers favors a certain dosage (e.g. 3 tablets per day). It would be necessary in order to confirm this hypothesis to compare the same drug at two different unitary dosages (e.g. diazepam 5 mg vs diazepam 10 mg).

(2) The criteria of adjustment which could be more favorable for one drug than for the other.

Besides the main analysis, it is of interest for future prescribers to know the results obtained with the different dosage for the same drug, but this analysis must remain descriptive.

A PRACTICAL EXAMPLE: ALPRAZOLAM VS DIAZEPAM

The details of this trial will be published elsewhere. The protocol was certainly not ideal: it was a 'compromise' resulting from discussions with the 12 participating psychiatrists. It is certainly not presented as a model to follow.

Patients were defined as chronic anxious outpatients with a minimal score on the Hamilton Anxiety Rating Scale and excluding clear depressive states.

On the basis of animal studies and preliminary human studies, we decided to compare identical capsules containing either alprazolam (0.25 mg) or diazepam (5 mg). Allocation of treatment was decided by randomization (random number table) and the whole study was performed under double-blind conditions.

The psychiatrists knew that each capsule contained either 5 mg of diazepam or an (expectedly) equi-active dose of another benzodiazepine. The initial dosage was a free decision according to the habits of the patient (and of the psychiatrist) and to the severity of anxiety. An initial dosage between 2 and 6 capsules per day was 'recommended'.

The dosage could be changed at the occasions of weekly consultations or consecutively by phone calls from the patient.

The schematic decision table shown in table 2 was proposed (and theoretically accepted by the 12 participants). In the absence of side-effects, the dosage had to be increased up to optimum efficacy. In presence of minor side-effects, the choice is more difficult and for 'the central case' we had to accept a free decision from the prescriber, which had to take into consideration efficacy and side-effects in the case of this particular patient. In the case of significant side-effects the decrease of dosage is imperative.

Table 2.

		Anxiety		
		Unchanged	Decreased	Suppressed
Side-effects	None	Increase dosage	Increase dosage (at a lesser degree)	Unchanged
	Minor	Increase dosage (at a lesser degree)	'Your decision'	Decrease dosage
	Serious	Stop (drop out)	Decrease dosage	Decrease dosage

The primary evaluations were performed at the beginning of the study and at its end (28 days):

(a) Hamilton Anxiety Rating Scale;
(b) global score of anxiety (on 1 to 10 scale);
(c) checklist of possible side-effects;
(d) global score of side-effects (on a 1 to 10 scale).

The results could be summarized as follows: 270 patients were included but only 222 observations were accepted (rejection before breaking the code); 77 men and 145 women, 107 received alprazolam and 115 diazepam. The initial dosages were the same in the two groups (4.24 vs 2.29 capsules with variations from 1 to 12!).

At the end of the trial, the mean numbers of daily capsules

were significantly different ($p<0.05$): alprazolam 6.45, diazepam 5.50 (corresponding respectively to 1.61 and 27.5 mg).

The percentages of 'good results' were not significantly different. For the final evaluations, alprazolam was superior to diazepam according to global evaluation of efficacy and of side-effects but identical when considering the Hamilton Anxiety Rating Scale. Finally, for the same efficacy, alprazolam appears to be less sedative than diazepam.

Possible Improvements for Future Trials

Is there a way to control the bias related to the variation of the number of capsules used and its psychological effects upon the investigator and the patient? When an evaluation is made, it should be as independent as possible from the number of capsules received by the patient at that time. For that reason, it would be desirable to keep the number of capsules constant during the trial and to modify only the unitary dosage of the capsules. This could be accomplished daily by the pharmacist for studies with inpatients.

It would be interesting to consider the different results of each patient at the times of the consultations or of the changes of dosage but (semi-) quantitative evaluations of efficacy and side-effects would be necessary. It would allow one to approach the 'individual therapeutic margin'.

Better training of the participating psychiatrists would be necessary (one full day was clearly insufficient).

CONCLUSIONS

During the study of a (new) drug, comparative clinical trials with realistic (naturalistic) adjustment of dosage must be performed. However, the ideal design of such studies is not yet sufficiently defined and a symposium on this subject would certainly be welcome.

In the field of psychotropic drugs, the adjustment of dosage depends mainly on side effects, especially for neuroleptics and for classical antidepressants. It can be used for antianxiety drugs, for hypnotics and also for neuroleptics when a sedative effect is wanted. For these drugs, such trials will certainly not replace classical ones but they will help to increase our knowledge and to improve the therapeutic use of these drugs.

Acknowledgements

Alprazolam was kindly supplied by Upjohn Laboratories. We thank for their contributions: Professor J. M. Alby, Dr S. Bornstein, Dr G. Clerc, Professor F. Gremy, Professor M. Porot and all the physicians who participated.

Improving reliability and validity of adverse drug reaction assessment in psychopharmacology

E.M.Sellers[1], C.A.Naranjo[1] and U.Busto[1]

INTRODUCTION

The assessment of adverse drug reactions* presents few unique
methodologic issues not shared with determination of drug efficacy
or trial methodology in general. For example, sample size is
always an important consideration. However, drug trial protocols,
drug trial methodology and published reports illustrate that
assessment of drug efficacy (benefit) receives detailed attention
but the counterpart assessment of risk is with few exceptions
given relatively cursory attention. Such a relative imbalance is
difficult to defend and far from ideal. Perhaps this imbalance
reflects the lesser intrinsic appeal of looking for problems
rather than therapeutic benefits. Such assessment is also difficult and hence time-consuming and expensive to do properly. *A
priori*, a full knowledge of benefit and risk is needed. Since the
additional margin of benefit of many newer neuropharmacologic
agents is relatively small, optimal therapy with most will be
determined by the burden of acute and chronic toxicity. The
assessment of adverse reactions due to psychotropic drugs includes
three methodologic components of particular importance: detection
of a potential drug-related event; establishment of the probability of a causal relationship; and evaluation of the severity
or clinical importance of the event in relation to the therapeutic
benefits.

---

[1]Clinical Pharmacology Program, Addiction Research Foundation, Clinical Institute;
and Departments of Pharmacology and Medicine, University of Toronto, Toronto,
Canada.

*An **adverse drug reaction** is any noxious, unintended and undesired effect of a
drug which is observed at doses usually administered in man. This definition
excludes cases of drug overdose, drug abuse or therapeutic errors.

DETECTING AND DISTINGUISHING DRUG-RELATED FROM NON-DRUG EVENTS

Signal-to-Noise Ratio

The probability of discovering an adverse reaction (or any event) depends upon: the actual or perceived relative frequency of the drug-induced event to the spontaneously occurring event in the patient population under study and to the non-patient control population; the sensitivity, validity and reliability of the method; the frequency and duration of observations for the event (intensity of observation); and to a lesser extent the mechanism of the drug-induced reaction (Feinstein, 1974).

The manifestations of adverse events are usually not unique and hence what is caused by the drug must be distinguished from other possible etiologies. Accordingly, the detection of adverse events depends on the relative characteristics and magnitudes of two factors, the frequency of the adverse event occurrence and its clinical importance, and the concurrent spontaneous baseline occurrence of the event in the absence of drug. Background noise is contributed by the symptoms and signs of primary illness. Such basal noise increases population variance and occasionally generates a signal that is identical and detectable as a possible drug-elicited signal (Jick, 1977). When a drug-induced event is frequent, it is usually recognized quickly in clinical trials. In contrast, when the drug-induced illness is less common, large prospective investigations of a cohort of patients receiving the drug and/or retrospective case-control studies are needed (Jick, 1977). If both drug-related and spontaneous events are rare or very common, no method exists for detection of drug-induced events (Jick, 1977). For example, detection of drug-induced depression in depressive illness may be difficult or impossible. In practice, since the frequency of drug-related and disease-related events is usually not known, selecting the ideal method for detecting specific reactions may be difficult. We usually have only a general idea of the true natural history of disease and treatment outcome in a specific group of patients and of other factors that may increase baseline variance, e.g. alcohol use, smoking, drug abuse, other drug use and non-compliance (Dirks and Kinsman, 1982). Large inter-individual variations in steady-state drug concentrations and variations in patient sensitivity to drug effects may also introduce further variations in risk. The detection of adverse reactions in such circumstances will be extremely difficult even with large patient samples; however, the use of within-subject design with multiple crossovers, sophisticated statistical techniques such as discriminant analysis and intensive patient monitoring can be powerful procedures to maximize the likelihood of detecting within-subject and group adverse drug events (Raskin, 1982). Such techniques, however, can only be effective for as long as the trial is conducted; hence adverse reactions which develop insidiously or long after exposure could be missed.

Normal subjects are often used for pharmacokinetic and inter-action studies. Since these subjects usually receive few drugs, a baseline free of spontaneously occurring adverse events could be determined and used as an absolute control. For infrequent events such a procedure has little advantage; however, for events that are common and which can be confused with symptoms of disease (e.g. depression, anxiety, sleep disorders), normal subjects may be suitable.

Required Sample Size

Clinical trials are usually short-term studies conducted in a few hundred or thousand patients before marketing a drug. Such limited exposure of patients to drug limits detection in the pre-marketing phase to those adverse events that are acute and common. The release of the new antipsychotic drug clozapine is an example (Anderman and Griffith, 1977; Idänpään-Heikkilä *et al.*, 1977; Idänpään-Heikkilä and Palva, 1977). Clozapine was introduced in Finland in 1975 when about 200 subjects had been studied in that country and 900 elsewhere. Within the first six months of post-marketing drug use, about 3200 patients received the drug and 17 cases of serious hematologic reactions (agranulocytosis 10; neutropenia 7) were reported to the Finnish National Drug Moni-toring Center. Because of these reactions, the drug was withdrawn from the market. The estimated frequency of developing agranulo-cytosis or severe granulocytopenia during clozapine treatment was 5.3 per 1000 (Anderman and Griffith, 1977; Idänpään-Heikkilä *et al.*, 1977; Idänpään-Heikkilä and Palva, 1977). This example illustrates the importance of post-marketing monitoring of any new drug, irrespective of the safety shown in clinical trials. It also indicates the role of physicians in detecting the serious toxicity of newly introduced drugs by voluntarily reporting ad-verse reactions to national drug monitoring centers. An inci-dental aspect of this example is that the observed frequency was between 8.8 and 21 times greater than observed in other countries and with other neuroleptics (0.47 per 1000). A pharmacogenetic determinant was suspected.

No available method for detecting adverse reactions could have predicted such events, only the administration of the drug to a sufficient number of subjects resulted in the discovery.

For dose-related adverse reactions, detection also depends on the administered dose of the drug. The sample sizes required for detecting three different adverse events (hepatitis, nausea, somnolence) which occur with varying probability depending on the dose of a hypothetical drug are shown in table 1. The assumptions made are that the adverse events are independent events; when giving 50 mg of the drug, the true probability of any one subject developing the adverse event is given for hepatitis ($p = 0.001$), nausea ($p = 0.004$) and somnolence ($p = 0.005$); the probabilities of the events increase linearly, and the chance to detect the event is 90% (power $1 - \beta = 0.90$).

Table 1. Number of subjects (N) needed to detect adverse events

Dose (mg)	Adverse events					
	Hepatitis		Nausea		Somnolence	
	p	N	p	N	p	N
50	0.001	2301	0.004	574	0.005	459
100	0.002	1150	0.008	286	0.01	229
200	0.004	574	0.016	142	0.02	113
400	0.008	286	0.032	70	0.04	56

Power = 90%
p = probability of event (power $1 - \beta = 0.90$)

To have a 90% chance of detecting one case of hepatitis induced by such a drug when 400 mg are given, a minimum of 286 patients exposed to the drug are required (table 1). This example illustrates why some adverse events are only detected when a large number of subjects have received the drug and why even with an actual frequency of 5.3 per 1000, the failure to observe the hematologic adverse events with clozapine after 200 patients is not surprising. Detection with greater assurance (e.g. power $1 - \beta$ = 0.95, 0.99) will require larger numbers of patients. Similarly, if patient monitoring is not intense enough to detect *all* drug-related events, more patients will be required.

Animal studies are helpful predictors of dose-related toxicity that must be looked for in humans. Observations in animals can be translated into anticipation and intensive monitoring for the possible reaction in the human. In contrast, dose-independent adverse events (e.g. drug allergy) are confined to individuals or patient subsets with particular genetic or immunologic characteristics. Therefore, these reactions are rarely predictable from toxicity studies in animals. If the reactions are infrequent, then large numbers of susceptible patients must receive the drug.

Since the absolute frequency of a reaction as well as the relationship to the dose are unknown, it is impossible to predict *a priori* the actual number of subjects required to detect a specific adverse reaction.

Current Monitoring Methods

Methods for collecting information on adverse reactions in clinical trials include unstructured and structured interviews, physical examination and laboratory tests. The procedures most commonly used are the open-ended unstructured interview, designed to eliminate suggestion of reactions to the patient, and a standardized list-of-symptoms checklist (Petrie and Levine, 1978). With the unstructured inquiry, the subject is asked at regular intervals about appearance of any symptoms or changes in body function. This method is of unknown reliability because of variable awareness in subjects of such symptoms, the difficulty in relating symptoms to the drug, and variation in patient motivation, affect, memory or judgement due to disease (e.g. dementia). Such unstructured inquiry may result in under-reporting or, in some situations, even over-reporting. For example, the use of a list of symptoms in neurotics was more likely to lead to the conclusion that a drug induced more side-effects (Downing *et al.*, 1970). Such simple questionnaires or observational methods may suffice for frequent and clinically important adverse reactions. However, the sensitivity, validity and reliability of such methods is unknown; hence, they are inadequate from a methodologic point of view.

In an attempt to standardize the assessments of adverse reactions in clinical trials, adverse drug reaction assessment scales, consisting of checklists of symptoms and signs, have been developed. However, the application of these scales is problematic because of inadequate operational definitions of terms and severity ratings, inclusion of a wide variety of symptoms and signs, and complex formats (Petrie and Levine, 1978). Examples of these procedures for assessing psychotropic drugs are the Treatment Emergent Symptoms Scales (Vinař, 1971; Guy, 1976). Guy's scale includes 33 symptoms, laboratory items and syndromes and has been widely used. A 'treatment emergent symptom' is defined as follows: the symptom was not present at pre-treatment, or if present was aggravated during the course of medication; and/or the symptom required some form of action or intervention as a consequence of its occurrence. The scale provides an eight-point action scale, the severity of the adverse reactions are classed as mild, moderate and severe, and the relationship between the drug and the adverse event is also recorded (none, remote, possible, probable, definite), but the definitions are vague and confusing. Many features of this scale have been utilized in transmuted form in many drug trials. The main difficulties of Guy's scale are the undefined or non-parallel items, the confusion that raters experience with the scale and the difficulty in data analysis (Petrie and Levine, 1978). In addition, the sensitivity, validity and reliability for different patient and racial populations is not established. The under-representation of females in pre-marketing trials suggests that adverse reaction information in that population is particularly sparse (Kinney *et al.*, 1981).

DETERMINATION OF CAUSALITY

The *causal association* between a drug and adverse events has usually been classified as definite, probable, possible or doubtful as follows:

(a) *definite* - a reaction which (i) follows a reasonable temporal sequence after administration of the drug, or in which the drug level has been established in body fluids or tissues; (ii) follows a known response pattern to the suspected drug; and (iii) is confirmed by improvement on dechallenge and by reappearance on rechallenge;

(b) *probable* - a reaction which (i) follows a reasonable temporal sequence after drug administration; (ii) follows a known response pattern; (iii) is confirmed on dechallenge but not on rechallenge; and (iv) cannot be explained by the known characteristics of the patient's disease;

(c) *possible* - a reaction which (i) follows a temporal sequence; (ii) may or may not follow a known response pattern; and (iii) could be explained by the known characteristics of the patient's clinical state; and

(d) *doubtful* - the event is more likely related to other factors than the suspected drug (Naranjo *et al.*, 1981).

The use of such standard definitions of probability of a causal relation generates wide variability in assessment (Karch and Lasagna, 1975; Koch-Weser *et al.*, 1977; Blanc *et al.*, 1979; Naranjo *et al.*, 1981). The suspected drug is usually confounded with other causes and often the adverse clinical event is not distinguishable from manifestations of the disease. Recently, the assessment of causality of adverse reactions has been systematized by using operational definitions such as those reported by Kramer *et al.* (1979) and those by Naranjo *et al.* (1981). The method proposed by Kramer *et al.* (1979) is a long and detailed questionnaire, which provides valid and reliable assessments. A simpler method, the Adverse Drug Reaction Probability Scale (APS) is also valid and reliable in a variety of clinical situations (Naranjo *et al.*, 1981). The APS is a 10-item questionnaire which systematically analyzes and scores the various components that must be assessed to establish a causal association between drug(s) and adverse events. The probability of the adverse reaction is given by the total score. The scores obtained with the APS are highly correlated with those obtained using the method of Kramer *et al.* (Busto *et al.*, 1982). Because reliable and valid assessment of the probability of a causal relation between drug and event is desirable, such techniques should be used.

ASSESSMENT OF SEVERITY

The *severity* of adverse reactions is usually classified as mild, moderate, severe or lethal as follows:

    (a) *mild* - no antidote, therapy or prolongation of hospitalization is necessary;

    (b) *moderate* - requires a change in drug therapy although not necessarily drug discontinuation; it may prolong hospitalization and requires specific treatment;

    (c) *severe* - potentially life-threatening; requires discontinuation of drug and specific treatment; and

    (d) *lethal* - directly or indirectly contributes to the death of the patient.

The validity, reliability and appropriateness of the definitions and application of this categorical approach are unknown. The classification lacks flexibility in the sense that many reactions are not uniquely classifiable, e.g. tardive dyskinesia. Attempts for systematizing the assessment of the drug benefit/risk ratio have been reported (Tallarida *et al.*, 1979). However, more refinement to assess the balance between the severity of the underlying disease and the adverse event are required. The severity or impact of the reaction must always be tested against benefit from the therapy. No interpretation of a 'severe' reaction is possible without information of expected and achieved improvement and the natural history of the disease. Similarly, the exclusion of 'mild' adverse events from reporting is not justified since the assumption is implicitly made that benefit is constant and substantial.

CONCLUSIONS

The methodologic principles for detection and evaluation of adverse reactions are theoretically well established, but are not fully operational. Some improvement would occur if more attention and scientific rigor were directed to assessing risk by ensuring that studies are conducted by trained clinical pharmacologists; incorporating an appropriate balance of spontaneous and elicited data gathering in all trials; inclusion of APS or similar methods to standardize the determination of causality; intense review of case report data during early trials with a high index of suspicion for possible adverse reactions; reporting of all clinical event data; use of newer data analysis techniques; including intense phase IV studies for all newly marketed drugs.

    Research is needed to develop primary validated and reliable instruments for adverse reactions assessment; to develop standardized operational methods to rate severity and compare it to benefit; to explore the feasibility of using normal subjects to establish the absolute range and severity of adverse events; and to develop trial monitoring techniques that will ensure that all organ systems in man receive equal attention in adverse event monitoring irrespective of drug class under investigation, and that intensity of monitoring in any trial can be characterized.

REFERENCES

Anderman, B. and Griffith, R.W. (1977). Clozapine-induced agranulocytosis: a situation report up to August 1976. Eur. J. Clin. Pharmacol., 11, 199–201.

Blanc, S., Leuenberger, P., Berger, J.-P., Brooke, E.M. and Schelling, J.-L. (1979). Judgments of trained observers on adverse drug reactions. Clin. Pharmacol. Ther., 25 (5), 493–7.

Busto, U., Naranjo, C.A. and Sellers, E.M. (1982). Comparison of two recently published algorithms for assessing adverse drug reactions. Br. J. Clin. Pharmacol., 13, 223–7.

Dirks, J.F. and Kinsman, R.A. (1982). Nondichotomous patterns of medication usage: the yes-no fallacy. Clin. Pharmacol. Ther. 31 (4), 413–17.

Downing, R.W., Rickels, K. and Meyers, F. (1970). Side reactions in neurotics. I. A comparison of two methods of assessment. J. Clin. Pharmacol. New Drugs, 10, 289–97.

Feinstein, A.R. (1974). Clinical biostatistics. XXVIII. The biostatistical problems of pharmaceutical surveillance. Clin. Pharmacol. Ther., 16 (1), 110–23.

Guy, W. (1976). ECDEU Assessment Manual for Psychopharmacology, revised 1976, DHEW Publication no. 76–338, National Institute of Mental Health, Washington.

Idänpään-Heikkilä, J., Alhawa, E., Olkimora, M. and Palva, I.P. (1977). Agranulocytosis during treatment with clozapine. Eur. J. Clin. Pharmacol., 11, 193–8.

Idänpään-Heikkilä, J. and Palva, I. (1977). Recent experiences concerning drug related blood dyscrasias in Finland. In Epidemiological Evaluation of Drugs (eds F. Colombo et al.), Elsevier/North-Holland, Amsterdam, pp. 241–8.

Jick, H. (1977). The discovery of drug-induced illness. New Engl. J. Med., 296, 481–5.

Karch, F.E. and Lasagna, L. (1975). Adverse drug reactions. A critical review. J. Am. Med. Assoc., 234 (12), 1236–41.

Kinney, E.L., Trautmann, J., Gold, J.A., Vesell, E.S. and Zelis, R. (1981). Under-representation of women in new drug trials. Ann. Intern. Med., 95, 495–9.

Koch-Weser, J., Sellers, E.M. and Zacest, R. (1977). The ambiguity of adverse drug reactions. Eur. J. Clin. Pharmacol., 11, 75–8.

Kramer, M.S., Leventhal, J., Hutchinson, T.A. and Feinstein, A.R. (1979). An algorithm for the operational assessment of adverse drug reactions. I. Background, description and instructions for use. J. Am. Med. Assoc., 242, 623-32.

Naranjo, C.A., Busto, U., Sellers, E.M., Sandor, P., Ruiz, I., Roberts, E.A., Janecek, E., Domecq, C. and Greenblatt, D.J. (1981). A method for estimating the probability of adverse drug reactions. Clin. Pharmacol. Ther., 30, 239-45.

Petrie, W.M. and Levine, J. (1978). The assessment of adverse drug reactions in clinical trials. Int. Pharmacopsychiat., 13, 209-16.

Raskin, A. (1982). Clinical trial methodology: issues for the psychopharmacologic treatment of anxiety disorders. In Int. Symp. on Guide-lines for the Use of Psychotropic Drugs: Anxiety Disorders, Toronto (eds P. Garfinkel, H. C. Stancer and V. Rakoff), in press.

Tallarida, R.J., Murray, R.B. and Eiben, C. (1979). A scale for assessing the severity of diseases and adverse drug reactions. Application to drug benefit and risk. Clin. Pharmacol. Ther., 25, 381-90.

Vinař, O. (1971). Scale for rating treatment emergent symptoms in psychiatry DVP. Activ. Nerv. Super., 13, 238-40.

Clinical evaluation of the cardiac effects of new psychotropic drugs

Graham D. Burrows[1], Trevor R. Norman[1], Jitu Vohra[2]
and Graeme Sloman[2]

INTRODUCTION

This paper briefly describes some methods for investigating the
cardiac effects of psychotropic drugs and describes some studies
with the newer antidepressant drugs - nomifensine and zimelidine.

Over recent years there appears to have been a growing
interest in the cardiotoxicity of psychotropic drugs. Nevertheless, there is still great controversy in this area.

A great variety of symptoms have been reported after the
ingestion of an overdose of a tricyclic compound. Typically these
include disorientation, ataxia, vomiting, coma, convulsions, ECG
changes and dysrythmias. Since some of the antidepressants show
an affinity for myocardial tissue, it is not surprising that a
large proportion of individuals experiencing overdoses of these
drugs show signs of cardiotoxicity. Even at therapeutic dose
levels there is compelling evidence that changes occur in cardiac
parameters.

Using surface ECG recordings and in other studies using His
bundle electrocardiography, we have shown that intracardiac conduction was prolonged in patients taking therapeutic doses of tricyclic antidepressants. Possible changes in cardiac function
occurring at therapeutic dose levels are highly relevant to the
treatment of depressed people with pre-existing cardiac problems.

Following tricyclic antidepressant overdose, the effects
produced by the cardiotoxicity of these drugs can be most dangerous and may be difficult to correct.

A frequent enquiry from clinicians responsible for the care
of people who have recently suffered a myocardial infarction and
are still receiving intensive inpatient care is whether it is safe

[1]Department of Psychiatry, University of Melbourne, Parkville, Victoria,
Australia.

[2]Department of Cardiology, Royal Melbourne Hospital, Parkville, Victoria,
Australia.

to prescribe an antidepressant drug when depressive disorder is prominent. What are the criteria? What drug should be prescribed?

At the Second International Meeting on Clinical Pharmacology in Psychiatry, Tromsø, 1980, we reviewed some of the clinical studies in this area (Burrows *et al.*, 1981b); a more detailed paper, including some animal studies, has also been reported (Burrows *et al.*, 1981a).

When applied to the study of cardiotoxicity of antidepressants, animal models may appear to measure effects dissimilar from those seen in man and may be totally divorced from clinical problems. No single animal method of testing for cardiotoxicity has become accepted, and a great variety of experimental approaches have been used by different workers. As a result, conflicting results and viewpoints occur, and comparisons between different research groups are almost impossible.

The same can be said of clinical studies in man; no single method is universally accepted, and a great variety of methods have been used (Glassman *et al.*, 1981).

TRICYCLIC ANTIDEPRESSANTS

The pharmacological activity of the older tricyclic compounds includes a number of actions: anticholinergic, norepinephrine re-uptake blockade, 5-HT re-uptake blockade, and quinidine-like action.

The quinidine-like actions are thought to be a direct action on the myocardium, probably due to the local cocaine-like anesthetic activity of these compounds. Quinidine, a class 1 antiarrhythmic agent, acts by affecting the action potential. Quinidine decreases the rate of rise of the action potential, thereby prolonging the effective refractory period. It delays conduction, as shown by prolongation of the QRS, QT and PR intervals on the electrocardiogram.

Quinidine also depresses contractility thought to be brought about by interfering with the fast initial inward current of sodium ions.

Tricyclic antidepressant drugs have been the pharmacological treatment of choice for most depressed patients in general and psychiatric practice. In recent years, psychiatrists have tended to use larger doses of these drugs, often giving them in a single nightly dose.

Because of this tendency, and because of the fact that the diagnosis of depression is being made more frequently in patients with ischemic heart disease (with tricyclic antidepressants being widely used in rehabilitation), an awareness of the pharmacology of the drugs, particularly their cardiac effects, is essential.

Tricyclic antidepressant pharmacological activity includes an anticholinergic action which is apparent at low drug concen-

trations. The tricyclic drugs block the re-uptake of norepinephrine and so raise the levels of circulating catecholamines. At
higher concentrations, myocardial contractility and heart rate are
depressed. Metabolic acidosis and respiratory depression, which
may occur especially in unconscious patients, may also affect the
cardiac state (Burgess and Turner, 1981).

In therapeutic doses of less than 200 mg per day in people
without heart disease there is usually no need for concern, but
the findings that therapeutic (and not only toxic) doses may cause
significant prolongation of distal atrioventricular conduction
indicate that these drugs should be used cautiously in people with
known heart disease. This would apply particularly to the elderly
or to young children.

Caution is necessary, but for the moderately to severely
depressed patient with persistent symptoms, the benefits of antidepressants should not be withheld since the risks are small.

Cardiotoxicity is a major feature of tricyclic antidepressant
overdosage where sinus tachycardia, conduction defects, supraventricular tachycardia, ST and T wave abnormalities, ventricular
arrhythmias, profound bradycardia and finally asystole may be
observed.

Before the tricyclic antidepressants are used, cardiological
assessment should be made, starting with a clinical history and
followed by a physical examination and an ECG. Chest X-ray and
exercise testing may be considered. Patients with heart failure
and/or angina may be made worse by the increase in heart rate
produced by tricyclic drugs. If the ECG is abnormal and shows
evidence of bundle branch block, the use of tricyclic drugs should
be reconsidered, since they may lead to complete heart block and
cardiac syncope. Dosage should be increased gradually and patients
seen at regular intervals (Burrows *et al.*, 1976).

These cardiovascular problems have stimulated the pharmaceutical industry to produce other antidepressants – ones that act
more quickly with few subjective side-effects, have fewer cardiovascular effects (both at therapeutic levels and in overdosage)
than the tricyclic group, and do not have the interactional problems of the monoamine oxidase inhibitors. Before discussing two
newer drugs, the methods used clinically to study cardiotoxicity
will be briefly described.

METHODS FOR CLINICAL EVALUATION OF CARDIAC EFFECTS

Electrocardiogram

Obviously the electrocardiogram (ECG) is the most readily available method for the clinician. It would seem that the first
report of tricyclic antidepressant ECG changes in man occurred 21
years ago in Scandinavia (Kristjansen, 1961), with descriptions of

ST-T changes and hypotension occurring following exercise, in depressed patients who had been prescribed imipramine.

Unfortunately, most of the numerous individual case reports of ECG abnormalities during tricyclic antidepressant therapy have been of patients receiving other multidrug administrations. The few studies of ECG changes occurring during pure tricyclic antidepressant therapy were reported elsewhere (Burrows *et al.*, 1981a).

The general pattern of ECG which emerges from these studies is of ST-T wave changes including ST deviation, increases in PR and QRS width, bundle branch block and sinus tachycardia, ventricular arrhythmias, profound bradycardia, supraventricular tachycardia and asystole. These changes appear reversible in patients without pre-existing heart disease when the drugs are withdrawn. Only a few studies have also monitored plasma levels along with the ECG changes and they have been reviewed elsewhere (Burrows *et al.*, 1981a; Burgess and Turner, 1981).

The results have been conflicting. Some studies have shown that there is an increase in ECG changes in patients with the higher plasma levels while others have shown no correlation between the plasma level and the extent of the QRS widening. The range of plasma levels, following overdose, overlap with those found in patients receiving chronic oral administration for therapeutic reasons, thus making the use of plasma levels alone an unreliable index of tricyclic overdosage.

Nevertheless, the most reliable and readily available clinical index of tricyclic overdosage is prolongation of the QRS width by 100 ms or more. QRS widening, arrhythmia and increased total plasma tricyclic antidepressant levels indicate major cardiotoxicity.

METHODS USED TO ASSESS THE EFFECT OF TRICYCLIC ANTIDEPRESSANTS ON THE HEART

Systolic Time Intervals

This is a non-invasive method for studying left ventricular function. The left ventricular pre-ejection period (PEP) is compared to the left ventricular ejection time (LVET). Simultaneous recording of ECG external carotid pulse and either phonocardiogram or apex cardiogram are needed to measure these intervals.

The PEP is measured from the onset of ventricular systole (beginning of first heart sound or from the apex cardiogram) to the onset of the carotid pulse. The LVET is measured from the onset of the carotid pulse to the carotid incisura. The PEP/LVET ratio is increased with impairment of left ventricular function.

The normal value of the PEP/LVET ratio is 0.345 ± 0.036 (S.D.). This ratio is inversely correlated with cardiac stroke volume. It is increased with heart disease and heart failure. The ratio is decreased with digitalis as a result of a positive inotropic effect.

Radioisotope Scanning

Images of the cardiac cavity may be obtained by intravenous injections of radionuclides, technetium-99 ($^{99}Tc_m$) albumin and photographing under ECG control.

This non-invasive method may be used to measure both left ventricular function and regional dysfunction.

Left Ventricular Systolic Ejection Fraction

This involves the angiographic estimate of the left ventricular ejection fraction. The left ventricular end-diastolic and end-systolic volumes are determined by angiography. The difference between the two volumes is divided by the end-diastolic volume giving the ejection fraction. The upper limit of normal ventricular end-diastolic volume is 99 ml.

The cardiac output may be measured by recording the time course of change in radioactivity, by radioscopic scanning following i.v. injection of the labeled radionuclide. This is an application of the indicator-dilution principle.

The use of this technique to study psychotropic drug effects is only just beginning.

His' Bundle Electrocardiography

The relationship between the His' bundle electrocardiography (HBE) and the standard ECG is shown in figure 1. This invasive technique involves cardiac catheterization facilities and professional personnel. Following local anesthesia, electrode catheters are percutaneously placed into a femoral vein, advanced under fluoroscopic and ECG control into the right ventricular cavity and slowly withdrawn to the region of the right tricuspid valve.

Tricyclic antidepressants have been shown in both therapeutic and toxic doses to prolong the H-V interval significantly. The effect on proximal or A-V conduction is variable.

We have suggested that prolongation of the H-V interval with some of these drugs may give a clue to the increased incidence of sudden deaths that have been reported in 'cardiac patients' taking tricyclic antidepressants.

Echocardiography

Echocardiography is perhaps the major diagnostic cardiological innovation in the past decade. It provides diagnostic information regarding structure and function in qualitative and quantitative form. This is as good as that obtained from invasive studies and,

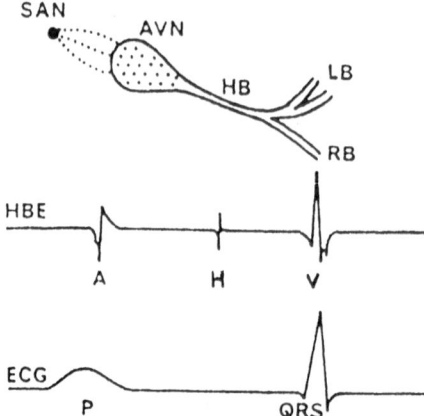

Figure 1. His' bundle electrogram (HBE) with the standard ECG.
An anatomical model of the conduction system at the top
of the figure is orientated to show the sites of origin
of the electrical waves. The A-H and H-V intervals
represent proximal and distal intracardiac conduction
respectively.

in some instances, better. The availability of ultrasound equipment is rapidly becoming widespread and, therefore, familiarity
with the technical equipment is necessary for both general practitioners and specialists.

The examination is performed with the patient recumbent in a
semi-left lateral position. A transducer is coupled to the chest
wall. A number of ultrasound positions may be used. The more
common are in the 3, 4 and 5 interfaces at the left sternal edge.
The echo beam is swept from the aortic root to the apex of the
heart.

Two-dimensional echocardiography is becoming increasingly
available and provides another useful technique for the assessment
of global and segmental myocardial function. Studies have been
carried out before and after tricyclic antidepressant drug administration.

NOMIFENSINE

Cardiological Effects

The structure of nomifensine is distinct from the tri- or tetracyclic antidepressants, monoamine oxidase inhibitors, or any of
the other existing groups of psychotropic agents. It is a deriva-

tive of tetrahydroisoquinoline. Double-blind controlled studies of nomifensine against placebo, imipramine, amitriptyline, nortriptyline and chlomipramine have shown it to be an effective antidepressant.

Studies in animals showed nomifensine to have slight and transient effects on the cardiovascular system. More recent studies on isolated guinea-pig atria, in the anesthetized rat, and on the right ventricular papillary muscle of the cat confirm that the effects of nomifensine in animals are less pronounced than those of other antidepressants.

Nomifensine did not cause significant changes in heart rate, cardiac output, mean arterial pressure, pulmonary artery pressure, or end-diastolic left ventricular pressure. There were no electro-cardiographic (ECG) changes. Non-invasive techniques of high-speed surface ECG and the measurement of systolic time intervals have shown that nomifensine does not appear to have a significant effect on the heart.

Reports of overdosage also indicate that nomifensine does not cause the serious cardiac arrhythmias which are present with tricyclic overdoses.

We investigated the effects of nomifensine on the CVS system. Preliminary results were reported at the 2nd IMCPP (Burrows *et al.*, 1981b).

Our study consisted of 10 patients suffering from primary unipolar depressive illness of moderate severity (Hamilton rating scores > 17). There was no clinical evidence of cardiac disease in any of the subjects.

A one-week drug-free period was allowed before patients were assigned to a graded dosage regimen, leading to a final daily dose of 100 or 200 mg nomifensine after seven days. There were five patients in both the 100 and 200 mg groups.

A full standard ECG was recorded prior to the commencement of nomifensine therapy and after three weeks of therapy. The parameters measured were heart rate, PR, QRS, corrected QT intervals, and repolarization changes. A His' bundle electrogram was also recorded prior to nomifensine and after three weeks of treatment. From this, values for A-H and H-V intervals could be obtained.

To check for possible side-effects of the drug, routine bio-chemical measurements were performed at the end of the pretreatment 'washout' period and after three weeks of therapy. These included hematocrit, hemoglobin, white blood cell count/differential, red blood cell count, alkaline phosphatase, bilirubin, SGOT, blood urea nitrogen, and urinalysis.

Besides routine clinical evaluation, the severity of the depression was assessed by the use of the Hamilton depression rating scale on days 0, 8, 15 and 22 of the study. Side-effects were also rated using a 12-point scale as described by Burrows *et al.* (1972).

Blood Sampling and Analysis

Samples (20 ml) of venous blood were collected on days 0, 8, 15 and 22. These samples were collected into cold lithium heparin tubes, immediately centrifuged at 4°C and the plasma separated, then stored frozen (– 20°C) in the dark until analysis. This method of collection and storage was found to be necessary in order to prevent significant degradation of the nomifensine samples. The analysis gave unconjugated nomifensine and total nomifensine (unconjugated plus an acid-labile *N*-glucuronide conjugate).

Results

Treatment with nomifensine was associated with an increase in heart rate in seven of the 10 patients (table 1), but this increase was not statistically significant ($p > 0.05$; Wilcoxon signed rank test). One patient showed an increase in PR interval of 0.01 s while on nomifensine.

The A-H interval, reflecting the time taken for the cardiac impulse to pass through the atrioventricular node, was within normal limits for the 10 patients (table 2). Nomifensine caused no significant change in the A-H interval

Interventricular Conduction

The H-V interval, representing the time taken for the cardiac impulse to travel through the His' bundle and bundle branches to the Purkinje fibers, was within normal limits for the 10 patients (table 2). Nomifensine caused no significant change in the H-V interval ($p > 0.05$; Wilcoxon signed rank test). Nomifensine also had no effect on the QRS width.

Corrected QT Interval and Repolarization Changes

Nomifensine caused no significant change in the corrected QT interval ($p > 0.05$; Wilcoxon signed rank test). There was no evidence of ST or T wave changes in the ECG.

Blood Pressure, Blood Chemistry and Urinalysis

Supine and standing blood pressure measurements were performed in all 10 patients on days 0 and 22. Nomifensine caused no significant change in supine and standing systolic and diastolic blood pressure ($p > 0.05$; Wilcoxon signed rank test). No consistent changes in the various hematological and biochemical factors monitored were observed.

Table 1. Effect of nomifensine on heart rate and PR interval
in the ECG

Patient no.	Age (years)	Sex	Dose (mg per day)	Heart rate (beats/min)		PR interval (s)	
				Before nomifen-sine	Day 22	Before nomifen-sine	Day 22
1	34	F	100	81	76	0.18	0.18
2	62	M	100	92	100	0.20	0.20
3	18	F	100	84	95	0.18	0.19
4	54	M	100	63	60	0.16	0.16
5	40	M	100	86	92	0.18	0.18
6	31	F	200	67	57	0.18	0.18
7	33	F	200	67	77	0.17	0.17
8	38	F	200	89	99	0.20	0.20
9	59	F	200	65	92	0.18	0.18
10	63	F	200	82	86	0.20	0.20

Table 2. Effect of nomifensine on A–H and H–V intervals
in the His' bundle electrogram*

Patient	A–H interval (ms)		H–V interval (ms)	
	Before nomifensine	Day 22	Before nomifensine	Day 22
1	80	85	48	50
2	100	100	60	60
3	104	100	50	55
4	70	70	40	40
5	85	80	45	45
6	70	70	45	45
7	70	80	40	40
8	110	95	45	50
9	80	90	45	45
10	95	75	60	60

* Normal values: A–H = 92 ± 38 ms; H–V = 43 ± 12 ms.

Nomifensine Plasma Concentrations

Plasma nomifensine concentrations were determined in all 10 patients (mean values are shown in table 3). These results reveal that the concentrations for day 22 of the trial were significantly lower than those of days 8 and 15. Day 22 samples were collected 12–15 h after the previous nightly dose of nomifensine, because a drug-free period at this time was required before the second His' bundle electrogram could be performed. The samples from days 8 and 15 were collected 2 h after the previous dose.

Table 3. Mean unconjugated and total nomifensine plasma concentrations in 10 patients receiving two dosage regimens (mean ± S.D.)

Dose	Unconjugated plasma concentrations (μg l^{-1})			Total plasma concentrations (μg l^{-1})		
	Day 8	Day 15	Day 22	Day 8	Day 15	Day 22
100(n = 5)	15± 8	13± 3	9± 3	289±143	246± 73	185± 68
200(n = 5)	36±36	35±26	19±15	753±618	590±422	370±272

No significant correlation between unconjugated or total plasma concentrations of nomifensine at day 22 and blood pressure (supine and standing), heart rate, PR, H-V, QRS, or corrected QT intervals was observed ($p>0.05$; Spearman rank order correlation coefficient). A significant negative correlation was found between unconjugated concentration (day 22) and A–H interval (r_s = – 0.62; $p>0.05$) and between total concentration (day 22) and A–H interval (r_s = 0.69; $p>0.05$).

Relationship Between Clinical Response and Plasma Concentrations

No significant correlation between unconjugated or total plasma concentrations of nomifensine at days 8, 15, or 22 and Hamilton ratings were found ($p>0.05$; Spearman rank order correlation coefficient).

Side-Effects

No severe adverse side-effects of nomifensine therapy were noted.

Discussion

Nomifensine has shown little influence on the cardiovascular system of the experimental animal. In the present study, 10 endogenously depressed patients, free of previous cardiovascular disease, revealed that nomifensine at a dose of up to 200 mg per day had no significant effect on blood pressure and heart rate, and the ECGs were unremarkable.

The present study revealed no intracardiac conduction defects with nomifensine therapy.

A significant negative correlation between the A-H interval and both unconjugated and total plasma concentrations at day 22 was observed. As nomifensine therapy did not cause a significant change in the A-H interval, the clinical relevance of the correlation remains to be elucidated in a larger patient population. None of the other cardiological parameters examined were found to correlate with nomifensine plasma concentrations.

The present study also showed no significant correlation between plasma concentrations and clinical response. This observation may not be generally applicable as only a small patient population was investigated. Further pharmacokinetic studies have shown the half-life of nomifensine to be 2-4 h, indicating that there should be a wide variation of plasma concentration within one day.

The cardiological data from this and previous studies suggest that, because of its relative lack of cardiotoxicity, nomifensine may be of value in the treatment of depressive syndromes, particularly those patients in whom the quinidine-like tricyclic antidepressants may not be desirable because of pre-existing disease of the cardiac system.

We previously reported (Vohra *et al.*, 1978) a 43-year-old woman with a bipolar affective disorder who took an overdose of nomifensine while receiving treatment for depression. She consumed 3.5 g nomifensine, 20 mg nitrazepam, and 200 mg chlorpromazine. On admission, approximately 4 h later, she was alert but her speech was slurred. She remained alert and conscious throughout her hospital stay. Her blood pressure on admission was 95/65 mmHg and pulse 90/min; ECG showed sinus rhythm and minor flattening of T waves. Throughout her hospital stay her ECG remained normal and the QRS width did not exceed 0.8 s. The corrected QT interval was also normal throughout. Plasma levels of nomifensine were measured every 4 h from 17 h after ingestion.

Montgomery *et al.* (1978) have also reported an overdose (1.5 g). Although their patient showed sinus tachycardia and ours did not, neither patient had any cardiovascular, ECG, or neurological abnormality.

These findings suggest that nomifensine is relatively free from cardiovascular side-effects. This drug may therefore have an advantage in the treatment of depression in cardiac patients,

particularly those in whom quinidine or quinidine-like drugs may
not be desirable because of pre-existing intracardiac conduction
defects (Burrows *et al.*, 1978; Dumovic *et al.*, 1979; McIntyre *et
al.*, 1980).

ZIMELIDINE

Zimelidine is a selective serotonin uptake inhibitor with a mono-
cyclic structure. Very few cardiovascular studies have been
reported.

We have just completed a double-blind trial, to compare
zimelidine and placebo in a group of 28 endogenously depressed
patients. Selection for the study was based on clinical judgement
and the Roth and Gurney scale. Patients with other psychiatric
conditions, concomitant physical illness or evidence of drug
dependence were excluded from the trial. After a five-day washout
period, patients who fulfilled the criteria were assigned to one
of the two treatment groups. Patients were matched for age, sex
and initial severity of depression. The efficacy of the treatment
was determined using the Hamilton rating scale for depression,
clinical global rating and Zung self-rating scale, administered on
days 0, 4, 7, 10, 14, 21, 28, 35 and 42. Side-effects and plasma
concentrations were determined on the same schedule. A sequential
analysis of the results showed zimelidine to be significantly
better than placebo ($p > 0.05$).

Cardiovascular Effects

There were no significant differences in blood pressure or pulse
between the two groups. Two patients (one zimelidine and one
placebo) developed persistent orthostatic hypotension. In three
other patients, all in the zimelidine group, orthostatic hypotension was observed in the first two weeks of treatment but did not
persist. One patient on zimelidine was withdrawn from treatment
because of an adverse reaction, which included intermittent hypertensive episodes.

Some changes in the ECG were noted in both groups, but none
were of the severity that required cessation of therapy. In the
zimelidine treated group ST-T wave changes (three patients),
ventricular extrasystoles (one patient) and sinus bradycardia (one
patient) were recorded. ST-T wave changes were present in two
patients before treatment and were unaltered throughout the trial
period. Individual and mean (± standard deviation) PR, QRS, ST
intervals and heart rate for the zimelidine treated patients are
presented in table 4. These parameters were not significantly
different after three or six weeks of zimelidine compared to
baseline measures ($p > 0.05$; Kruskal-Wallis analysis of variance for

Table 4. ECG parameters for patients on zimelidine*

Patient no.†	Baseline				Week 3				Week 6			
	PR	QRS	ST	HR§	PR	QRS	ST	HR§	PR	QRS	ST	HR§
2	0.18	0.10	0.34	69	0.18	0.10	0.28	70	0.14	0.10	0.30	72
8	0.14	0.10	0.26	84	0.18	0.10	0.56	71	0.16	0.10	0.38	72
10	0.14	0.08	0.32	65	0.18	0.10	0.32	78	-	-	-	-
12	0.18	0.08	0.30	76	-	-	-	-	0.18	0.08	0.28	77
13	0.18	0.10	0.30	74	0.18	0.10	0.36	76	0.18	0.12	0.30	69
18	0.14	0.12	0.32	56	0.14	0.12	0.30	57	0.14	0.10	0.30	56
20	0.16	0.10	0.28	66	0.16	0.08	0.28	90	0.18	0.10	0.32	62
23	0.16	0.10	0.36	54	0.20	0.08	0.36	54	0.18	0.08	0.36	53
28	-	-	-	75	-	-	-	52	-	-	-	55
Mean	0.16	0.098	0.31	68.7	0.17	0.097	0.35	68.5	0.17	0.097	0.32	64.5
± S.D.	0.02	0.013	0.03	9.7	0.02	0.014	0.10	13.3	0.02	0.014	0.04	9.2

* Normal ranges (s): PR, 0.12-0.20; QRS, 0.08-0.12; ST, 0.27-0.35
† ECGs were not taken for patients 6, 16 and 28
§ HR = heart Rate

repeated measures), and are not significantly different from normal values. In the placebo group, sinus tachycardia (two patients) and ventricular extrasystoles (one patient) were recorded.

There were no significant correlations between plasma zimelidine or norzimelidine concentrations and clinical response (as judged by the Hamilton scores or the amelioration scores) at weeks 2, 3, 4, 5 or 6 ($p>0.05$; Spearman rank order correlations). Similarly, there were no significant correlations between zimelidine or norzimelidine concentrations and side-effects (or corrected side-effects scores; obtained by subtracting the base-line values from side-effects scores at weeks 2, 3, 4, 5 and 6) ($p>0.05$; Spearman rank order correlations).

The present study did not confirm the finding that patients with high plasma norzimelidine concentrations (above 1000 nmol l^{-1}) show poor response to treatment (Montgomery *et al.*, 1981). Although one patient with high plasma norzimelidine levels did not respond to zimelidine therapy, two others showed a significant improvement. The present study could not confirm the finding that patients with high norzimelidine concentrations (above 1000 nmol l^{-1}) had a higher incidence of anticholinergic side-effects (Montgomery *et al.*, 1981), or a higher incidence of sleep disturbance. The incidence of anticholinergic side-effects and sleep disturbance was no different between the three patients with norzimelidine concentrations greater than 1000 nmol l^{-1} and those with lower concentrations.

Plasma zimelidine concentrations at week 6 were found to be significantly negatively correlated with ST interval ($r = -0.8827$, $p>0.01$; Spearman rank order correlation), and significantly positively correlated with heart rate ($r = 0.7714$, $p>0.05$; Spearman rank order correlation). These parameters, however, did not show a significant correlation or a similar trend after three weeks of zimelidine treatment: zimelidine concentrations and ST interval, $r = 0.1273$, $p>0.05$, Spearman rank order correlation; zimelidine concentrations and heart rate, $r = -0.4286$, $p>0.05$, Spearman rank order correlation. As all cardiovascular parameters are within the normal range and not significantly altered by zimelidine therapy, the above correlations are not clinically significant.

Zimelidine concentrations were not significantly correlated with other cardiovascular parameters, and norzimelidine concentrations were not significantly correlated with any cardiovascular parameters at weeks 3 or 6 ($p>0.05$; Spearman rank order correlations).

It should be emphasized that patients with cardiac conditions who have organic psychiatric illnesses should be capable of being treated with appropriate psychiatric drugs. In general the cardiovascular side-effects of psychiatric drugs given in therapeutic doses are minimal. Self-poisoning will always be a problem.

The techniques that are currently available for evaluating the side-actions of psychotropic drugs are really the major investigation tools that are currently available for assessing myocardial function and intracardiac conduction.

It is important to stress that the *resting values* have limited application whereas measurements taken under physical and emotional stress are more relevant to the 'real life' situation. This is the area of future development.

In a recent study (Veith *et al.*, 1982), 24 depressed patients with heart disease were treated with antidepressants. The tricyclic antidepressants doxepin and imipramine had no effect on left ventricular ejection fraction at rest or during maximal exercise as measured by radionuclide ventriculograms obtained before and after treatment. These researchers under-scored the need for reappraisal of the cardiovascular risks of tricyclic antidepressants. They also suggest that in the absence of severe impairment of myocardial performance depressed patients with pre-existing heart disease could be effectively treated, without an adverse effect on ventricular rhythm or hemodynamic function. Obviously, if the depression is severe enough active treatment with antidepressants is warranted.

Perhaps initially lower doses of the drugs are required and there would be some value, possibly, in monitoring both cardiovascular parameters and plasma antidepressant levels.

REFERENCES

Burgess, C. and Turner, P. (1981). Cardiovascular effects of antidepressants: clinical implications. In Stress and the Heart (ed. D. Wheatley), Raven Press, New York, pp. 173-91.

Burrows, G., Davies, B. and Scoggins, B. (1972). Plasma concentration of nortriptyline and clinical response in depressive illness. Lancet, ii, 619-23.

Burrows, G., Hughes, I. and Norman, T. (1981a). Cardiotoxicity of antidepressants: experimental background. In Stress and the Heart (ed. D. Wheatley), Raven Press, New York, pp. 131-71.

Burrows, G., Norman, T. and Hughes, I. (1981b). Cardiovascular effects of antidepressants. In Clinical Pharmacology in Psychiatry: Neuroleptic and Antidepressant Research (eds E. Usdin, S.G. Dahl, L.F. Gram, and O. Lingjaerde), Macmillan, London and Basingstoke, pp. 319-41.

Burrows, G., Vohra, J., Dumovic, P., Scoggins, B. and Davies, B. (1978). Cardiological effects of nomifensine, a new antidepressant. Med. J. Aust., 1, 341-3.

Burrows, G., Vohra, J., Hunt, D., Sloman, J., Scoggins, B. and Davies, B. (1976). Cardiac effects of different tricyclic antidepressant drugs. Br. J. Psychiatry, 129, 335-41.

Dumovic, P., Burrows, G., Vohra, J. and Freeman, S. (1979).
    Cardiological studies with nomifensine, a new antidepressant.
    Clin. Exp. Pharmacol. Physiol., 6, 229-30.
Glassman, A., Walsh, T. and Roose, S. (1981). Cardiovascular
    effects of the tricyclic antidepressants: implications for
    new research. In Clinical Pharmacology in Psychiatry: Neuro-
    leptic and Antidepressant Research (eds E. Usdin, S.G. Dahl,
    L.F. Gram and O. Lingjaerde), Macmillan, London and
    Basingstoke, pp. 343-9.
Kristjansen, E. (1961). Cardiac complications during treatment
    with imipramine (Tofranil). Acta Psychiat.Neurol., 36, 427.
McIntyre, I.M., Burrows, G.D., Norman, T.R., Dumovic, P. and
    Vohra, J. (1980). Plasma nomifensine concentration. Cardio-
    logical effects and clinical response. Int. Pharmaco-
    psychiatry, 15, 325-33.
Montgomery, S., Crome, P. and Braithwaite, R. A. (1978).
    Nomifensine overdosage. Lancet, ii, 828-9.
Montgomery, S., McAuley, R., Rani, S., Roy, D. and Montgomery, D.
    (1981). A double-blind comparison of zimelidine and
    amitriptyline in endogenous depression. Acta Psychiat.
    Scand., 63 (Suppl 290), 314-27.
Veith, R., Murray, M., Raskind, A., Caldwell, J., Barnes, R.,
    Gumbrecht, G. and Ritchie, J. (1982). Cardiovascular effects
    of tricyclic antidepressants in depressed patients with
    chronic heart disease. New Engl. J. Med., 306, 954-9.
Vohra, J., Burrows, G.D., McIntyre, I.M. and Davis, B. (1978).
    Cardiovascular effects of nomifensine. Lancet, ii, 902-3.

The implications of left ventricular performance for tricyclic antidepressant drug treatment

Alexander H. Glassman[1], Steven P. Roose[1], B. Timothy Walsh[1],
Thomas Cooper[1], Elsa V. Giardina[2] and J. T. Bigger Jr[2]

INTRODUCTION

Early animal work with the tricyclic antidepressants indicated that these drugs are cardiotoxic and, more specifically, that they adversely affect cardiac contractility. This has been a consistent finding across a large number of clinical studies looking at a variety of tricyclic drugs in a variety of test animals (Kaumann *et al.*, 1965; Laddu and Somani, 1969; Langslet *et al.*, 1971). However, as is so commonly the problem with such data, these studies implied, but in no way could definitively establish, what these drugs would do in humans. An uncertainty remained because of the difficulty in interpreting concentration and metabolic differences between man and various experimental animals. During the 1960s a number of investigators reported cases of tricyclic overdose where myocardial failure was a major clinical problem (Laddu and Somani, 1969; Sigg *et al.*, 1963). These reports cite the animal data as evidence to explain the clinical symptomatology of these patients and then concluded that the clinical symptomatology of these patients was *prima facie* evidence for the existence of a direct negative inotropic effect from tricyclic drugs. Unfortunately, these reports did not include direct measurements of left ventricular performance. In fact, the first study to examine direct measurements of left ventricular performance was published in 1974 (Thorstrand, 1974), almost 20 years after the tricyclics were first introduced.

EARLIER CLINICAL STUDIES

When the cardiovascular effects of tricyclic antidepressants are reviewed, the discussion is almost always limited to the effects

[1]Department of Psychiatry, and [2]Department of Medicine and Pharmacology, College of Physicians and Surgeons, Columbia University, New York, USA.

of the tricyclic antidepressant drugs on the electrical activity of the heart. This is because the electrocardiogram (ECG) is such a readily available tool and the ECG measures electrical activity. The mechanical activity, or pumping function of the heart, is more difficult to evaluate. Only since the mid-1970s have investigators begun to look at the effects of tricyclic drugs on the mechanical function of the heart. Muller, Burckhardt and Raeder were among the first to attempt a systematic investigation of the effect of tricyclic drugs on left ventricular performance (Muller and Burckhardt, 1974; Burckhardt *et al.*, 1978). Over the course of several years they studied a group of 66 depressed patients receiving an assortment of tricyclic and tetracyclic antidepressant drugs. Although it was difficult to ascertain if there were any differences between the drugs examined, there was a clear overall negative inotropic effect from the tricyclic drugs. A few years later, Taylor and Braithwaite examined eight depressed patients before and after receiving nortriptyline and reached the same conclusion (Taylor and Braithwaite, 1978); the tricyclic drug showed an adverse effect on cardiac contractility. Several other investigators have subsequently reached similar conclusions. Burgess *et al.* (1979) studied a normal group of volunteers given a single dose of amitriptyline, and Camp *et al.* (1979) reported on a series of 12 hyperactive children treated with 5 mg kg^{-1} of imipramine hydrochloride. In both cases there was evidence of a negative inotropic effect of the tricyclic antidepressant.

A perplexing contradiction to this apparent unanimity of opinion came from the original overdose study by Thorstrand (1974) in Scandinavia. About the same time that Muller published his first studies of contractility during therapeutic treatments with tricyclics, Thorstrand published a study of 10 patients with tricyclic antidepressant overdose, comparing them to patients with barbiturate overdose. Using direct cardiac catheterization techniques Thorstrand found no evidence of impairment of the heart's mechanical performance. Even when the patients were comatose, Thorstrand found evidence of high, not low, cardiac output.

The studies of Muller, Burckhardt, Camp, Taylor and Burgess all used systolic time intervals as a measure of left ventricular function. The systolic time interval is an indirect measure of ventricular performance that is dependent, in part, on the QRS duration. Because QRS lengthening is a characteristic induced by the tricyclic drugs, we were concerned that these drugs might spuriously alter the systolic time interval so that it would no longer be an accurate measurement of left ventricular performance in the presence of these compounds. In order to examine this possibility, we studied the effects of both imipramine and desipramine on left ventricular performance in a group of depressed patients using both echocardiographic fractional shortening and systolic time interval measures (Giardina *et al.*, 1982). Consistent with the earlier studies, both drugs altered the systolic time interval by increasing the pre-ejection period and consequently pre-ejection period/left ventricular ejection time ratio. However, as we had postulated, the echocardiographic fractional shortening remained unchanged with either drug. Recently, Langou *et al.* (1980) have published additional overdose data that also would argue against the conclusion implied by systolic time interval measurements.

RADIONUCLIDE ANGIOGRAPHY

The paucity of data involving the effects of tricyclic drugs on the mechanical action of the heart is not accidental. The most reliable method for measuring left ventricular performance involves the direct catheterization of the heart. These techniques, although accurate, are not without risk and hard to justify in a patient without overt heart disease, where the only purpose of catheterization is to examine drug effects. As a result, it has been traditional to measure drug effects with indirect measures of left ventricular performance such as systolic time intervals, echocardiography, or ballistocardiograms. These measures are all complex and, while they are not invasive, they are subject to a number of inherent pitfalls. For that reason the recent development of radionuclide angiography represented a significant advance in both clinical cardiology and clinical pharmacology. It supplies a reliable measure of left ventricular performance that is non-invasive and reliable, even in patients with serious heart disease. As a result it can readily be used to study drug effects on left ventricular function.

In 1981, Giardina *et al.* first published data using radionuclide angiography to examine the effects of tricyclic drugs on left ventricular performance (Giardina *et al.*, 1981). The primary focus of the study was the anti-arrhythmic activity of tricyclics in cardiac patients who were not depressed. They studied 10 patients treated with imipramine and 12 with nortriptyline and found no effect of either drug on left ventricular performance. This further confirmed our original suspicion that the systolic time interval data were systematically flawed. Recently, Veith *et al.* (1982) published data on 17 depressed patients, eight treated with imipramine and nine with doxepin, studied both before and after drug and in both the resting and exercise condition. They also found no evidence that tricyclics impair left ventricular performance. However, they cautioned that only limited conclusions should be drawn from their data because they only studied a very limited number of patients who had a significant degree of left ventricular impairment as a baseline condition. They suggested that those patients with severe pre-existing left ventricular impairment may be more vulnerable to any negative inotropic effect that a drug might possess. We have recently ex-

amined a group of patients selected because they had pre-existing
left ventricular impairment and found no evidence of any further
impairment in left ventricular function while on tricyclics even
in this significantly impaired group (Glassman *et al.*, in press).

PHARMACOKINETICS AND LEFT VENTRICULAR PERFORMANCE

However, it became apparent that, even though tricyclic drugs do
not adversely affect left ventricular performance, it does not
follow that it is either safe or, in any sense, ordinary to administer these drugs to those depressed patients with compromised
ventricular performance. The collection of a group of depressed
patients with impaired left ventricular performance also allowed
an examination of drug clearance in these patients. In spite of
the large inter-individual variability in metabolism characteristic of these compounds (Glassman *et al.*, in press), the plasma
concentrations of imipramine and its demethylated metabolite were
dramatically higher in those patients with impaired left ventricular function than would be predicted on the basis of oral dose
given. In this group an average oral dose of less than 3.5 mg
kg^{-1} resulted in a mean plasma level of 388 ng ml^{-1} of imipramine
and its demethylated metabolite (imipramine + desipramine). In a
previous study of 60 depressed patients essentially free of heart
disease, this same oral dose of imipramine produced a mean imipramine + desipramine steady-state plasma concentration of 200 ng
ml^{-1}. This represents a highly significant statistical difference
($p < 0.001$) even though the magnitude of the difference in plasma
concentrations is understated because three of the patients with
impaired left ventricular function stopped the drug before they
reached steady state. In addition to the difference in total
steady-state plasma concentrations of the drug, impaired left
ventricular function would seem to alter the normal distribution
of imipramine and its metabolites. In these patients, both imipramine and 2-OH-imipramine are far more common than one ordinarily
would expect. In a large number of patients without cardiac
disease, Cooper reported that desipramine is present in higher
concentration in plasma than its parent compound, and Potter has
found desipramine and 2-OH-desipramine to be present in higher
concentrations (Cooper and Prien, personal communication; Potter
et al., 1982). In patients with left ventricular failure the
opposite was true; imipramine concentrations were almost twice
those of its demethylated metabolite (see figure 1). Similarly it
has been shown that in depressed patients free from cardiac
disease, 2-OH-imipramine is readily demethylated to 2-OH-desipra-
mine and the concentrations of the demethylated metabolite usually
are four or five times those of 2-OH-imipramine. However, in the
depressed patient with left ventricular impairment the concentrations of 2-OH-imipramine were essentially equal to those of the

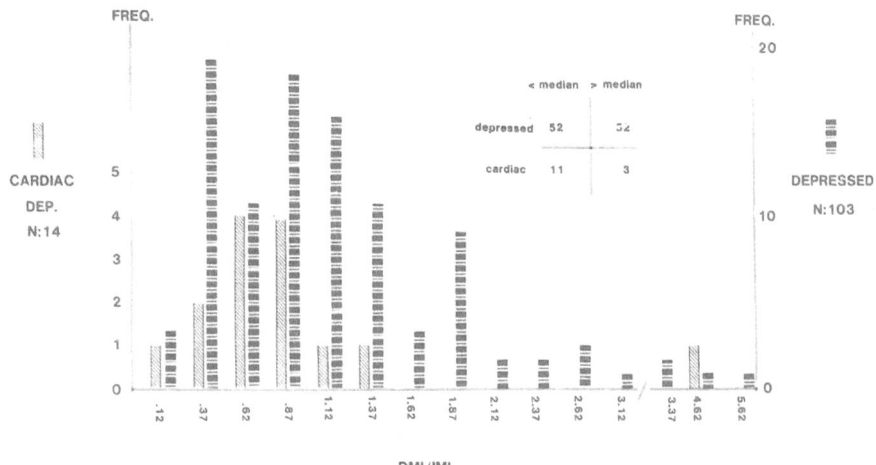

Figure 1. The frequency distribution of the ratio desipramine/
imipramine (DMI/IMI) in two groups of depressed
patients. The dark bars represent the ratios of 104
depressed patients free of cardiovascular disease,
treated with 150 mg per day of imipramine. The lighter,
hatched bars represent the ratios of 15 depressed
patients with impaired left ventricular function. The
chi-square measures the distribution of these ratios
above and below the median ratio for the entire sample
in the cardiac and non-cardiac patients. The difference
is significant at the level $p < 0.05$.

hydroxylated demethylated compound. The pattern of alterations in
metabolism suggest that they result from inadequate demethylation.
This would not be surprising given that demethylation is a flow-
dependent process and these patients would be expected to have
reduced hepatic blood flow secondary to their impaired left ventricular function. However, because these patients all have
significant left ventricular impairment, the vast majority of them
are simultaneously receiving cardiovascular medication. Thus, one
cannot say unequivocally whether the observed differences in
metabolism between this group and control populations are because
of decreased hepatic blood flow, decreased renal blood flow or the
cardiovascular drugs to which they are usually exposed. The
reason for this difference in metabolism remains to be clarified.

ORTHOSTATIC HYPOTENSION

Although it is in no way obvious that it is causally connected
with the metabolic differences just discussed, patients with
impaired left ventricular function have a dramatic increase in the

frequency of severe orthostatic hypotension. Among the 15 imipramine treated patients with clinical evidence of impaired left ventricular performance, seven developed orthostatic hypotension so severe that they fell and the drug had to be discontinued. Two additional patients had their drug discontinued at the end of the protocol period because of measured drop in blood pressure averaging 33 mmHg. Although they did not fall, these drops in measured pressure were considered precarious in this population. This intolerance to imipramine is a dramatic increase over any rate previously reported.

There is an interesting question if the falls experienced by this group of patients were due entirely to the orthostatic drop in systolic pressure or if these patients may also have a pre-existing vulnerability to postural changes in blood pressure. Ordinarily, brain blood flow is maintained at a constant rate independent of systemic blood pressure, when systemic pressure is between 70 and 180 mmHg. If, however, the systemic blood pressure is above or below that range, then brain blood flow is directly related to systemic pressure. There is now evidence that tricyclic antidepressants decrease the range of brain blood flow independence (Preskorn *et al.*, 1982). It may be that heart failure in some way further restricts this independence. If so, it is possible that patients with heart failure treated with tricyclics are at risk to fall because small changes in systemic pressure will affect brain blood flow.

In order to examine further the relationship between orthostatic hypotension and cardiovascular disease, we reviewed data collected from 39 consecutive admissions to the research unit having both a diagnosis of major affective disorder and heart disease. The cardiovascular disease varied in type and severity although the more severe grades of functional impairment were likely to occur in those patients with impaired left ventricular performance because we recruited patients with left ventricular impairment regardless of severity. Depressed patients with functional impairment related to angina were not actively recruited and were undoubtedly under-represented in this population.

We identified those patients who fell and had the drug stopped (eight patients) and those patients who had the drug stopped or dose decreased because of orthostatic hypotension but did not fall (three patients). Thus, 11 of our 39 cardiac depressives had trouble due to orthostatic hypotension. The most striking observation is that 11 of the 25 males given imipramine had orthostatic trouble but none of the 14 female patients experienced serious difficulty. This difference is significant at the $p < 0.003$ level. In addition, clinical evidence of impaired left ventricular performance (a large heart on X-ray and/or a history of congestive heart failure), the number of cardiovascular medications, or the degree of functional impairment as measured by the New York Heart Association classification, were also significant variables and were equally associated with the likelihood of developing orthostatic 'trouble'. Interestingly, neither age, pre-drug orthostatic change, nor plasma concentration of imipramine or its demethylated metabolite predicted that a patient would have orthostatic difficulties when treated with imipramine.

SUMMARY AND CONCLUSION

For two decades there has been an impression that tricyclic drugs adversely affect left ventricular performance. This initially arose out of animal studies and was subsequently supported by a series of systolic time interval studies. Though it is easily understood how that impression gained wide acceptance, the impression is nonetheless erroneous. The overdose data of Thorstrand (1974) and Langou *et al.* (1980) and the radionuclide studies of Giardina *et al.* (1981), Veith *et al.* (1982) and our own recent radionuclide studies at usual therapeutic levels, leave little reason to believe that tricyclic antidepressants, in any usual situation, have an adverse effect on left ventricular performance.

Ironically, although it was this concern about the effects of tricyclic antidepressants on left ventricular performance that prompted us to study patients with ventricular impairment, it turns out that the clinical problem in treating these patients probably results from the effect of impaired left ventricular performance on their metabolism. It is now clear that, in depressed patients with impaired left ventricular performance, the clearance of the drug is altered and the chances of orthostatic hypotension with serious consequences is vastly increased – certainly this is true in depressed males. It would seem that the occurrence of an apparently simple adverse event, i.e. falling secondary to orthostatic hypotension, is related to the patient's cardiac condition – impaired left ventricular performance – sex and, perhaps, even his psychiatric diagnosis. It is intriguing to note that the data of Giardina *et al.* (1981) obtained in cardiac patients without depression showed no evidence of orthostatic hypotension compared to the severe orthostatic hypotension in our depressed, cardiac population. Although it remains to be clarified why this high rate of orthostatic hypotension occurs and whether it occurs with tricyclics other than imipramine, it is clear that the treatment of depressed patients with impaired left ventricular performance is a complex and, at least with imipramine, a potentially dangerous undertaking.

Acknowledgement

This work was supported in part by Grant MH 32592, The National Institute of Mental Health and by the Taub Foundation.

REFERENCES

Burckhardt, D., Raeder, E., Muller, V., Imhof, P. and Neubauer, H. (1978). Cardiovascular effects of tricyclic and tetracyclic antidepressants. J. Am. Med. Assoc., 239 (3), 213-16.

Burgess, C.D., Montgomery, S., Wadsworth, J. and Turner, P. (1979). Cardiovascular effects of amitriptyline, mianserin, zimelidine and nomifensine in depressed patients. Postgrad. Med. J., 55, 704-8.

Camp, J.A., Winsberg, B.G. and Goldstein, S. (1979). Effects of imipramine on left ventricular performance in children. In Biological Psychiatry Today (eds J. Obiols, C. Ballus, E. Gonzalez Monclus and J. Pujol), Elsevier/North-Holland Biomedical Press, New York, pp.849-51.

Cooper, T.B. and Prien, R.F. (personal communication). NIMH - Psychopharmacology Branch, Collaborative study of the prophylactic effect of imipramine hydrochloride.

Giardina, E.G.V., Bigger, J.T., Jr and Glassman, A.H. (1982). Comparison between imipramine and desmethylimipramine on the electrocardiogram and left ventricular function. Clin. Pharmacol. Ther., 31, 230.

Giardina, E.G.V., Bigger, J.T., Jr and Johnson, L.L. (1981). The effect of imipramine and nortriptyline on ventricular premature depolarizations and left ventricular function. Circulation, 64 (IV), 316.

Glassman, A.H., Johnson, L.L., Giardina, E.G.V., Walsh, B.T., Roose, S.P., Cooper, T.B. and Bigger, J.T., Jr (in press). The use of imipramine in depressed patients with impaired left ventricular function. Ann. Int. Med., submitted for publication.

Kaumann, A., Basso, N. and Aramendia, P. (1965). The cardiovascular effects of *N*-(gamma-methyl-aminopropyl-iminodibenzyl)-HCl (desmethylimipramine) and guanethidine. J. Pharmacol. Exp. Ther., 147, 54-64.

Laddu, A.R. and Somani, P. (1969). Desipramine toxicity and its treatment. Toxicol. Appl. Pharmacol., 15, 287-94.

Langou, R.A., Van Dyke, C., Tahan, S.R. and Cohen, L.S. (1980). Cardiovascular manifestations of tricyclic antidepressant overdose. Am. Heart J., 100, 458-64.

Langslet, A., Johansen, W.G., Ryg, M., Skomedal, T. and Øye, I. (1971). Effects of dibenzepine and imipramine on the isolated rat heart. Eur. J. Pharmacol., 14, 333-9.

Muller, V. and Burckhardt, D. (1974). Die Wirkung tri- und tetrazyklischer Antidepressiva auf Herz und Kreislauf. Schweiz. Med. Wochenschr., 104, 1911-13.

Potter, W.Z., Calil, H.M., Sutfin, T.A., Zavadil, A.P., III, Jusko, W.J., Rapoport, J. and Goodwin, F.K. (1982). Active metabolites of imipramine and desipramine in man. Clin. Pharmacol. Ther., 31, 393-401.

Preskorn, S.H., Raichle, M.E. and Hartman, B.K. (1982). Anti-depressants after cerebrovascular permeability and metabolic rate in primates. *Science*, 217, 250-2.

Sigg, E.B., Osborne, M. and Korol, B. (1963). Cardiovascular effects of imipramine. *J. Pharmacol. Exp. Ther.*, 141, 237-43.

Taylor, D.J. and Braithwaite, R.A. (1978). Cardiac effects of tricyclic antidepressant medication: a preliminary study of nortriptyline. *Br. Heart J.*, 40, 1005-9.

Thorstrand, C. (1974). Cardiovascular effects of poisoning with tricyclic antidepressants. *Acta Med. Scand.*, 195, 505-14.

Veith, R.C., Raskind, M.A., Caldwell, J.H., Barnes, R.F. Gumbrecht, G. and Ritchie, J.L. (1982). Cardiovascular effects of tricyclic antidepressants in depressed patients with chronic heart disease. *New Engl. J. Med.*, **306**, 954-9.

Registration of antidepressant drugs - views of a regulatory agency

Kjell Strandberg[1]

INTRODUCTION

The prime objective of a national drug policy is to provide the community with reasonably priced, safe and efficacious drugs of high pharmaceutical quality. To achieve this objective, a number of regulatory activities have to be carried out constantly, among which are: inspection of pharmaceutical plants and laboratories; analytical and biological control; assessment of clinical trial protocols and safety documentation; assessment of new drug applications (NDAs); post-marketing surveillance, including drug promotion activities; drug consumption surveys; drug prescribing patterns; and adverse reaction reporting. Society expects its drug regulatory agency to take actions promptly whenever a drug hazard is identified. Similarly, it expects the introduction of new valuable drugs with the minimum of delay caused by the regulatory handling of the application.

REGISTRATION

To be licensed, a new drug must prove efficacy beyond doubt and its side-effects must not be disproportional to its intended effect. Controlled clinical trials are mandatory for most drugs in order to provide acceptable data for claims of efficacy. Ideally, safety data should be collected similarly but, for long-term risk assessment, data from open studies usually suffice. More importantly, risk assessment studies should be guided by results of prior appropriate animal pharmacology and toxicology studies as well as by human pharmacokinetic and pharmacodynamic data indicating possible risks in patients with, for example, hepatic or renal failure, low-capacity drug metabolism, or treatment with other drugs subject to possible interactions. The data

[1]Department of Drugs, National Board of Health and Welfare, Box 607, S-751 25 Uppsala, Sweden.

submitted to prove efficacy and safety must be scientifically valid and should meet the standards of contemporary first-line research. As progress is made, obsolete drugs should be phased out by industry and little action should be needed from regulatory agencies. However, commercial interests prevail and, hence, regulatory agencies must also act in this area. It is important to note that actions taken in order to remove a drug from the market should similarly rest on scientifically valid grounds, whether related to efficacy or safety problems.

Applying these criteria to the Swedish drug market, presently around 2500 pharmaceutical specialities are registered, representing about 900 substances and a variety of dosage forms and different strengths. Psychotropic drugs constitute less than 10% of the total number of drugs. There are 24 neuroleptics, 11 antidepressants, seven benzodiazepines, six barbiturates and less than 20 combination products available. Partly as a result of regulatory activities, the number and use of barbiturates and combination products have been falling drastically over the last few years, the centrally acting anorectic drugs being removed from the market almost two years ago.

Swedish drug regulatory control is in practice executed as a joint activity between professionals in the regulatory body and external experts. The necessity of keeping a qualified staff within the divisions of pharmacy, animal pharmacology and toxicology, pharmacotherapeutics and clinical research in order to respond to the goals of the health program and ongoing progress in the field is recognized by recruiting staff on scientific merit and allotting budgeted time for research and clinical activities. Recognizing this as extraordinary in comparison to the situation in most other regulatory agencies, the fact remains that efficient drug control calls for quality in order to meet the demands of society and the challenge by industry. To make up the gap, it is mandatory that experts in university positions contribute to the decision making. There will never exist a regulatory body staffed to cope fully with the wide range of activities expected from it. There are also good reasons to question the cost/benefit of striving in that direction. The participation of external experts in regulatory work is, thus, vital and the overall quality of drug use will depend on it. This view must be recognized and leading clinicians and scientists insisting on improvement in drug utilization can serve the cause by taking part in regulatory activities.

With regard to new drugs, true innovative drugs have become increasingly sparse. The majority of the recent introductions by pharmaceutical companies have been improvements to existing compounds yielding compounds with, for example, improved bioavailability, sustained duration of action, less dependence on metabolism, improved receptor selectivity with consequences also for side-effects. Some of these new drugs have indeed provided means for better pharmacotherapy; others seem to indicate doubtful gains of prolonged efficacy and improved compliance. The case has been made many times that innovative research is extremely expensive and risky. Hence, to some extent, the industry must play it safe. Indeed, Lasagna (1982) has recently voiced the possibility that innovative research might be arrested altogether due to non-profitability. Are all really new drugs to be orphan drugs?

It is not my task to look into the future. Yet, the scope and format of pharmaceutical research relates strongly to drug regulatory activities. Indeed, it is important to both parties to engage in constructive cost/benefit analyses of current animal toxicology testing, methodology of clinical trials, post-marketing surveillance schemes, etc. It would be extremely helpful to determine in advance reasonable levels of security as to, for example, impurities in extraction of biosynthetic polypeptides, animal toxicology studies required for new classes of compounds, as well as the strategy for clinical trials. In this way, planning will be less time-consuming, operational procedures streamlined, and regulatory work optimized. Recent international attempts to seek more exchange of information between regulatory authorities and to standardize the control procedures are encouraging.

ANTIDEPRESSANT DRUGS

To illustrate this point more concretely, it seems appropriate to discuss some problems that we have experienced in reviewing clinical data for antidepressant drugs. Over the last five years our regulatory agency has received six NDAs for this class of drug. So far only two drugs have been cleared; namely, lofepramine, essentially a prodrug of desipramine and accordingly assessed more by pharmacokinetic standards than by clinical ones, and zimelidine, a selective 5-HT uptake inhibitor. Doxepine was rejected primarily, owing to a poor submission failing to prove efficacy.

The submissions for the antidepressants raised a number of methodological problems, some of which were shared with drugs of different therapeutic classes. Two different types of antidepressants were distinguished, one claiming to possess a novel mechanism of action and one showing a higher degree of receptor selectivity than available tricyclic compounds, with possible consequences for clinical efficacy as well as side-effects.

In either case the main problem related to proof of efficacy (table 1). For most of the drugs, a number of small, unrelated clinical trials were submitted in which the new drug had been compared on a fixed-dose basis with standard doses of amitriptyline, imipramine, etc., in 20-50 patients during 4-6 weeks trials, many of which were open. The selection of patients and dropouts was too often poorly accounted for. In some studies, patients with endogenous depression were included together with patients with other types of depression. The selection of dose was infrequently supported by appropriate studies, either by re-uptake inhibition

Table 1. Problems in clinical documentation

Efficacy
    Lack of appropriate animal models
    Inadequate extent of human pharmacology studies including
       dose-finding studies and plasma concentration-effect
       relations
    Poor definition of patient inclusion and exclusion criteria
    Unsatisfactory accounts of dropouts
    Lack of calculations of appropriate sample size and, hence,
       frequently too small patient materials
    Inadequate or lacking description of how representative the
       study population is
    Too many uncontrolled studies
    Too many fixed-dose comparative studies
    Lack of predefined criteria for effect

Safety
    Poor registration and follow-up of adverse effects
    Too few controlled studies of adequate duration

---

models or pharmacological studies with regard to biological markers or possible side-effects, e.g. sedation or anticholinergic effects. In fact, the lack of stringent explorative phase I studies was distressing. Likewise, the design of many clinical studies was poor.

RECOMMENDATIONS

Information about the state of affairs was passed on to our Board of Drugs, the advisory board on licensing of new drugs. It was decided to form a small task force with the mandate to work out guidelines for clinical documentation of antidepressant drugs. That work is still ongoing but I would like to share with you some suggestions made by the task force (table 2). Thus, it was felt that the diagnostic criteria must be stringent and acknowledged and validated rating scales should be employed. Early clinical studies with new antidepressant drugs should be done in patients with primary major depression (endogenous depression, melancholia) in order to prove the antidepressant properties of the drug. The patient material should be well characterized as to age, sex, duration and severity of disease, prior or ongoing treatment, hospitalization or outpatients, etc. It is important to include elderly patients in the trial program since this patient category will be a target group for therapy upon release of the drug.

    For inclusion, the severity of disease in terms of rating scores should be specified. For therapeutic effect, the required reduction in rating scores should be stated prior to commencing

Table 2. Recommendations for clinical trials

Stringent diagnostic criteria utilizing acknowledged and
　validated rating scales
Adequate characterization of patient material with regard to
　other factors such as age, sex, duration and severity of
　disease, prior or ongoing treatment, hospitalization or
　outpatients, etc.
Ensure that the study program is representative of clinical
　therapy, e.g. inclusion of old patients
Inclusion of statistical analysis of patient numbers to meet
　the objective of the study
Use of washout periods prior to study treatment to reduce
　placebo response
Predefined criteria for effect recordings
Need to establish *early* efficacy of a new compound
　necessitating placebo-controlled studies, plasma
　concentration-effect studies and/or large controlled
　comparative studies

---

the study. To reduce the placebo response, a preceding washout
period should be included.

The number of patients needed to make a study worthwhile is
truly important to consider. It is our experience that the numbers
often are inadequate to meet the objectives of the study. Too
frequently the studies include no statistical analysis of power
justifying the design of the study. It must be borne in mind that
30-40% of the patients may respond to a placebo and that tricyclic
antidepressants may have a therapeutic effect in 60-75% of the
patients, all depending on the severity of disease. With this
setting, handbooks in statistics show that in order to prove a new
agent's efficacy of the mentioned order of magnitude in comparison
to placebo, a study of more than 50 patients on either agent must
be undertaken to assure significance. Conversely, it is evident
that using too small patient populations and comparing the efficacy of two drugs with one another may result in no difference,
and a Type II error.

For antidepressant drugs, small fixed-dose studies have
dominated the scene during recent years. In addition to the
reduced possibility of identifying a difference in efficacy between drugs, such a design may introduce non-comparability with
regard to side-effects. Thus, when a drug is used in a non-equi-
potent dose, this might not be revealed in a small study whereas a
low dose might well be associated with a low incidence of side-
effects. The overall result will inevitably read: 'This drug is
as efficacious but gives fewer side-effects.'

With the developments in this field, there are reasons to
demand proofs of efficacy as well as comparative studies of incidence of side-effects. To achieve this, multicenter trials or

multiple independent trials with identical study protocols seem to be unavoidable. Theoretically, the effect of a new drug may be established initially in placebo-controlled clinical trials or by demonstration of a plasma concentration-effect relationship. Current discussions in our country bring attention to the problem of conducting conventional placebo-controlled trials in depressed patients. It has been suggested that such studies may replace plasma concentration-effect studies or the use of long washout periods in comparative studies. It has also been suggested that placebo techniques should only be used in patients resistant to available antidepressant treatment or in withdrawal studies. Apparently, the ethical problems are handled differently, judging from the fact that placebo-controlled studies are undertaken in the US. From the scientific point of view, placebo studies provide excellent means for assessment of efficacy and side-effects of a new therapeutic agent.

Controlled comparative studies are needed to provide a firm basis for judging a new drug's merits against established therapy. As has been pointed out, it is mandatory that such studies are planned to yield the information required, again pointing to large studies in well-characterized patients. In advocating such an approach, it is realized that clinics must cooperate rather than act on an individual basis. Such collaboration would hopefully eliminate some trials of non-innovative drugs, since resources would be directed towards developing areas, thereby also guiding pharmaceutical company research. Concentration is likely to yield more interest in and impact on the trial protocol by the participants. Today, too many trials seem to be carried out to collect a desired overall number of patients, whereas fewer but larger and better designed trials would advance scientific knowledge as well as meeting regulatory requirements.

It should however be understood that with this type of study the results may not be representative of the patient population, and this may be a sacrifice in exchange of trial quality. Thus, subsequent studies will have to face the fact that the overall patient population with depressive disorders likely to benefit from drug treatment may well present a spectrum of characteristics and responses with consequences for the trial protocols. Yet, to provide a solid basis of knowledge for such studies to follow seems to be highly recommendable and necessary for regulatory decision. It is also pertinent to point to this development in other areas, such as cardiovascular research. From a regulatory point of view, it is desirable that the professionals in the field address the problem of how clinical trials should best be conducted.

REFERENCE

Lasagna, L. (1982). Will all new drugs become orphans? <u>Clin. Pharmacol. Ther.</u>, 31(3), 285-9.

Phase-4 studies in psychopharmacology - new antidepressant drugs

P.Kragh-Sørensen[1], P.Christensen[1], L.F.Gram[2], C.B.Kristensen[2], M.Møller[3], O.L.Pedersen[1] and P.Thayssen[3]

INTRODUCTION

The well known 'phase system' used in evaluation of new drugs consists of phases 1, 2 and 3 which are performed before marketing and phase 4 which is carried out after marketing. The pre-marketing phases (1, 2 and 3) aim at describing intended and unintended drug effects in well defined, but rather small, groups of subjects or patients. In contrast, the phase-4 study aims at describing the events following the use of the drug in a larger, more heterogeneous and less well defined population. This system is generally accepted and used in all countries having a modern drug regulatory system, and has generally served its purpose well.

The relatively rigid but variable framework of phases 1, 2 and 3 should be considered when defining the content of phase-4 studies and the research methods to be used. This problem can best be examined by studying the limitations of the phase-3 investigations. The phase-3 investigations cover a limited number of patients; the duration of treatment is often short; and the indications for the treatment are strict and often not commensurate with real life. Phase-3 studies are increasingly often carried out in a special research regimen by particularly interested researchers, but still the designs of many studies are not always comparable and many trials suffer from obvious methodological deficiencies. All these factors point to the necessity of further studies of the new drug after marketing.

Several problems are to be solved in the phase-4 study. Focus should be not only on safety problems and side-effects but also on further registration of therapeutic effect. New indications for use of the compound should be kept in mind. Clinical pharmacological investigation should be continued and the need for

The Clinical Psychopharmacology Research Unit, Departments of [1]Psychiatry, [2]Clinical Pharmacology, and [3]Clinical Physiology, Odense University, DK-5000 Odense C, Denmark.

114

therapeutic drug level monitoring should be thoroughly examined (Hvidberg, 1980; Morselli, 1981). These studies should end with a sort of cost/benefit analysis of the new therapy relative to existing therapy.

NEW ANTIDEPRESSANTS AND PHASE-4 STUDIES

During the past few years several new compounds (e.g. iprindole, viloxazine, mianserin and nomifensine) have been marketed in several countries as effective antidepressants. These drugs have already been widely used and are probably also accepted in clinical practice.

Since these drugs are relatively devoid of effects on the monoamine re-uptake mechanisms, their introduction has created doubt about the validity of the amine hypothesis of depression and mechanism of action of tricyclic antidepressants (Zis and Goodwin, 1979). However, their clinical antidepressant effect has been questioned (Brogden *et al.*, 1978, 1979; Zis and Goodwin, 1979; Hollister, 1981), and as discussed by Strandberg (1983) these difficulties in proving the therapeutic effect are associated with the design of the clinical studies. The many methodological problems and especially the criteria for patient selection make it difficult to conclude that these new drugs really are antidepressants.

It is generally accepted that response to tricyclic antidepressants has been scientifically established only in endogenously depressed patients (Kiloh *et al.*, 1962; Greenblatt *et al.*, 1964; Morris and Beck, 1974; Bielski and Friedel, 1976). The therapeutic effects reported in the published studies on new antidepressants have often been insufficiently demonstrated, and the possible differences from conventional tricyclic antidepressants have not been sufficiently examined. This may, at least partly, be because the studies deal with heterogeneous patient populations. The criteria for diagnostic classification of patients are often poorly defined and not always given, and endogenously depressed patients are not always separated from patients with other depressive states. A conclusion concerning the therapeutic effect in different patient populations is, therefore, impossible.

Perusal of the literature on phase-3 studies on new antidepressants thus points to a need for re-examination of their therapeutic effects in the phase-4 studies. In addition, phase-4 studies should yield extensive information with regard to unintended effects, in particular serious adverse reactions that occur infrequently and therefore have not been detected in the pre-marketing studies. Several new antidepressants have been introduced with claims of fewer cardiovascular side-effects, and such claims ought to be challenged in the phase-4 studies. Depending on the particular aim of the study, phase-4 studies may concentrate either on collection of limited information in a large patient population, or on more intensive studies in smaller patient populations.

Studies of the latter type should be carried out in comparison with standard drugs, ideally in randomized parallel groups, but this is often not feasible. The usual blinding procedure can often be eliminated, while the number of patients and duration of observation period should be realistic. An alternative to parallel groups may be the prospective comparison of sequential treatment series with new antidepressants alternating with established antidepressants. The inherent weakness of this design is that the patient population may change over time, and therefore it is important to include treatment periods with standard drug at regular intervals. This design has been used by us in studies on antidepressant treatment in the elderly and has also been adopted by other groups (von Zeersen and Cording-Tömmel, 1981; Cording-Tömmel, 1982).

DESIGN OF PHASE-4 STUDIES ON ANTIDEPRESSANTS - AN EXAMPLE

Psychiatrists generally believe that antidepressant treatment of elderly patients (>60 years) is troublesome and in many cases contraindicated (Burrows *et al.*, 1983) in relation to the expected increase in undesired effects, in particular cardiovascular reactions. Many clinicians, therefore, prefer electroconvulsive treatment in elderly endogenously depressed patients.

Until recently, our knowledge about the cardiovascular effects of tricyclic and other antidepressants in the elderly has been rather limited, and the practical value of plasma concentration monitoring has not been studied systematically in this age group.

At the Clinical Psychopharmacology Research Unit at Odense University, we have therefore established a standard research program for treatment of elderly endogenously depressed patients. This program has been designed in accordance with earlier plasma level/effect studies in which heed was given to the methodological problems in question (Gram *et al.*, 1981). To date, studies with imipramine, nortriptyline and mianserin (recently marketed in Denmark) have been carried out.

Methods and Patients

Patients over 60 years of age with endogenous depression are examined in a prospective research program that includes the following:

(1) Open plasma level monitored treatment, one week on

placebo followed by at least five weeks on active treatment.

(2) Patients classified as endogenously depressed on a diagnostic scale (Newcastle Diagnostic Index: Gurney *et al.*, 1972; Kragh-Sørensen *et al.*, 1976; Bech *et al.*, 1980) and scoring more than 17 points on the Hamilton Depression Rating Scale (HDRS: Hamilton, 1967) are included. During active treatment, weekly registration of therapeutic effect (HDRS) and side-effects (Asberg *et al.*, 1971) are carried out.

(3) Orthostatic blood pressure reaction (lying and 1-6 min standing) and standard electrocardiogram (ECG) are recorded weekly. Systolic time intervals and 24 h ECT monitoring are carried out in the placebo week and in the second and third weeks of active treatment (Thayssen *et al.*, 1981; Møller *et al.*, 1983).

In each of the completed studies, 14-18 patients were started on placebo and 11-15 patients were started on active treatment (table 1).

Only oxazepam for sedation and already instituted treatment for heart disease (e.g. diuretics, digoxin) were allowed. Some patients had mild cardiac disease, but all patients were cardiovascularly well compensated.

Imipramine and nortriptyline were given twice daily at 8 a.m. and 8 p.m., and the dose was adjusted to give therapeutic plasma concentrations (imipramine + desipramine >200 μg l^{-1}; nortriptyline 60-150 μg l^{-1}).

In the mianserin study, a fixed-dose regimen was used. The first 11 patients were treated with 60 mg daily and 20 mg daily was given to the last four patients. The dose was given in a single dose at 8 p.m.

Results and Discussion

The primary aim of these studies has been to examine adverse reactions; in particular, the cardiovascular effects of the three antidepressants and possible pharmacokinetic differences between them.

The therapeutic effect was examined concurrently and evaluated on the basis of comparison between the consecutive studies. As shown in table 1, the different compounds were given to similar patient populations and in almost identical settings.

With this background, it is interesting that distinct and clinically relevant differences between the three drugs were demonstrated. In the following, a brief outline of the pharmacodynamic, pharmacokinetic and therapeutic differences will be given (for further details, see Thayssen *et al.*, 1981; Bjerre *et al.*, 1981; Kragh-Sørensen *et al.*, 1981; Møller *et al.*, 1983).

Table 1. Imipramine, nortriptyline and mianserin treatment in elderly ($\geqslant$ 60 years) endogenously depressed patients: clinical data

Drugs	Patients initially included	Excluded during placebo	Sex	Patients given active treatment		
				Age (mean and range)	HDRS at the end of placebo period (mean ± S.D.)	
Imipramine	15	4	3M, 8F	73 (63–83)	25 ± 4 (N = 11)	
Nortriptyline	14	2	5M, 7F	70 (60–78)	23 ± 4 (N = 12)	
Mianserin	18	3	4M, 11F	68 (60–86)	25 ± 5 (N = 15)	

Cardiovascular Effects

Both imipramine and mianserin caused significant orthostatic blood pressure drop, whereas nortriptyline caused only a slight and clinically insignificant drop (figure 1) (Thayssen *et al.*, 1981; Kragh-Sørensen *et al.*, 1981; Møller *et al.*, 1983). The effect on orthostatic blood pressure was very pronounced during treatment with imipramine and in two patients it was associated with fall and fracture of the collum femoris. The pronounced drop in orthostatic blood pressure during imipramine treatment necessitated cautious dosage which, in turn, meant that several patients did not reach therapeutic plasma concentrations within the five-week treatment period. The orthostatic blood pressure reaction after mianserin did not give rise to similar pronounced problems, perhaps due to a compensatory increase in heart rate not seen during imipramine treatment (figure 1).

Some patients with hypotensive reactions both in the imipramine and the mianserin groups were subsequently treated with nortriptyline in therapeutic plasma concentrations (60-150 μg 1^{-1}) without any noticeable effect on orthostatic blood pressure.

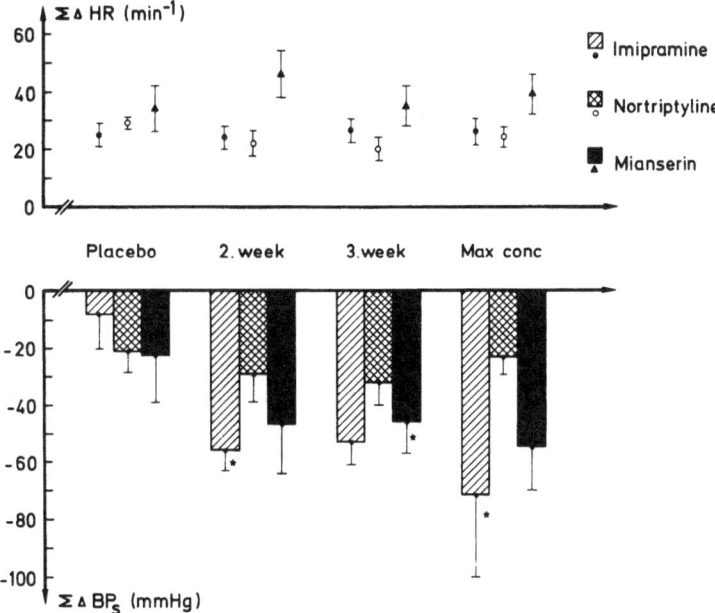

Figure 1. The cumulative changes in heart rate (HR) and systolic blood pressure (BP_s) from supine position to 1, 3 and 5 min in the standing position during treatment with imipramine (N=10), nortriptyline (N=10) and mianserin (N=10). Values are given as mean ± S.E.M. *p<0.05 for differences between placebo and active treatment.

Cardiac ventricular performance evaluated by systolic time interval measurement showed changes in the ratio pre-ejection period/left ventricular ejection time (PEP/LVET) indicating impairment of the left ventricular performance during nortriptyline and mianserin treatment, but not during imipramine treatment, probably due to the relatively low plasma levels in our imipramine patients (*vide supra*).

It has been suggested (Glassman *et al.*, 1983) that the changes seen in PEP and PEP/LVET during antidepressant therapy may be induced by alteration in intraventricular conduction. However, as no prolongation of the electrocardiographic intervals was found in our study, the significant changes in PEP/LVET ratio most likely reflect impairment of left ventricular function. Another possible mechanism is that the antidepressants cause vein dilatation (α_1 adrenoceptor blockade) resulting in reduced cardiac preload and increased PEP/LVET ratio. In any case, the changes in PEP/LVET ratio were modest and not associated with signs of cardiac decompensation.

The 24 h ECG monitoring showed that nortriptyline increases the supine heart rate, whereas neither imipramine, nortriptyline nor mianserin induced changes in the cardiac conduction time or arrhythmias.

From these results it can be concluded that during plasma level controlled therapy in elderly patients, imipramine, nortriptyline and mianserin have modest effects on myocardial contractility, no significant influence on the cardiac conductance, and no arrhythmogenic effect. The clinically most important cardiovascular effect is the orthostatic hypotension, which is pronounced with imipramine, moderate with mianserin and slight or insignificant with nortriptyline.

Pharmacokinetics

The imipramine treatment in the elderly was complicated by dose-dependent kinetics resulting in disproportional rise in desipramine concentrations with increasing dose of imipramine (Bjerre *et al.*, 1981). Proportionality between dose and steady-state plasma levels was found with nortriptyline (Kragh-Sørensen and Larsen, 1980; Bjerre *et al.*, 1981) and with mianserin (unpublished data). Dose adjustment in order to obtain therapeutic drug levels was thus more difficult with imipramine than with nortriptyline and mianserin.

Interaction between tricyclic antidepressants and neuroleptics is a well known phenomenon (Gram, 1977). In these series of investigations, this interaction was observed for all three compounds at relatively low perphenazine doses given late in the treatment period (fourth to eighth week) (Bjerre *et al.*, 1981). The interaction between perphenazine and mianserin resulted in a rise in the plasma concentration of both mianserin and the main metabolite desmethylmianserin when perphenazine was added to the treatment (figure 2).

Steady-state plasma levels of imipramine and nortriptyline on conventional doses have been shown to be higher in elderly than younger patients (Gram *et al.*, 1977; Nies *et al.*, 1977; Kragh-Sørensen and Larsen, 1980). The mianserin dose given in this investigation was 30-60 mg per day and corresponded to plasma concentrations of 25-70 µg l^{-1}. This plasma level range is the same as that found in younger patients (Coppen *et al.*, 1976; Montgomery *et al.*, 1978; Perry *et al.*, 1978; Russell *et al.*, 1978).

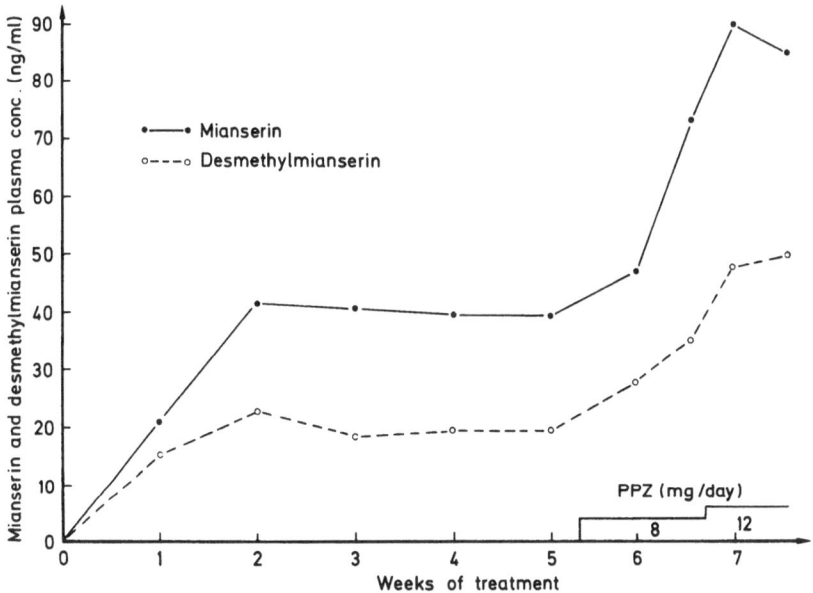

Figure 2.   Drug interaction between mianserin and perphenazine (PPZ) in a hospitalized 72-year-old male patient.

Therapeutic Outcome

The analysis of the data concerning the therapeutic effect was particularly interesting in relation to the results with mianserin, although mianserin was selected primarily because it was marketed as an antidepressant having no or few cardiovascular effects.

As shown in table 1, the patient materials in the three studies were comparable in terms of selection criteria, placebo

Table 2.   Imipramine, nortriptyline and mianserin treatment in
elderly (⩾60 years) endogenously depressed patients:
therapeutic outcome (responders = sum of HDRS ⩽7 points)

Drug and no. of patients (N)*	Responders within 5 weeks	Responders 5-8 weeks	Total no. of Responders
Imipramine (N = 9)	2 (22%)	5 (56%)	7 (78%)
Nortriptyline (N = 11)	7 (64%)	2 (18%)	9 (82%)
Mianserin (N = 12)	1† (8%)	0 (-)	0 (-)

* Dropouts before week 4 not included
† Depressive relapse in week 6

dropouts, initial severity (HDRS), age and sex; 15 patients
entered the active treatment with mianserin.

Surprisingly, it was found that nine patients on mianserin
treatment did not respond at any time to the treatment (table 2).
Four of these patients deteriorated to such an extent that electroconvulsive therapy was required. The other five patients subsequently responded on treatment with nortriptyline.   In six
patients mianserin had some therapeutic effect according to HDRS.
Two of these patients were followed on continued mianserin treatment, but within 5-8 weeks their condition worsened and nortriptyline treatment was instituted.   In two other patients, mianserin
was discontinued in the fifth week due to poor effect.   In two
patients (partial responders on HDRS) the mianserin treatment was
stopped because of severe drowsiness after week 5, and both could
be discharged from hospital without specific antidepressive treatment, and with few or no symptoms of depression.

Assuming that our design permits comparison of the results
from the three studies, it can be seen (table 2) that the therapeutic effect after eight weeks in both the imipramine and nortriptyline groups was clearly superior (∿ 80% recovery).   This
recovery rate is comparable with the therapeutic effect seen in
younger patient populations (Glassman, 1981).

The poor results after five weeks' treatment for the group of
patients treated with imipramine was due to the difficulties in
adjusting the dose to yield therapeutic plasma concentrations
because of orthostatic hypotension and dose-dependent kinetics.

A possible explanation for the unexpected poor therapeutic
result with mianserin could be that elderly patients with endogenous depression generally react poorly to antidepressive drug
treatment.   However, nine of the mianserin patients responded
satisfactorily on subsequent nortriptyline treatment.

Other reasons for inconsistency in therapeutic effect between mianserin and imipramine and nortriptyline could be disparity in sex, age, severity of disease, polarity of depression, diagnostic selection, etc., but these factors were not disparate in our investigation, and possible differences in exclusion criteria, particularly in the placebo washout period, were unlikely (table 1).

In only one study (Montgomery *et al.*, 1978) has therapeutic plasma concentration ranges of mianserin been suggested (15-70 µg l^{-1}). In our study, the 11 patients who completed four weeks on active mianserin treatment all had steady-state plasma concentrations lying within this range (25-60 µg l^{-1}). All patients showed stable steady-state concentrations after two weeks' treatment (cf. figure 2). We have, therefore, no pharmacokinetic or clinical explanation of the poor therapeutic effect of mianserin. The dosage chosen and the plasma concentration achieved are the same as those used in phase-3 studies (Brogden *et al.*, 1978).

It seems unlikely that mianserin, in contrast to imipramine and nortriptyline, should be particularly ineffective in elderly patients.

Conclusion

The described design of this prospective phase-4 study in elderly endogenously depressed patients fulfills all requirements for clinical psychopharmacological research on antidepressants with regard to selection and stratification of patient material and measurement of pharmacokinetic variables (Gram *et al.*, 1981). In a phase-4 study, procedures involving randomization and control therapy usually are not feasible.

Because of the negative therapeutic findings in the mianserin study, the design of phase-4 studies and research on therapeutic drug monitoring becomes pertinent. In particular, it is essential to establish the validity of phase-4 studies carried out as sequential single-drug studies without use of control therapy. Using a design quite similar to ours, von Zeersen and Cording-Tömmel (1981) and Cording-Tömmel (1982) have also questioned the antidepressant effect of mianserin in a younger patient population suffering from severe endogenous depression.

We cannot conclude from these results that mianserin does not have antidepressant properties. However, we can question the value of previously published phase-3 investigations, by far the greatest part of which did not satisfy requirements for controlled clinical trials with antidepressants (Brogden *et al.*, 1978; Zis and Goodwin, 1979; Strandberg, 1983). Therefore, the logical consequence of this study and the study from the Munich group (von Zeersen and Cording-Tömmel, 1981; Cording-Tömmel, 1982) must be that further controlled studies with mianserin should be carried out. The many methodological problems not sufficiently dealt with in many recent studies (phases 2 and 3) on new antidepressant drugs indeed have the perspective that inactive compounds possibly can be marketed as antidepressants.

From a theoretical point of view these results, if replicable, will question the value of many new theories concerning the mechanism of action of antidepressants that were proposed after the introduction of these new compounds, and perhaps bring some new support to the monoamine hypotheses. Also, the validity of quantitative electroencephalographic measurements (Itil *et al.*, 1972) to predict the antidepressant efficacy in patients accordingly can be questioned. Indeed, all new theories need clinical justification before being accepted.

REFERENCES

Asberg, M., Cronholm, B, Sjöqvist, F. and Tuck, D. (1971). Correlation of side-effects with plasma concentrations of nortriptyline. Br. Med. J., 3, 331-4.

Bech, P., Gram, L.F., Reisby, N. and Rafaelsen, O.J. (1980). The WHO depression scale: relationship to the Newcastle scales. Acta Psychiatr. Scand., 62, 140-3.

Bielski, R. J. and Friedel, R. O. (1976). Prediction of tricyclic antidepressant response: a critical review. Arch. Gen. Psychiatry, 23, 164-73.

Bjerre, M., Gram, L.F., Kragh-Sørensen, P., Kristensen, C.B., Pedersen O.L., Møller, M. and Thayssen, P. (1981). Dose dependent kinetics of imipramine in elderly patients. Psychopharmacology, 75, 354-7.

Brogden, R.N., Heel, R.C., Speight, T.M. and Avery, G.S. (1978). Mianserin: a review of its pharmacological properties and therapeutic efficacy in depressive illness. Drugs, 16, 273-301.

Brogden, R.N., Heel, R.C., Speight, T.M. and Avery, G.S. (1979). Nomifensine: a review of its pharmacological properties and therapeutic efficacy in depressive illness. Drugs, 18, 1-24.

Burrows, G.D., Norman, T.R., Vohra, J. and Sloman, G. (1983). Clinical evaluation of the cardiac effects of new psychotropic drugs. This volume, pp. 83-98.

Coppen, A., Gupta, R. and Montgomery, S. (1976). Mianserin hydrochloride: a novel antidepressant. Br. J. Psychiatry, 129, 342-5.

Cording-Tömmel, C. (1982). Zur wirksamkeit von Mianserin und Maprotilin in Vergleich zu Amitriptylin bei schwerer endogener depression. Thesis, Hamburg.

Glassman, A. H. (1981). Plasma levels. Pitfalls and power. In Clinical Pharmacology in Psychiatry (ed. E. Usdin), Elsevier, New York, pp. 277-86.

Glassman, A.H., Roose, S.P., Walsh, B.T., Cooper, T., Giardina, E.V. and Bigger, J. T., Jr (1983). The implications of left ventricular performance for tricyclic antidepressant drug treatment. This volume, pp. 99-107.

Gram, L.F. (1977). Factors influencing the metabolism of tricyclic antidepressants. Dan. Med. Bull., 24, 81-9.

Gram, L.F., Bech, P., Reisby, N. and Jørgensen, O. S. (1981). Methodology in studies on plasma level/effect relationship of tricyclic antidepressants. In Clinical Pharmacology in Psychiatry (ed. E. Usdin), Elsevier, New York, pp. 155-69.

Gram, L.F., Søndergaard, I., Christiansen, J., Petersen, G.O., Bech, P., Reisby, N., Ibsen, I., Ortmann, J., Nagy, A., Dencker, S.J., Jacobsen, O. and Krautwald, O. (1977). Steady-state kinetics of imipramine in patients. Psychopharmacology, 54, 255-61.

Greenblatt, M., Grosser, G.H. and Wechsler, H. (1964). Different response of hospitalized depressed patients to somatic therapy. Am. J. Psychiatry, 120, 935-43.

Gurney, C., Roth, M., Garside, R.F., Kerr, T.A. and Schapera, K. (1972). Studies on the classification of effective disorder. Br. J. Psychiatry, 121, 162-6.

Hamilton, M. (1967). Development of a rating scale for primary depressive illness. Br. J. Soc. Clin. Psychol., 6, 278-96.

Hollister, L.E. (1981). 'Second generation' antidepressant drugs. Psychosomatics, 22, 872-9.

Hvidberg, E.F. (1980). Monitoring drug plasma levels in clinical practice? A procedure for evaluation is needed. Eur. J. Clin. Pharmacol., 17, 317-19.

Itil, T.M., Polvan, N. and Hsu, N. (1972). Clinical and EEG effects of GB 94, a tetracyclic antidepressant. Curr. Ther. Res., 14, 395-414.

Kiloh, L.H., Ball, J.R.B. and Garside, R.R. (1962). Prognostic factors in treatment of depressive states with imipramine. Br. Med. J., 1225-57.

Kragh-Sørensen, P., Hansen, C.E., Bastrup, P.C. and Hvidberg, E.F. (1976). Self inhibiting action of nortriptyline's anti-depressi ve effect at high plasma levels. Psychopharmacologia, 45, 305-16.

Kragh-Sørensen, P., Kristensen, C.B., Pedersen, O.L., Bjerre, M., Benjaminsen, S., Møller, M., Thayssen, P. and Gram, L.F. (1981). Antidepressant treatment with imipramine and nortriptyline in elderly patients. In Clinical Pharmacology in Psychiatry: Neuroleptic and Antidepressant Research (eds E. Usdin, S.G. Dahl, L.F. Gram and O. Lingjaerde), Macmillan, London, pp. 351-7.

Kragh-Sørensen, P. and Larsen, N.-E. (1980). Factors influencing nortriptyline steady-state levels. Plasma and saliva levels. Clin. Pharmacol. Ther., 28, 796-803.

Møller, M., Thayssen, P., Kragh-Sørensen, P., Pedersen, O.L., Kristensen, C.B., Bjerre, M., Benjaminsen, S. and Gram, L.F. (1983). Mianserin: cardiovascular effects in elderly patients. Psychopharmacology, in press.

Montgomery, S., McAuley, R. and Montgomery, D.B. (1978). Relationship between mianserin plasma levels and antidepressant effect in a double blind trial comparing a single night-time and divided daily dose regimen. Br. J. Clin. Pharmacol., 5, Suppl. 71-6.

Morris, J.B. and Beck, A.J. (1974). The efficacy of antidepressant drugs: a review of research (1958 to 1972). Arch. Gen. Psychiatry, 30, 667-74.

Morselli, P.L. (1981). Clinical significance of neuroleptic plasma level monitoring. In Clinical Pharmacology in Psychiatry. Neuroleptic and Antidepressant Research (eds E. Usdin, S. G. Dahl, L. F. Gram and O. Lingjaerde), Macmillan London, pp. 199-209.

Nies, A., Robinson, D.S., Friedman, M.J., Green, R., Cooper, T.B., Ravaris, C.L. and Ives, J.O. (1977). Relationship between age and tricyclic antidepressant plasma levels. Am. J. Psychiatry, 134, 790-3.

Perry, G.F., Fitzsimmons, B., Shapiro, L. and Irwin, P. (1978). Clinical study of mianserin, imipramine and placebo in depression: blood level and MHPG correlations. Br. J. Clin. Pharmacol., 5, Suppl. 1, 35-41.

Russell, G.F.M., Niaz, U., Wakeling, A. and Slade, P.D. (1978). Comparative double-blind trial of mianserin hydrochloride (Organon GB 94) and diazepam in patients with depressive illness. Br. J. Clin. Pharmacol., 5, Suppl. 1, 57-65.

Strandberg, K. (1983). Registration of antidepressant drugs - views of a regulatory agency. This volume, pp. 108-13.

Thayssen, P., Bjerre, M., Kragh-Sørensen, P., Møller, M., Pedersen, O.L., Kristensen, C.B. and Gram, L.F. (1981). Cardiovascular effects of imipramine and nortriptyline in elderly patients. Psychopharmacology, 74, 360-4.

von Zeersen, D. and Cording-Tömmel, C. (1981). Is mianserin a potent antidepressant? Paper presented at III World Congress on Biological Psychiatry, Stockholm 1981, Abstract no. F. 534.

Zis, A.P. and Goodwin, F.K. (1979). Novel antidepressants and the biogenic amine hypothesis of depression. Arch. Gen. Psychiatry, 36, 1097-107.

Section Three

Clinical Pharmacokinetics of Neuroleptics

Overview: measuring plasma concentrations of psychotherapeutic drugs

Leo E. Hollister[1]

INTRODUCTION

Determining plasma concentrations of psychotherapeutic drugs is still relatively new, most of the studies having been done in the past 10–15 years. The idea of such monitoring is not new; when bromides were widely used in psychiatry and neurology, monitoring serum concentrations was recommended although seldom done. Technological advances have made routine monitoring possible. The only question that remains is when it is worth doing, assuming that the laboratories doing such work provide accurate determinations at a reasonable cost.

As experience with measuring plasma concentrations of psychotherapeutic drugs is of variable duration, I shall consider each group in terms of the length of the past experience.

LITHIUM

This ion has a relatively narrow therapeutic margin and fairly well defined range of serum concentrations of 0.9–1.4 mEq 1^{-1}. The lower limits of concentration for its prophylactic use are still being investigated but may be as low as 0.5 mEq 1^{-1}. Lithium is an unusual therapeutic agent, however, as it is distributed in body water for the most part, undergoes no protein binding, is not metabolized and is virtually totally excreted unchanged. Thus, the proven value of measuring serum lithium concentrations may be difficult to extend to drugs with high volumes of distribution, high protein binding, varying degrees of lipid solubility, extensive metabolism, and sometimes active metabolites.

[1] Stanford University School of Medicine and Veterans Administration Medical Center, 3801 Miranda Ave., Palo Alto, California 94304, USA.

The convention is to measure lithium levels as close to 12 h
after the last dose as possible (Amdisen, 1977). Such measurements
should not be done until the patient has been on a given dose of
lithium for about five days, when steady-state concentrations are
reached.   Ordinarily, measurements are made at intervals of one
week during the first month of treatment but as infrequently as
once every month or two during maintenance treatment. Measurements
should be repeated shortly after another drug has been added to
the   therapeutic   program   (diuretics   and   non-steroidal   anti-
inflammatory agents increase levels) or whenever some intercurrent
illness appears.   One should pay heed to toxic symptoms even if
plasma concentrations are reported to be in the therapeutic range.
     Abundant experience has indicated that good clinical results
are sometimes obtained in some patients treated with 'subthera-
peutic' concentrations of lithium while toxicity has occurred when
serum levels were within the therapeutic range.   Accordingly, such
determinations can be used only as guides to dosing and should not
take precedence over clinical observations.

TRICYCLIC ANTIDEPRESSANTS

Despite extensive study, controversy still exists as to whether a
range of therapeutic plasma concentrations can be defined.   Part
of the problem is due to the heterogeneity of depressions, for the
specific antidepressant effect of tricyclics is largely limited to
depressions   characterized   as   'endogenous',   a   minority   of   all
depressions.
     Another difficulty is that some of these drugs produce active
metabolites, often in greater abundance than the parent drug, that
have   either   the   same   or   somewhat   different   pharmacological
actions.   Failure to take into consideration significant amounts
of demethylated or hydroxylated metabolites may confound the
issue.
     Some ranges of reported therapeutic plasma concentrations for
various   tricyclics   are   shown   in   table 1.   Greatest   agreement
centers   around   nortriptyline.   Recent   work   indicated   that   the
10-hydroxy metabolite of nortriptyline has a significant pharmacological activity and this metabolite is usually more abundant
than the parent drug.   Yet virtually all studies attempting to
relate plasma concentrations to clinical effects of this drug have
ignored this metabolite.
     Evidence is highly suggestive, although far from conclusive,
that too low a concentration of tricyclic antidepressant may be
associated with a suboptimal clinical response, while concentrations that are very high may be associated with serious side-
effects (mental confusion or cardiac disturbances).   Such a relationship seems to be entirely logical.   The issue to be settled
is whether the present guides can be translated into improved
clinical practice.

Table 1. Proposed therapeutic ranges for antidepressants
(μg l^{-1})

Nortriptyline	50–150 (Kragh-Sorensen *et al.*, 1976)
	200 (poorer response) (Montgomery *et al.*, 1978)
Imipramine	45 imipramine/75 desipramine (Reisby *et al.*, 1977)
	180 total (Glassman *et al.*, 1977)
Amitriptyline	60–230 total (Vandel *et al.*, 1978)
	200 total (Kupfer *et al.*, 1977)
Desipramine	up to 145 (Amsterdam *et al.*, 1979)
Protriptyline	70–170 (Biggs and Ziegler, 1977)
Clomipramine	240–700 desmethyl clomipramine (Della Corte *et al.*, 1979)
	100–250 clomipramine (Stern *et al.*, 1980)
Maprotiline	200–300 (Pinder *et al.*, 1977)

When might it be appropriate to monitor plasma concentrations of tricyclics? The following are a few suggestions.

(1) The most important indication by far is when a patient has received what could be an adequate dose and has failed to respond. A low plasma concentration might be construed as some abnormality of the drug kinetics in that patient or, more likely, failure to take medication as prescribed. Advising patients with low plasma levels to take their medication exactly as prescribed often results in an increase in plasma concentration, even with no change in dose. On the other hand, if the plasma concentration is in the therapeutic range, but not excessively high, one might feel encouraged to increase the dose so long as clinical toxicity was not evident.

(2) Higher than usual doses of tricyclics merit measurement of plasma concentrations. Doses of 300 mg per day or more of amitriptyline and imipramine seem to show altered kinetics with a non-linear increase in plasma concentrations. Monitoring might help to avoid problems with toxicity and would demonstrate a degree of prudence.

(3) When treating very old or very young patients one might wish to check plasma concentrations to keep them low. The reason for doing so is that protein binding of these highly protein-bound drugs is impaired at the extremes of age. Thus, more drug is present in the unbound, or pharmacologically active, form. The usual interpretation of plasma concentrations will not hold under these circumstances, so that one may wish to keep them at about 50% of what one might wish in a robust patient in the middle years of life.

(4) The presence of intercurrent illness may be a reason to lower plasma concentrations to the lower limits of potential therapeutic efficacy, as drug kinetics may be altered in complex ways during illness.

(5) In cases of drug overdose, plasma concentrations may be particularly useful late in the course when making a decision about when to relax vigilance. A plasma concentration that has returned to the therapeutic range, as well as clinical evidence of remission, would make one feel secure in removing the patient from intensive care. Such determinations would not be especially useful in the course of intoxication, for the level of drug has relatively little bearing on the subsequent clinical course of the intoxication; that is best judged by the prevailing clinical appearance of the patient.

NEUROLEPTICS

Neuroleptics have been used longer than tricyclics in clinical practice, but fewer investigators have tried to define a range of therapeutic plasma concentrations. Some of the limitations on these data are due to technical problems. Chlorpromazine has many potentially active metabolites so that it is really uncertain that simply measuring levels of the parent drug is adequate. The same is true for thioridazine. Some piperazinylphenothiazines, such as fluphenazine, produce only very low steady-state levels, so close to the level of sensitivity of the measuring technique that chances for error are large. Thiothixene has two isomers, one of which contains most of the therapeutic activity. These are somewhat difficult to separate using techniques other than mass spectrometry. Further, steady-state concentrations of this drug also tend to be very low. The relatively sparse data are summarized in table 2.

Haloperidol has emerged as a very popular neuroleptic. It has the advantage that its only active metabolite is present only in inconsequential amounts. Consequently, a great deal of interest has focused on trying to delineate its range of therapeutic plasma concentrations. As can be seen in table 2, neither the lower nor the upper limits have been clearly defined. One might assume that a concentration of 8–10 μg 1^{-1} might represent a suitable lower limit for such a range.

In summary, the data are too sparse and contain too many possible sources of error to accept claims about a range of therapeutic plasma concentrations for neuroleptic drugs. Laboratories can provide numbers, at least for some of these drugs, but their meaning is unclear.

Table 2.   Proposed therapeutic ranges for neuroleptics
(μg l^{-1})

Chlorpromazine	50–300 adults (Rivera-Calimlin *et al.*, 1976)
	40–80 children (Rivera-Calimlin *et al.*, 1979)
Thioridazine	740 total (Cohen *et al.*, 1980)
Butaperazine	400–300 (plasma) (Garver *et al.*, 1977)
	20–60 (erythrocyte) (Garver *et al.*, 1977)
Haloperidol	8–18 (Magliozzi *et al.*, 1981)

BENZODIAZEPINE ANXIOLYTICS

The pharmacokinetics of almost every one of these drugs has been extensively described. Yet no investigator has proposed that measurement of plasma concentrations be adopted in clinical practice. A very early study suggested that minimal plasma concentrations of diazepam for clinical efficacy should be in the region of 400 μg l^{-1} for total diazepam and its active metabolite, nordiazepam (Dasberg *et al.*, 1974). Patients being treated with the drug have shown, however, a very wide range of plasma concentrations, often seemingly doing well at concentrations less than 400 μg l^{-1}.

As the margin of safety with benzodiazepines is very large, it seems unlikely that clinicians will change their present habits of adjusting doses on the basis of clinical response rather than on the basis of plasma concentrations. Still, monitoring of plasma concentrations might detect poor compliance with the treatment program, or possible abuse of the drug.

CONCLUSIONS

The present practice of monitoring serum lithium concentrations is well established, valuable and inexpensive. Arguments for the cost-efficacy for measuring plasma concentrations of other psychotherapeutic drugs are far from persuasive. Particular situations may arise in which such monitoring could be useful. One must remember that not all laboratories provide accurate estimates and that such information might be more of a hindrance to good medical practice than a help.

REFERENCES

Amdisen, A. (1977). Serum level monitoring and clinical pharmacokinetics of lithium. Clin. Pharmacokinetics, 2, 73–92

Amsterdam, J., Brunswick, D.J. and Mendels, J. (1979). High dose
desipramine plasma drug levels and clinical response. J.
Clin. Psychiatry, 40, 141–3

Biggs, J.T. and Ziegler, V.E. (1977). Protriptyline plasma levels
and antidepressant response. Clin. Pharmacol. Ther., 22,
269–73

Cohen, B.M., Lipinski, J.F., Pope, G., Harris, P.Q. and Altesman,
R.K. (1980). Neuroleptic blood levels and therapeutic
effects. Psychopharmacologia, 70, 191–3

Dasberg, H.J., van der Kleijn, E., Guelen, P.J.R. and van Praag,
H.M. (1974). Plasma concentrations of diazepam and of its
metabolite N-desmethyl-diazepam in relation to anxiolytic
effect. Clin. Pharmacol. Ther., 15, 473–83

Della Corte, L., Broadhurst, A.D., Sgaragli, G.P., Filippini, S.,
Heeley, A.F., James, H.D., Faravelli, C. and Pazzogli, A.
(1979). Clinical response and tricyclic plasma levels during
treatment with clomipramine. Br. J. Psychiatry, 134, 390–400

Garver, D.L., Dekirmenjian, H., Davis, J.M., Casper, R. and
Ericksen, S. (1977). Neuroleptic drug levels and therapeutic
response: preliminary observations with red blood cell bound
butaperazine. Am. J. Psychiatry, 134, 304–7

Glassman, A.H., Perel, J.M., Shostak, M., Kantor, S.J. and Fliess,
J.L. (1977). Clinical implications of imipramine plasma
levels for depressive illness. Arch. Gen. Psychiatry, 34,
197–204

Kragh-Sørensen, P., Hansen, C.E., Baastrup, P.C. and Hvidberg,
E.F. (1976). Self-inhibiting action of nortriptyline's
antidepressive effect at high plasma levels: a randomized
double-blind study controlled by plasma concentrations in
patients with endogenous depression. Psychopharmacologia,
45, 305–12

Kupfer, D.J., Hanin, I., Spike, D.G., Grau, T. and Coble, P.
(1977). Amitriptyline plasma levels and clinical response in
primary depression. Clin. Pharmacol. Ther., 22, 904–11

Magliozzi, J.R., Hollister, L.E., Kathryn, A.V. and Earle, G.M.
(1981). Relationship of serum haloperidol levels to clinical
response in schizophrenic patients. Am. J. Psychiatry, 138,
365–7

Montgomery, S., Braithwaite, R.A., Dawling, S. and McAuley, R.
(1978). High plasma nortriptyline levels in the treatment of
depression. Clin. Pharmacol. Ther., 23, 309–14

Pinder, R.M., Brogden, R.N., Speight, T.M. and Avery, G.S. (1977).
Maprotiline: a review of its pharmacological properties and
therapeutic efficacy in mental depressive states. Drugs, 13,
321–52

Reisby, N., Gram, L.F., Bech, P., Nagy, A., Petersen, G.O., Ortmann, J., Ibsen, I., Dencker, S.J., Jacobsen, O., Krautwald, O., Sondergaard, I. and Christiansen, J. (1977). Imipramine clinical effects and pharmacokinetic variability. Psychopharmacology, 54, 263-7

Rivera-Calimlim, L., Nasrallah, H., Strauss, J. and Lasagna, L. (1976). Clinical response and plasma levels: effects of dose, dosage schedules, and drug interactions on plasma chlorpromazine levels. Am. J. Psychiatry, 133, 646-52

Rivera-Calimlin, L., Griesbach, P.H. and Perlmutter, R. (1979). Plasma chlorpromazine concentrations in children with behavioral disorders and mental illness. Clin. Pharmacol. Ther., 26, 114-21

Stern, R.S., Marks, I.M., Wright, J. and Luscombe, D.K. (1980). Clomipramine plasma levels, side effects and outcome in obsessive-compulsive neurosis. Postgrad. Med. J., 56, Suppl. 1, 134-9

Vandel, S., Vandel, B., Sandoz, M., Allers, G., Bechtel, P. and Volmat, R. (1978). Clinical response and plasma concentration of amitriptyline and its metabolite nortriptyline. Eur. J. Clin. Pharmacol., 14, 185-90

Possible role of hydroxymetabolites in the action of neuroleptics

Svein G. Dahl[1], Petter-Arnt Hals[1], Helge Johnsen[1], Eliane Morel[2] and Kenneth G. Lloyd[2]

INTRODUCTION

A major cause of the rapid growth of clinical pharmacokinetics as a discipline was the observation that the same dose of a drug may give very different plasma drug levels in individual patients. Pharmacokinetic variation could thus explain part of the individual variation in drug response, and therapeutic monitoring of plasma drug levels has since become a useful tool in the management of treatment with various drugs.

Further development of chemical techniques has made possible the measurement of plasma levels of drug metabolites together with the parent compound. From this it has been found that the ratio between the plasma concentrations of a metabolite and the parent drug may show large variations between individual patients.

Active drug metabolites may have a pharmacodynamic profile and toxicity different from that of the parent drug, and therefore it may be expected that the contribution from an active metabolite to the effects of a drug may be different between individual patients. Monitoring of plasma levels of active metabolites in addition to the levels of the parent compound should, at least in theory, provide additional information which may be useful in the management of individual patients.

METABOLITES OF NEUROLEPTIC DRUGS

Plasma Levels

Oral administration of neuroleptics often results in an especially large range of plasma drug levels (Dahl, 1979, 1981). As discussed

---

[1]Department of Pharmacology, Institute of Medical Biology, University of Tromsø, N-9000 Tromsø, Norway.
[2]Department of Biology, L.E.R.S. Synthélabo, Paris, France.

earlier (Dahl, 1979), it seems likely that for the phenothiazines inter-individual variation in the extent of pre-systemic metabolism may be a major reason for the observed variation in the plasma drug levels. There have been relatively few studies comprising plasma level measurement of neuroleptic drug metabolites, but those which have been published have reported a 7- to 20-fold variation in the plasma concentration ratios of metabolite to parent drug at steady state within small groups of patients (Dahl, 1982).

Chemical and pharmacological problems concerning the large number of different phenothiazine drug metabolites which may be formed have previously received much attention (Kaul *et al.*, 1974). As discussed recently (Dahl, 1982), the number of phenothiazine drug metabolites which are formed in such amounts that they may be expected to contribute to the effects of the drug in man is, however, usually much lower than the total number of identified or postulated metabolites. An example of this is given in figure 1, which shows the formulas of the metabolites of levomepromazine which have been identified in urine (Dahl and Garle, 1977; Johnsen and Dahl, 1982) and in plasma (Dahl and Garle, 1977; Dahl *et al.*, 1982c) from psychiatric patients, after repeated oral doses of the drug. As shown in figure 1, at least 10 different levomepromazine metabolites are formed in man. The five metabolites which are formed by a single phase I reaction were, however, found in much higher concentrations than the other metabolites in the urine, and only these five metabolites could be identified in the plasma.

Another study demonstrated that the steady-state blood levels of two of these metabolites were above the concentrations of unmetabolized levomepromazine in four out of five patients (Dahl *et al.*, 1982a). The three other levomepromazine metabolites which have been identified in plasma, namely 3-hydroxy, 7-hydroxy and *O*-desmethyl levomepromazine (figure 1), have not yet been assayed in plasma or whole blood from patients. It was found, however, that each patient had about the same plasma concentration of 3-hydroxy levomepromazine as that of 7-hydroxy levomepromazine, at steady state (Dahl *et al.*, 1982c). This demonstrates that the pattern of aromatic hydroxylation of levomepromazine in man is different from that of the congener chlorpromazine, which appears to be hydroxylated only in the 7-position.

Molecular Structure and Biological Activity of Chlorpromazine Metabolites

7-Hydroxy chlorpromazine has been demonstrated to be clinically active in a crossover trial against chlorpromazine, in five patients (Kleinman *et al.*, 1980). As shown in figure 2, the

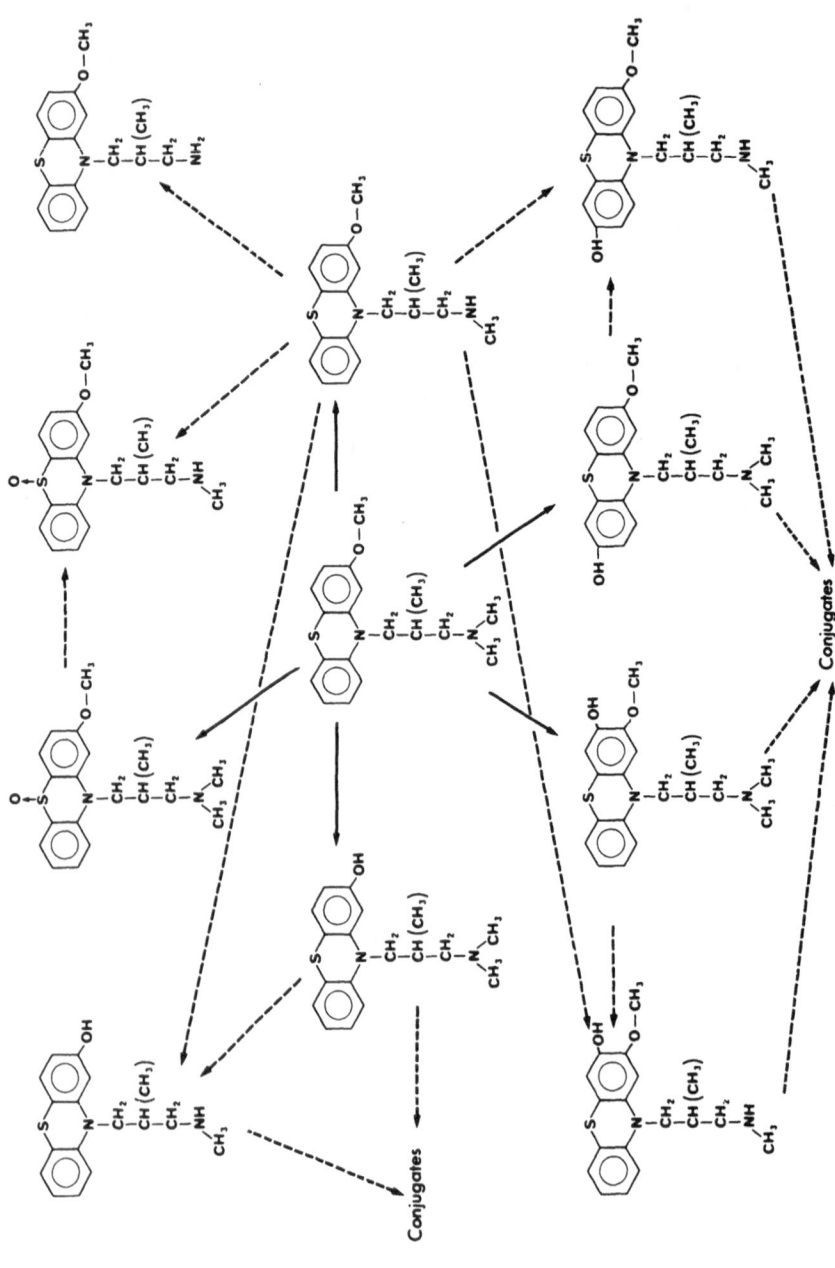

Figure 1. Metabolic scheme of levomepromazine in man. Arrows drawn using solid lines point to the five metabolites which have been identified in the plasma; the other metabolites have been identified in urine only.

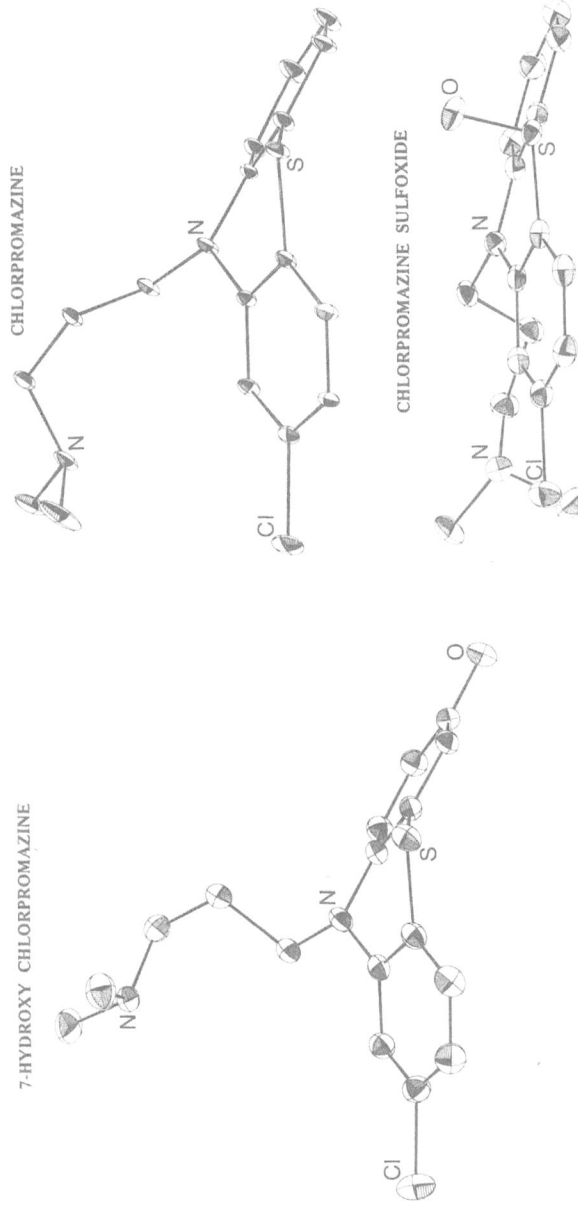

Figure 2. Molecular structures of chlorpromazine and two of its metabolites in the solid state. Computerized drawings were made by the ORTEP program (Johnson, 1971), from previously published atomic coordinates for chlorpromazine (McDowell, 1968), 7-hydroxy chlorpromazine (McDowell, 1977) and chlorpromazine sulfoxide (Dahl *et al.*, 1982b). Hydrogen atoms are not drawn. Carbon and other atoms, the latter of which are marked by their chemical symbol, are represented by ellipsoids. The size and orientation of the ellipsoids indicate the magnitude and directions of the thermal vibration of the atoms in the molecule.

Table 1. Biological activity of chlorpromazine and some of its metabolites (+, active; -, inactive). Relative potencies of metabolites, compared to chlorpromazine, are given in parentheses

Test system	CPZ	7-OH CPZ	N-DCPZ	N-DDCPZ	CPZNO	CPZSO	Reference
EEG, isolated perfused rat brain	+	+ (0.50)				-	Krieglstein et al. (1980)
Inhibition of MAO activity, human brain	+	+ (0.95)	+ (1.06)	+ (1.01)		- (0.03)	Roth et al. (1979)
Inotropic effect, isolated rat or guinea-pig atrium	+ (negative inotropic)	+ (positive inotropic)					Dahl and Refsum (1976), Temma et al. (1977)
Plasma prolactin, male rats	+	+ (0.85)				-	Meltzer et al. (1977)
Amphetamine-induced stereo-typed behavior, rats	+	+	+	-	+	-	Lal and Sourkes (1972)
Various pharmacological tests, mice	+	+					Manian et al. (1965)

CPZ, chlorpromazine; 7-OH CPZ, 7-hydroxy chlorpromazine; N-DCPZ, N-monodesmethyl chlorpromazine; N-DDCPZ, N-didesmethyl chlorpromazine; CPZNO, chlorpromazine N-oxide; CPZSO, chlorpromazine sulfoxide.

solid-state molecular structure of 7-hydroxy chlorpromazine resembles that of chlorpromazine itself, while chlorpromazine sulfoxide has another conformation of the side chain in the solid
state. As discussed earlier (Dahl *et al.*, 1982b), it is possible
that the different molecular conformations of the two metabolites
in the solid state may have biological significance.

The biological activities of 7-hydroxy chlorpromazine and
chlorpromazine sulfoxide have been examined in various systems, as
summarized in table 1. Figure 3, which is reproduced from one of
these studies, represents a typical example of the results.
Chlorpromazine caused a significant increase in the percentage of
delta waves in isolated perfused rat brain, and the same effect,
although of a smaller magnitude, was observed for 7-hydroxy chlorpromazine (figure 3).   Chlorpromazine sulfoxide, in the same
concentrations, had no significant effect in this preparation.

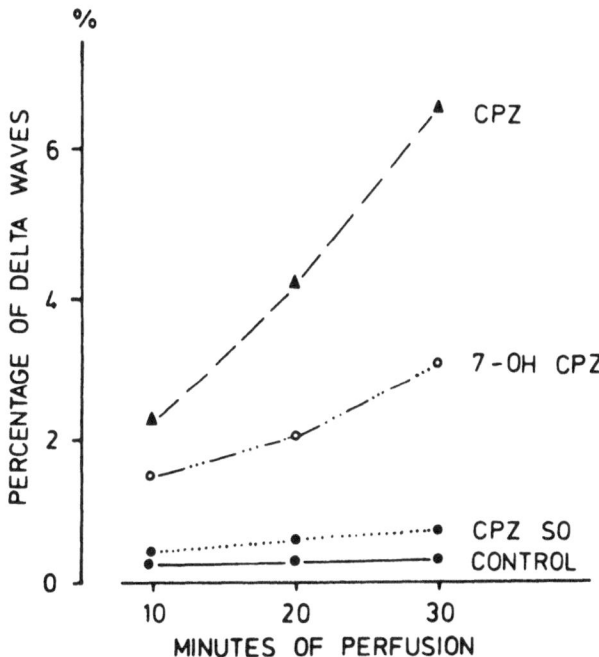

Figure 3. EEG effects of chlorpromazine (CPZ), 7-hydroxy chlorpromazine (7-OH CPZ) and chlorpromazine sulfoxide
(CPZSO) in isolated perfused rat brain: increase of
delta activity. Reproduced from Krieglstein *et al.*
(1980), with kind permission from Pergamon Press Ltd.

The positive inotropic effect of 7-hydroxy chlorpromazine in isolated guinea-pig atrium, which is mentioned in table 1, is an example of a pharmacological effect of a drug metabolite which is qualitatively different from that of the parent compound. Chlorpromazine itself is generally 'cardiodepressive', and a negative inotropic effect of chlorpromazine has been demonstrated in isolated rat atria (Dahl and Refsum, 1976).

BINDING AFFINITIES OF NEUROLEPTIC DRUG METABOLITES TO DOPAMINERGIC AND ALPHA-ADRENERGIC RECEPTORS IN THE BRAIN

The binding affinities to three different receptor types in rat brain have been examined for the major metabolites of chlorpromazine and levomepromazine in man (P.A. Hals and S.G. Dahl, unpublished results). Preliminary data from this study are given in table 2, together with the results of a previous study by Dahl and Hall (1981).

Reference samples of 3-hydroxy levomepromazine, 7-hydroxy levomepromazine and O-desmethyl levomepromazine were synthesized from levomepromazine in our laboratories. Reference samples of the other levomepromazine metabolites and of the chlorpromazine metabolites used in the receptor binding assays were generously donated by Rhône-Poulenc Industries, France.

N-Monodesmethyl levomepromazine was the most potent levomepromazine derivative both in dopaminergic (DA_2) and in alpha$_1$-adrenergic receptor binding (table 2). 3-Hydroxy levomepromazine was relatively active, compared to levomepromazine itself, in dopaminergic (DA_2) receptor binding but not in alpha$_1$-adrenergic binding. As may be noted from table 2, the 3-hydroxy derivative of both drugs was 3-4 times more active than the corresponding 7-hydroxy derivative, in dopaminergic (DA_2) receptor binding.

It appears from table 2 that N-monodesmethyl chlorpromazine is nearly twice as active as chlorpromazine in alpha$_2$-adrenergic binding. It should be emphasized, however, that the results from the alpha$_2$-adrenergic binding experiments which are given in table 2 are preliminary, and have to be confirmed by a larger number of experiments.

7-Hydroxy fluphenazine has been identified as a metabolite of fluphenazine in the dog (Dreyfuss and Cohen, 1971), but conclusive data identifying this compound as a metabolite of fluphenazine in man have not yet been published. 7-Hydroxy fluphenazine has relatively low affinity in dopaminergic (DA_2) receptor binding, compared to fluphenazine itself, but had 41% of the potency of the parent drug in alpha$_1$-adrenergic binding in rat cortex (table 3).

Table 2. Receptor binding affinities in rat brain: Potencies* of major metabolites† of chlorpromazine and levomepromazine, relative to that of the parent drug

Compound	Relative potencies (parent drug=1.00)		
	Receptor type, Brain region, Ligand		
	Dopaminergic(DA_2) Striatum ^{3}H-Spiroperidol	α_1-Adrenergic Cortex ^{3}H-WB4101	α_2-Adrenergic Cortex ^{3}H-Para-amino-clonidine
Levomepromazine (LM)	1.00	1.00	1.00
7-Hydroxy LM	0.17	0.08	0.22
3-Hydroxy LM	0.51	0.04	0.22
O-Desmethyl LM	0.04	0.03	0.05
N-Monodesmethyl LM	0.71	0.62	0.24
LM sulfoxide	0.05	0.19	0.03
Chlorpromazine (CPZ)	1.00	1.00	1.00
7-Hydroxy CPZ	0.53	0.31	0.19
3-Hydroxy CPZ	2.04	0.34	0.63
N-Monodesmethyl CPZ	0.37	0.52	1.92
CPZ sulfoxide	0.02	0.06	0.05

*The potency ratios were obtained by comparing the IC_{50}'s of the metabolites to that of the parent compound (P.A. Hals and S.G. Dahl, unpublished results; Dahl and Hall, 1981).
†Although the 3-hydroxy derivative has been identified as a major metabolite in man for levomepromazine but not for chlorpromazine, 3-hydroxy chlorpromazine was included in this study for comparison.

Table 3. Potencies* of 7-hydroxy fluphenazine relative to fluphenazine in receptor binding

Compound	Relative potency		
	Dopaminergic (DA_2) ^{3}H-Spiroperidol Sheep caudate	Dopaminergic (DA_2) ^{3}H-Spiroperidol Calf caudate	α_1-Adrenergic ^{3}H-WB4101 Rat cortex
Fluphenazine	1.00	1.00	1.00
7-Hydroxy fluphenazine	0.014†	0.15§	0.41†

*Relative potencies were obtained by the comparison of the IC_{50} of 7-hydroxy fluphenazine to that of fluphenazine.
†Data from Bylund (1981).
§Data from Wiles (1981).

Loxapine is a relatively new neuroleptic of the same chemical group (dibenzoxazepine) as clozapine. Loxapine has two major metabolites in man, both of which attain higher steady-state plasma levels than the parent drug after oral doses of loxapine: 8-hydroxy loxapine and 8-hydroxy-N-desmethyl loxapine (Cooper and Kelly, 1979). These metabolites have 13% and 6%, respectively, of the potencies of loxapine in DA_2 receptor binding in rat striatum (Coupet and Rauh, 1979).

IN VIVO TEST OF NEUROLEPTIC POTENCY OF PHENOTHIAZINE DRUG METABOLITES

A substantial body of evidence has suggested that neuroleptic drugs exert their clinical effects mainly through antagonism of DA_2 receptors in the brain (Snyder, 1981). *In vitro* assessment of DA_2 receptor binding affinity is generally not sufficient to predict the clinical potency of a potential neuroleptic, since this also depends on its distribution in the brain and other pharmacokinetic variables. Inhibition of apomorphine-induced climbing in mice is a behavioral test, based on blockade of a DA receptor mediated event, which may be used as an *in vivo* test of neuroleptic potency (Worms *et al.*, 1982).

The potencies of the compounds which are included in tables 2 and 3 have been examined in this test (E. Morel, S.G.Dahl and K.G. Lloyd, unpublished results), using male albino mice weighing 23-25 g. Reference samples of fluphenazine and 7-hydroxy fluphenazine were generously donated by E.R. Squibb and Sons, Inc., New Jersey, USA. The results are summarized in table 4, in terms of relative potencies of the metabolites compared to the parent compound.

As may be noted from table 4, the data from the climbing test are generally in agreement with the results of the receptor binding studies (tables 2 and 3). 3-Hydroxy levomepromazine was slightly more potent than the parent compound, and levomepromazine sulfoxide was virtually inactive, in the climbing test. As discussed by Pinder (1983), the alpha$_1$-adrenergic binding affinities of antidepressant drugs are correlated with their sedative effects. Levomepromazine is known as a neuroleptic with very pronounced sedative effects, and as mentioned by Bergman (1983), in a recent Swedish survey 46% of the levomepromazine prescriptions were for sleep disturbances. It is interesting to note, therefore, that N-monodesmethyl levomepromazine had both relatively high potency in alpha$_1$-adrenergic receptor binding (table 2) and a strong muscle relaxant or sedative effect in mice, as judged by the grip test which was performed immediately after the climbing test.

It may also be noted that the relative potencies of 7-hydroxy chlorpromazine, 3-hydroxy chlorpromazine and 7-hydroxy fluphena-

Table 4. Inhibition of apomorphine-induced climbing in mice: potencies* of metabolites relative to the parent drug

Compound	Relative potency
Levomepromazine (LM)	1.0
7-Hydroxy LM	<0.5
3-Hydroxy LM	1.4
O-Desmethyl LM	<0.5
N-Monodesmethyl LM	- †
LM sulfoxide	<0.05
Chlorpromazine (CPZ)	1.0
7-Hydroxy CPZ	0.7
3-Hydroxy CPZ	3.1
N-Monodesmethyl CPZ	0.6
CPZ sulfoxide	<0.05
Fluphenazine (FPZ)	1.0
7-Hydroxy FPZ	0.12

*Relative potencies were obtained by the comparison of the ED_{50}'s of the metabolites to that of the parent drug (E. Morel, S.G. Dahl and K.G. Lloyd, unpublished results).
†Pronounced muscle relaxant activity.

zine were of similar orders of magnitude in DA_2 receptor binding in rat brain (tables 2 and 3) and in inhibition of apomorphine-induced climbing in mice (table 4).

Together with the available relevant pharmacokinetic data, the results of these studies could indicate that 3-hydroxy levomepromazine may contribute to the neuroleptic effects of levomepromazine in man while N-monodesmethyl levomepromazine may contribute significantly to the sedative effects of this drug. Further, they could indicate that both 7-hydroxy chlorpromazine and N-monodesmethyl chlorpromazine may possibly contribute to the neuroleptic effects of chlorpromazine. Although 3-OH CPZ is relatively more potent in both binding and behavioral tests, it is not found in measurable quantities in man (see below). It is still an open question whether significant amounts of 7-hydroxy fluphenazine are formed in man during fluphenazine treatment. This metabolite appears to have low pharmacological activity, and probably does not contribute to the effects of fluphenazine in man.

COMMENTS

Compared to the substantial amount of information concerning its pharmacology and toxicology that is required before a new drug is introduced on the market, the available information about the possible effects of identified drug metabolites is, in most cases, minimal.

As mentioned in a recent review (Dahl, 1982), a relationship between plasma drug levels and clinical effects and certain side-effects have now been demonstrated, more or less convincingly, for six different neuroleptic drugs. The presence of relatively high plasma levels of some neuroleptic drug metabolites in some patients raises the following questions which should be solved for each drug:

(1) Which compounds (administered drug, metabolites) may contribute to the therapeutic effects?
(2) Which compounds may contribute to the known side-effects?
(3) Which compounds should be assayed in plasma by therapeutic monitoring and in studies of plasma level-effect relationships?

Problems (1) and (2) can only be resolved by studying the effects of each known metabolite separately. Once this is known, the answer to question (3) is, of course, also given.

Although metabolic hydroxylation of other psychotropic drugs often yields active metabolites (see, for example, Bertilsson *et al.*, 1983), one cannot generally assume that this is the case, as demonstrated by the results given in the present article. Also within a related chemical class of compounds such as the phenothiazines, hydroxylation in the corresponding position on the molecule may lead to more or less potent metabolites, as shown in tables 2, 3 and 4 for the 7-hydroxy derivatives of chlorpromazine, levomepromazine and fluphenazine.

The pattern of enzymatic hydroxylation in man may also be different for compounds belonging to the same chemical class. The appearance of relatively high concentrations of 7-hydroxy chlorpromazine in plasma after chlorpromazine treatment does not necessarily imply that all other phenothiazine drugs are converted to significant amounts of 7-hydroxy metabolites. The formation of comparatively large amounts of 3-hydroxy levomepromazine, but not of 3-hydroxy chlorpromazine, after treatment with these drugs, is another example of the same principle.

It should be underlined that inference of the possible impact of a derivative of a drug on the effects of the drug in man cannot be made only from information about the biological activity of the compound. It must also have been demonstrated that the compound in question really is formed in man in more than trace amounts, after therapeutic doses of the drug. The literature contains several examples of authors suggesting that 3-hydroxy chlorpromazine and 7,8-dihydroxy chlorpromazine, which are both pharmacologically active, may contribute to the effects and toxicity of chlorpromazine. There is, however, no evidence that significant amounts of these compounds are formed in man.

Acknowledgements

The donation of reference compounds from Rhône-Poulenc Industries, Paris, France, and from E.R. Squibb & Sons, Inc., Princeton, New Jersey, USA, is gratefully acknowledged.

REFERENCES

Bergman, U., Agenäs, I. and Dahlström, M. (1983). Utilization of psychotropic drugs in Sweden and the other Nordic countries. This volume, pp.3-17

Bertilsson, L., Mellström, B., Nordin, C., Siwers, B. and Sjöqvist, F. (1983). Stereospecific 10-hydroxylation of nortriptyline - genetic aspects and importance for biochemical and clinical effects. This volume, pp. 217-26

Bylund, D.B. (1981). Interactions of neuroleptic metabolites with dopaminergic, alpha adrenergic and muscarinic cholinergic receptors. J. Pharmacol. Exp. Ther., 217, 81-6

Cooper, T.B. and Kelly, R.G. (1979). GLC analysis of loxapine, amoxapine, and their metabolites in serum and urine. J. Pharm. Sci., 68, 216-9

Coupet, J. and Rauh, C.E. (1979). ^{3}H-Spiroperidol binding to dopamine receptors in rat striatal membranes: influence of loxapine and its hydroxylated metabolites. Eur. J. Pharmacol., 55, 215-8

Dahl, S,G. (1979). Monitoring of phenothiazine plasma levels in psychiatric patients. In Neuropsychopharmacology, (ed. B. Saletu, P. Berner and L. Hollister), Pergamon Press, Oxford, pp.567-75

Dahl, S.G. (1981). Pharmacokinetic aspects of new antipsychotic drugs. Neuropharmacology, 20, 1299-302

Dahl. S.G. (1982). Active metabolites of neuroleptic drugs: possible contribution to therapeutic and toxic effects. Ther. Drug Monit., 4, 33-40

Dahl, S.G., Bratlid, T. and Lingjaerde, O. (1982a). Plasma and erythrocyte levels of methotrimeprazine and two of its non-polar metabolites in psychiatric patients. Ther. Drug Monit., 4, 81-7

Dahl, S.G. and Garle, M. (1977). Identification of nonpolar methotrimeprazine metabolites in plasma and urine by GLC - mass spectrometry. J. Pharm. Sci., 66, 190-3

Dahl, S.G. and Hall, H. (1981). Binding affinity of levomepromazine and two of its major metabolites to central dopamine and α-adrenergic receptors in the rat. Psychopharmacology, 74, 101-4

Dahl, S.G., Hjorth, M. and Hough, E. (1982b). Chlorpromazine, methotrimeprazine and metabolites: structural changes ac-

companying the loss of neuroleptic potency by ring sulf-
oxidation. Mol. Pharmacol., 21, 409-14

Dahl, S.G., Johnsen, H. and Lee, C.R. (1982c). Gas chromatographic mass spectometric identification of O-demethylated
and mono-hydroxylated metabolites of levomepromazine in blood
from psychiatric patients by selected ion recording with high
resolution. Biomed. Mass Spectrom., 9, 534-8

Dahl, S.G. and Refsum, H. (1976). Effects of levomepromazine,
chlorpromazine and their sulfoxides on isolated rat atria.
Eur. J. Pharmacol., 37, 241-8

Dreyfuss, J. and Cohen, A.I. (1971). Identification of 7-hydroxy-
fluphenazine as major metabolite of fluphenazine-^{14}C in the
dog. J. Pharm. Sci., 60, 826-8

Johnsen, H. and Dahl, S.G. (1982). Identification of O-demethylated and ring-hydroxylated metabolites of methotrimeprazine
(levomepromazine) in man. Drug. Metab. Dispos., 10, 63-7

Johnson, C.K. (1971). ORTEP. Report ORNL-3794, Oak Ridge
National Laboratory, Tennessee.

Kaul, P.N., Conway, M.W. and Clark, M.L. (1974). Pharmacokinetics
of chlorpromazine metabolites - a colossal problem. In Phenothiazines and Structurally Related Drugs, (ed. I.S. Forrest,
C.J. Carr and E. Usdin), Raven Press, New York, pp. 391-8

Kleinman, J.E., Bigelow, L.B., Rogol, A., Weinberger, D.L.,
Nazrallah, H.A., Wyatt, R.J. and Gillin, J.C. (1980). A
clinical trial of 7-hydroxychlorpromazine in chronic schizo-
phrenia. In Phenothiazines and Structurally Related Drugs:
Basic and Clinical Studies, (ed. E. Usdin, H. Eckert and I.S.
Forrest), Elsevier/North-Holland, Amsterdam. pp. 275-8

Krieglstein, J., Rieger, H. and Schütz, H. (1980). Comparative
study on the activity of chlorpromazine and 7-hydroxychlor-
promazine in the isolated perfused rat brain. Biochem.
Pharmacol., 29, 63-7

Lal, S. and Sourkes, T.L. (1972). Effect of various chlorpromazine metabolites on amphetamine-induced stereotyped behaviour
in the rat. Eur. J. Pharmacol., 17, 283-6.

McDowell, J.J.H. (1968). Crystal and molecular structure of
chlorpromazine. Acta Cryst. B, 25, 2175

McDowell, J.J.H. (1977). The structure of the metabolite 7-
hydroxy chlorpromazine. Acta Cryst. B, 33, 771-4

Manian, A.A., Efron, E.D. and Goldberg, M.E. (1965). A comparative pharmacological survey of a series of monohydroxylated
and methoxylated chlorpromazine derivatives. Life Sci., 4,
2425-38

Meltzer, H.Y., Fang, V.S., Simonovich, M. and Paul, S.M. (1977).
Effect of metabolites of chlorpromazine on plasma prolactin
levels in male rats. Eur. J. Pharmacol., 41, 431-6

Pinder, R.M. (1983). Antidepressants and α-adrenoceptors. This
volume, pp.268-287

Roth, J.A., Whittemore, R.M., Shakarjian, M.P. and Eddy, B.J. (1979). Inhibition of human brain type A and B monoamine oxidase by chlorpromazine and metabolites. Commun. Psycho-pharmacol., 3, 235-43

Snyder, S.H. (1981). Dopamine receptors, neuroleptics, and schizophrenia. Am. J. Psychiatry, 138, 460-4

Temma, K., Akera, T., Brody, T.M. and Manian, A.A. (1977). Hydroxylated chlorpromazine metabolites: positive inotropic action and the release of catecholamines. Mol. Pharmacol., 13, 1076-85

Wiles, D. (1981). Preliminary assessment of a calf caudate radioreceptor assay for the estimation of neuroleptic drugs in plasma: comparison with other techniques. In Clinical Pharmacology in Psychiatry - Neuroleptic and Antidepressant Research, (ed. E. Usdin, S.G. Dahl, L.F. Gram and O. Lingjaerde), Macmillan, London, pp. 111-21

Worms, P., Broekkamp, C.L.E. and Lloyd, K.G. (1982). Behavioural effects of neuroleptics. In Neuroleptics: Neurochemical, Biochemical, Behavioural and Clinical Perspectives, (ed. J.T. Coyle and S.J. Enna), Raven Press, New York, in press

Radioreceptor assay for measurement of anticholinergic drugs in serum

Joseph T. Coyle[1] and Larry E. Tune[1]

INTRODUCTION

Extrapyramidal side-effects (EPS) including Parkinsonian symptoms, dystonic reactions and akathisia frequently complicate use of neuroleptic drugs (Ayd, 1961; Donlon and Stenson, 1976). These iatrogenic symptoms, which are both stigmatizing as well as uncomfortable, deter many patients from compliance with neuroleptic treatment (Van Putten, 1974). Thus, the management of EPS must be considered an essential part in the effective treatment of psychotic disorders with neuroleptics. Reduction in neuroleptic dosage is usually not the primary strategy in controlling these side-effects because EPS correlate poorly with neuroleptic dose or therapeutic response (Alpert *et al.*, 1978). Rather, co-treatment with the classical anti-Parkinsonian drugs, all of which block muscarinic receptors with the exception of amantadine, is the accepted approach for reducing EPS. Nevertheless, many patients persist in suffering from EPS in spite of treatment with recommended doses of anticholinergics (DiMascio, 1971). Clinicians generally avoid high doses of anticholinergic drugs to treat refractory EPS because of concerns about the confusional states and impaired peripheral parasympathetic function including dry mouth, blurred vision, constipation and urinary retention that can occur with toxic doses of anticholinergic drugs. In light of the marked variation in the disposition of psychotropic medications, we have undertaken studies to clarify the relationship between serum levels of anticholinergics measured by a radioreceptor assay technique and the therapeutic as well as noxious effects of these drugs.

[1]Division of Child Psychiatry, Departments of Psychiatry and Behavioral Sciences, Neuroscience, Pharmacology and Experimental Therapeutics, and Pediatrics, Johns Hopkins University, School of Medicine, Baltimore, Maryland 21205, USA.

SITE OF ACTION OF ANTICHOLINERGIC DRUGS

In recent years, the mechanisms whereby anticholinergic drugs reduce the acute EPS caused by neuroleptics has been reasonably well characterized by neuroanatomic and neurophysiologic studies (Calne *et al.*, 1975). Current evidence suggests that the therapeutic effects of neuroleptics derive from their blockade of dopamine receptors, particularly the D-2 subtype (Creese *et al.*, 1976; Kebabian and Calne, 1979) within the striatum; these receptors mediate the inhibitory effects of dopamine on cholinergic interneurons (figure 1). Blockade of the striatal D-2 receptors results in disinhibition of the cholinergic neurons; and the increased turnover and release of acetylcholine causes an excessive stimulation of their postsynaptic striatal muscarinic cholinergic receptors (Racagni *et al.*, 1976). Fortunately, the dopaminergic-cholinergic synaptic sequence appears to be unique to the extrapyramidal system and therefore pharmacologic restitution of cholinergic tone by co-administration of muscarinic receptor antagonists does not disturb the therapeutic action of neuroleptics that presumably occurs at dopamine synapses in the cortico-limbic projections. While this description of striatal cholinergic-dopaminergic neuronal synaptic relationships appears operationally valid, it does not adequately reflect the emerging evidence of the topographic organization of the striatal connections or the second-order interactions between striatal neurons and dopaminergic afferents.

Recent studies have uncovered major cholinergic projections from the magnocellular nuclei in basal forebrain including the nucleus basalis of Meynert, diagonal band of Broca and medial septal nucleus that innervate the cerebral cortex and hippocampal formation (Johnston *et al.*, 1981). Evidence is emerging that this cholinergic system appears to play a critical role in higher cognitive functions. Destruction of the hippocampal cholinergic pathway in experimental animals profoundly impairs recent memory (Olton and Feustle, 1981). And the basal forebrain cholinergic pathways selectively degenerate in Alzheimer's dementia, a disorder characterized by a profound deterioration of higher cognitive functions in man (Whitehouse *et al.*, 1982). Since anticholinergic drugs impair recent memory (Drachman, 1971) and, at high doses, cause more global disruptions of cognitive functions (Longo, 1966), interference with neurotransmission at the cortico-hippocampal cholinergic synapses is the likely site of this effect of anticholinergics.

The muscarinic receptors, the predominant population of receptors mediating the central effects of acetylcholine, have been well characterized by means of ligand-binding techniques (Birdsall and Hulme, 1976). These receptors exhibit relatively uniform characteristics with regard to antagonist interactions throughout major brain regions (Birdsall *et al.*, 1980). Displace-

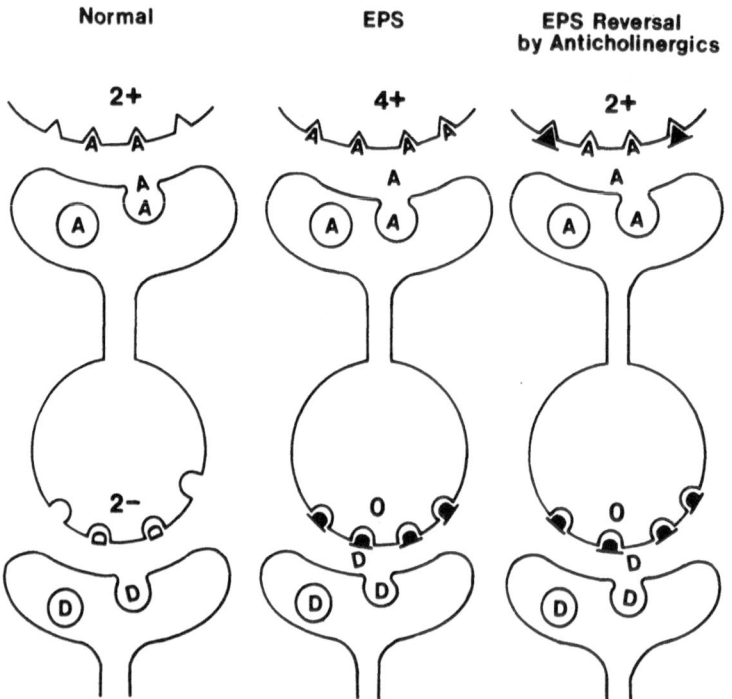

Figure 1.   Schematic representation of the interaction between
             neuroleptics and anticholinergics at striatal dopamin-
             ergic synapse. Dopaminergic terminals in the striatum
             release dopamine (D) that inhibits the activity of
             cholinergic interneurons. Neuroleptics (▲), by block-
             ing the D-2 receptor, disinhibit the cholinergic
             neurons, resulting in increased stimulation of musca-
             rinic receptors by acetylcholine (A). Muscarinic
             antagonists (▲) can normalize muscarinic receptor
             activation and thereby reduce EPS.

ment studies with agonists reveal a subpopulation of sites uniformly labeled by antagonists that can be resolved into low, high
and 'super' high affinity compounds (Birdsall *et al.*, 1978). The
most commonly used antagonist ligand to label the muscarinic
receptors is [³H]-quinuclidinyl benzilate (QNB); this ligand
exhibits a subnanomolar affinity for the receptors with an extremely slow rate of dissociation that results in a very favorable
ratio of specific to non-specific binding. The compelling correlation between the affinity of muscarinic antagonists for the
[³H]-QNB labeled sites and their ability to antagonize the physiologic effects of cholinergic agonists has established that this

ligand is an excellent probe for the antagonist conformation of central muscarinic receptors (Yamamura and Snyder, 1974). Furthermore, cross-species studies indicate a high degree of conservancy of muscarinic receptor characteristics as revealed by the specific binding of [^{3}H]-QNB.

CHARACTERIZATION OF THE RADIORECEPTOR ASSAY FOR ANTICHOLINERGICS

Since several radioreceptor assays for psychotropic medications have been developed to detect these drugs on the basis of their interactions with specific receptor sites (Ferkany and Enna, 1982), we felt that the muscarinic receptor labeled with [^{3}H]-QNB might serve as an effective probe for detecting drugs on the basis of their anticholinergic properties. Preliminary experiments indicated that the addition of 200 µl of drug-free human serum to the 2 ml buffer mix used for measuring the specific binding of [^{3}H]-QNB to suspensions of membranes prepared from the rat forebrain caused a 29 ± 2% inhibition of total binding and a 30 ± 5% inhibition of non-specific binding of [^{3}H]-QNB (0.3 nM) to the receptor sites (Tune and Coyle, 1980). Thus, the ratio of total to non-specific binding remained constant at 8.5:1. Displacement curves generated by the addition of increasing concentrations of drugs known to have varying potency as anticholinergics revealed comparable K_I's in the absence or in the presence of 200 µl of drug-free human serum. Notably, the assay detected the classical muscarinic antagonists such as benztropine as well as the anticholinergic properties of drugs with other primary effects such as diphenhydramine, amitriptyline and thioridazine. In order to have a norm against which individual displacement values for serum could be compared, inhibition curves with atropine in the presence of drug-free human serum were run for each assay. Thus, values for serum samples could be expressed in terms of the equivalent amount of atropine that produced comparable inhibition of the specific binding of [^{3}H]-QNB.

To validate the assay, serum levels of nortriptyline in patients receiving this drug as an antidepressant were measured both by the muscarinic receptor assay and by gas-liquid chromatography (Tune and Coyle, 1981). Since the gas chromatographic method measures total serum levels of nortriptyline, the nortripytline was extracted from serum in heptane-isoamyl alcohol (99:1) and then back-extracted in 0.1 N HCl for its detection on the basis of its muscarinic blocking properties (figure 2). Although the serum levels of nortriptyline ranged over 10-fold in seven patients (25 – 305 µg l^{-1}), there was an excellent correlation between the values obtained with the radioreceptor assay and those determined by gas-liquid chromatography (r = 0.99; p < 0.001).

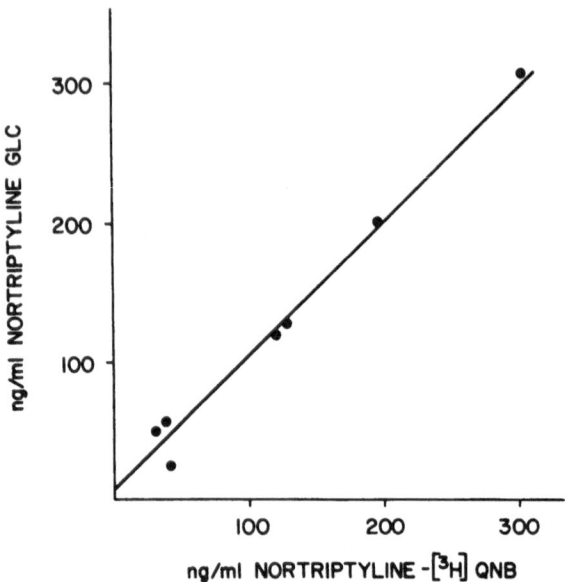

Figure 2.   Correlation between serum nortriptyline levels measured
by gas chromatography (GLC) and by the radioreceptor
assay. Nortriptyline was extracted from serum obtained
from seven patients being treated for unipolar depression ($r = 0.99$; $N = 7$; $p < 0.001$).

Since whole serum has been used in the assay, only anticholinergic drugs dissociated from serum proteins are free to
compete with [^{3}H]-QNB at the muscarinic receptors. Because the
serum is diluted 10-fold with the assay buffer, the equilibrium
between free and protein-bound drug is shifted, resulting in a
constant increase in the unbound drug. To assess the degree of
protein binding of benztropine, we examined the relationship
between the values measured with whole serum added and the levels
obtained in split samples, in which the serum proteins were first
precipitated by treatment with perchloric acid. The values for
whole serum, as a percent of the total amount of anticholinergic
in the perchloric extract of the serum, varied from 1.4 to 10% in
samples from 34 patients receiving benztropine. Nevertheless, the
two values correlated significantly ($p < 0.05$) and an average of
95% of the benztropine was bound to serum proteins under the
conditions of the assay. Since free drug represents that available to interact with receptors *in vivo*, we felt that the measurements of whole serum gave a better insight to the physiologically
active component of the anticholinergic drugs.

ACUTE EXTRAPYRAMIDAL SYMPTOMS AND SERUM NEUROLEPTIC AND
ANTICHOLINERGIC LEVELS

In a cross-sectional study, the relationship between serum levels
of anticholinergics and the total daily dose of benztropine was
examined in 49 patients who were receiving this drug in addition
to neuroleptics. No correlation was observed between the serum
levels of the anticholinergics and total daily doses of benz-

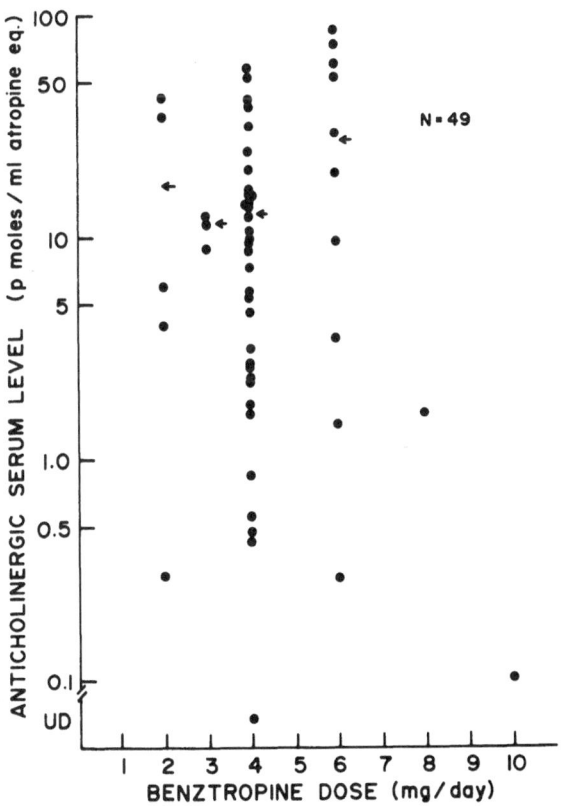

Figure 3. Relationship between total daily dose of benztropine
and serum levels of free anticholinergics. Serum
samples were obtained from 49 inpatients who were
receiving a fixed dose of benztropine for at least 4
days prior to phlebotomy. Results for the radioreceptor assay are expressed in terms of the amount of
atropine (pmol) that produced the same amount of inhibition. Arrows indicate the mean level for each daily
dose.

tropine. To the contrary, serum anticholinergic activity varied on the average of 10-fold from the lowest to the highest level in patients receiving 2, 4 and 6 mg per day of benztropine (figure 3). In six patients, who were followed serially with increasing oral doses of benztropine, a markedly non-linear relationship between daily dose and serum anticholinergic levels was observed. In most cases, 2 mg increments in oral dose were associated with several-fold increases in the serum level of anticholinergic activity.

A cohort of 109 patients, who were receiving at least 400 mg per day of chlorpromazine equivalents (Davis, 1976) were evaluated for the presence and severity of EPS with the DiMascio scale; and serum levels of neuroleptics were determined by the radioreceptor assay of Creese and Snyder (1977). In this cross-sectional study, the patients' drug doses were determined by their treating physician; and the majority of these patients were receiving haloperidol as the neuroleptic. Notably, a poor and non-significant correlation between serum levels of neuroleptics and the severity of EPS was observed ($r = 0.029$; $N = 109$; $p > 0.1$). This finding is consistent with clinical observations that the development of EPS is a poor predictor of therapeutic doses of neuroleptics (Alpert *et al.*, 1978) and that individuals vary in vulnerability to the EPS-inducing effects of neuroleptics (Chase *et al.*, 1970).

For 76 of these patients, whose serum levels of anticholinergics had been measured in the same samples, there was a highly significant inverse relationship between the severity of EPS and the serum levels of anticholinergics (figure 4) detected by the radioreceptor assay ($r = 0.441$; $p < 0.005$). Of patients with serum levels less than 10 pmol ml^{-1} of atropine equivalents, 44 experienced EPS with a DiMascio score greater than or equal to 2 while only 9% of patients with serum levels in excess of 10 nmol l^{-1} of atropine equivalents experienced significant EPS ($\chi^2 = 8.9$; $N = 76$; $p < 0.005$). The value, 10 nmol l^{-1} atropine equivalents, is approximately five times the K_I of atropine for the muscarinic receptor in the assay and thus reflects a serum level associated with substantial blockade of muscarinic receptors. To rule out an artifactual skew in the serum neuroleptic levels that might account for the low incidence of EPS in patients with higher serum anticholinergic levels, the relationship between serum neuroleptic and serum anticholinergic levels was plotted. However, no significant correlation was observed in the whole population ($r = 0.16$) or in those patients experiencing EPS ($r = -0.21$) or free of EPS ($r = 0.25$).

Since the mechanism of action of anticholinergics in reversing EPS involves correcting the neuroleptic-induced cholinergic dysfunction in the striatum (Calne *et al.*, 1975), we were curious whether the ratio of anticholinergic activity to dopamine receptor

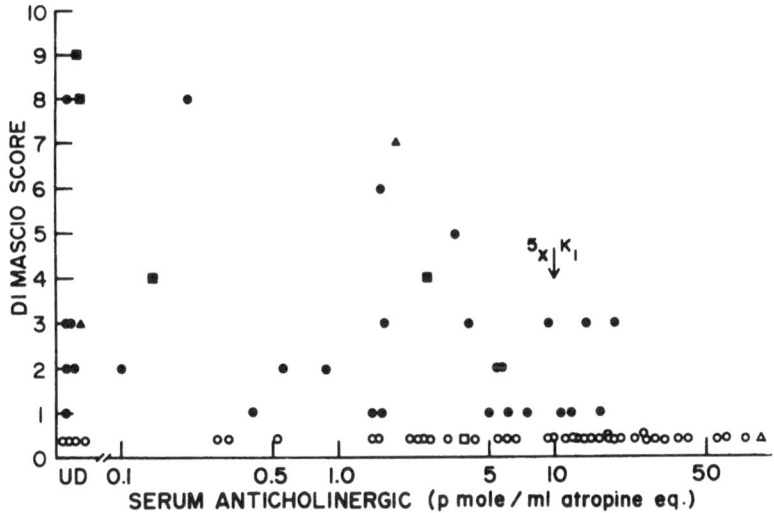

Figure 4.   Correlation between acute extrapyramidal side-effects
and serum anticholinergic levels. Seventy-six patients,
who were receiving both neuroleptics (at least 400 mg
per day of chlorpromazine or its equivalent) and anticholinergic medication for at least 4 days of constant
dosage, were rated for EPS with the DiMascio scale and
a blood sample was obtained.   Results for the radioreceptor assay are presented in terms of the amounts of
atropine (pmol) that produce the same degree of inhibition of specific binding of $[^3H]$-QNB. Open symbols
are EPS-negative and closed symbols are EPS-positive
patients. UD, undetectable serum levels. Circles,
benztropine; squares, trihexyphenidyl; triangles,
diphrenhydramine. 5 x K_I indicates the concentration
of atropine equivalent to five times the K_I for atropine (r = 0.441; N = 76; p < 0.005).

blocking activity might play a critical role in control of EPS.
In other words, we wondered whether EPS resulting from low serum
neuroleptic levels might be corrected by low anticholinergic
levels whereas high serum neuroleptic levels would require high
anticholinergic levels (figure 5). However, plotting the relationship between EPS and the ratio of serum anticholinergics to serum
neuroleptics, both measured by the radioreceptor assay techniques,
did not reveal a significant inverse correlation (r = 0.257; 0.1 >
p > 0.05; N = 76).   Nevertheless, patients with serum anticholin-
ergic/neuroleptic ratios of 0.5 or greater had a significantly

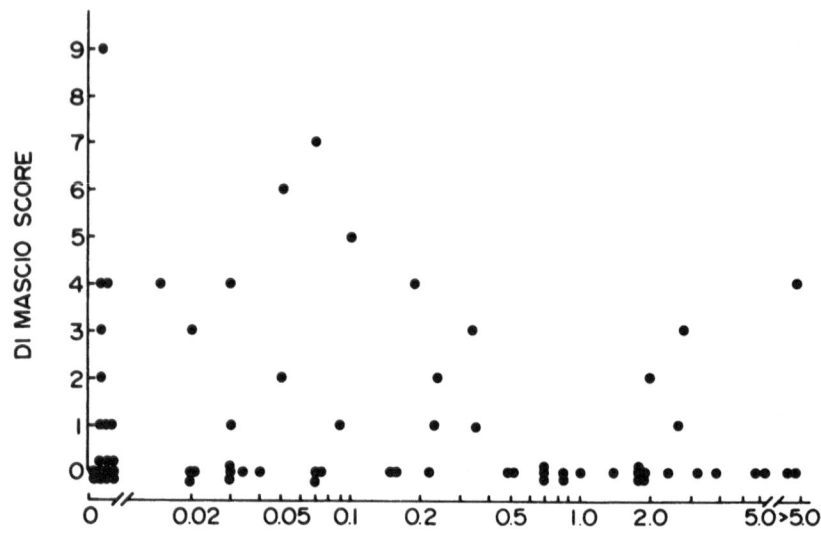

RATIO ANTI-ACH/Neuroleptic

Figure 5. Correlation between acute extrapyramidal side-effects
and the ratio of anticholinergic to neuroleptic drug
levels. The results from 76 patients were used to
examine the relationship between EPS and the ratio of
serum anticholinergic to neuroleptic levels. Anticholinergic and neuroleptic levels were converted to
similar units (μg l^{-1} atropine equivalents and μg l^{-1}
chlorpromazine equivalents) to calculate the ratio (r =
0.257; 0.2> p > 0.05; N = 76).

lower incidence of EPS as compared to those with a lower ratio (χ^2
= 7.5; p < 0.02). Thus, an 'ideal ratio' between anticholinergics
and neuroleptics does not appear to be involved in EPS control
although an excess of anticholinergic is associated with a more
favorable response.

COGNITIVE EFFECTS OF ANTICHOLINERGIC DRUGS

As discussed above, the anticholinergic drugs not only interfere
with cholinergic neurotransmission in the striatum but also with
the function of the cholinergic projections to the cerebral cortex
and hippocampal formation, which are thought to play an important
role in cognitive functions. Accordingly, we wondered whether the
serum levels of anticholinergics associated with reduction in EPS

Table 1. Effects of anticholinergics on recent memory function in
schizophrenic patients

| Parameter | Mean ± S.E.M. | Correlation coefficients | | |
		Atropine equivalents	Chlorpromazine equivalents	Recent memory
Mini PSE	4.7 ± 0.8	0.05	0.07	− 0.29
Atropine equivalents (nmol l⁻¹)	12.0 ± 2.5	−	0.12	− 0.51*
Chlorpromazine equivalents (µg l⁻¹)	32.0 ± 10	−	−	0.20
Recent memory	7.2 ± 0.2	−	−	−

The correlation coefficients for the various parameters measured
in 24 patients are presented. Recent memory refers to the average
number of correct responses for 15 trials (Tune *et al.*, 1982).
* $p < 0.01$.

might also result in impairments in recent memory. A cohort of 24
patients, all of whom were receiving neuroleptics and satisfied
Research Diagnostic Criteria (Spitzer *et al.*, 1975) for schizophrenia, were examined with regard to the severity of schizophrenic symptoms as measured by the Mini-Present State Exam of
Wing (1974), verbal intelligence quotient (verbal IQ) as measured
by the Wexler Adult Inventory Scale (WAIS) and performance on a
recent memory task (Tune *et al.*, 1982). Serum levels of neuroleptics and anticholinergics were measured by the radioreceptor
assay techniques. All of the patients were in remission; and none
of the patients were disoriented to person, place or time. No
significant correlation was observed between the serum levels of
anticholinergics or neuroleptics with regard to the severity of
schizophrenic symptoms (table 1). However, a significant inverse
correlation between serum levels of anticholinergics and performance on the recent memory test was demonstrated ($r = 0.51$; $p <
0.01$; $N = 24$). Notably, the serum levels of anticholinergics
measured in these patients were within the range associated with
control of EPS; thus, it appears that serum levels of anticholinergics effective in reducing EPS may also cause subtle but significant impairments in higher cognitive functions in the absence
of frank delirium.

These findings have received additional support from a pro-spective study of post-operative delirium in patients undergoing cardiac surgery (Tune *et al.*, 1981). In this study, patients were examined for cognitive function by the Mini-Mental Status Exam (Folstein *et al.*, 1975) and were rated for delirium by clinical assessment. After surgery, blood was obtained at the time of clinical evaluation for measurement of serum anticholinergic levels. When all the samples taken throughout the course of the study were analyzed, 14 out of 16 samples obtained from patients who were rated as clinically delirious had serum anticholinergic levels greater than 7.5 nmol 1^{-1} of atropine equivalents while only five of 33 samples obtained from cognitively intact patients had serum levels greater than this (χ^2 = 23.8; p < 0.001). Com-parison of the change in Mini-Mental State Examination from before surgery with serum anticholinergic levels revealed a highly sig-nificant inverse correlation (r = 0.83; N = 24; p < 0.01). Thus, as serum levels of anticholinergic drugs increased, there was a progressive impairment in higher cognitive functions as assessed by the difference in scores before and after surgery. While multiple factors contribute to post-operative delirium in patients undergoing cardiac surgery, these results suggest that drugs with anticholinergic effects may play a significant contributory role.

CONCLUSION

Radioreceptor assays have attracted increasing interest because of their purported ability to detect drugs on the basis of their receptor site specific mechanisms of action (Ferkany and Enna, 1982). In addition, these assays are relatively inexpensive and technically easy to perform. The radioreceptor assay based upon muscarinic antagonist inhibition of the specific binding of [^{3}H]-QNB clearly has important advantages. Extensive studies carried out to characterize the binding site for [^{3}H]-QNB have demon-strated that this ligand labels a homogeneous population of sites, with regard to antagonist interactions, that correlates well with regard to physiologic affinity of antagonist to block muscarinic receptor activation (Birdsall and Hulme, 1976; Birdsall *et al.*, 1978, 1980). And the muscarinic antagonist activities of a host of drugs including neuroleptics, antihistamines and antidepress-ants, whose primary mechanism of action likely does not involve the cholinergic system, have been well described (Richelson and Divinitz-Romero, 1977). Thus, a serum assay utilizing the [^{3}H]-QNB labeled muscarinic receptor will detect drugs regardless of chemical structure on the basis of their ability to block musca-rinic receptors. Finally, the high affinity of [^{3}H]-QNB for the muscarinic receptor and the favorable ratio of specific to non-specific binding ensures that the assay is not only specific but also extremely sensitive.

Results obtained thus far with the muscarinic radioreceptor assay for anticholinergic drugs in serum indicate a marked variation among patients in their disposition of anticholinergic drugs used to treat neuroleptic-induced acute EPS; thus, serum levels vary over a range of 10-fold or more in patients given the same dose of benztropine, a finding consistent with other psychotropic drugs including anticonvulsants and antidepressants (Eadie and Tyrer, 1974; Rish *et al.*, 1979). The variation in serum levels attained with standard doses of anticholinergics may explain, in part, the variability in clinical response of EPS to anticholinergic treatment. Furthermore, dose-response studies in individual patients indicate a non-linear relationship between oral dose and serum levels of anticholinergics with small increments in dose often associated with large increases in serum levels. These dose-level curves are reminiscent of those reported for phenytoin (Eadie and Tyrer, 1974).

Clinical experience indicates that individuals vary considerably in their susceptibility to developing EPS when treated with neuroleptics. In our cross-sectional study, serum level of neuroleptic measured by radioreceptor assay correlated poorly with the presence and severity of EPS. It is important to note that fluphenazine decanoate is associated with quite low constant serum levels of neuroleptic but a moderately high level of EPS (Tune *et al.*, 1979). One source of variation in susceptibility to EPS may involve differences among individuals in the ability of their nigro-striatal dopaminergic pathway to increase in activity to compensate for striatal D-2 receptor blockade (Chase *et al.*, 1970). Nevertheless, a highly significant inverse correlation was demonstrated between serum levels of anticholinergics in patients receiving neuroleptics and EPS severity. A serum level of anticholinergic which would be associated with substantial muscarinic receptor blockade (10 nmol 1^{-1} of atropine equivalents) was associated with a low incidence of EPS. When these data were expressed in terms of the ratio of muscarinic receptor blocking activity to dopamine receptor blocking activity, it was apparent that a high ratio favored EPS control. The results of these studies suggest that for those patients who develop EPS, oral doses of anticholinergics that result in serum levels approaching 10 nmol 1^{-1} of atropine equivalents should eliminate or markedly attenuate EPS.

Current evidence suggests that the muscarinic receptors in the striatum are identical to those in the cortex with regard to antagonist characteristics. Thus, it would be expected that muscarinic receptor blockade, which may be optimal for attenuating EPS, may nevertheless significantly impair cortico-hippocampal cholinergic neurotransmission. The results of a cross-sectional study support this concern since serum anticholinergic levels correlated significantly with impairments in performance on a recent memory test but were unrelated to psychiatric symptom severity in schizophrenic outpatients (Tune *et al.*, 1982). Impairments in cognitive functions were also observed in surgical patients in serum ranges of anticholinergics that were near those associated with reduction in EPS (Tune *et al.*, 1981). While the results of our studies have pointed to a critical level of serum anticholinergics which is effective in eliminating or attenuating EPS, this level encroaches upon that associated with impairments in higher cognitive functions. Thus, one must consider both the benefits as well as the liabilities associated with anticholinergic drug use to control neuroleptic-induced EPS.

Acknowledgements

We thank Carol Kenyon for secretarial assistance and the staff of the Henry Phipps Psychiatric Clinic for their cooperation. This research was supported by the National Institute of Mental Health (NIMH RSDA MH-00125) and by the Interdisciplinary Training Program in Neurosciences (MH-15330).

REFERENCES

Alpert, M., Diamond, F., Weisenfreund, J., Talepros, E. and Friedhoff, A. J. (1978). The neuroleptic hypothesis: a study of the co-variation of extrapyramidal and drug effects. Br. J. Psychiatry, 133, 169–75

Ayd, F. J. (1961). A survey of drug-induced extrapyramidal reactions. J. Am. Med. Assoc., 175, 1054–60

Birdsall, N. J. M., Burgen, A. S. V. and Hulme, E. C. (1978). The binding of agonists to brain muscarinic receptors. Mol. Pharmacol., 14, 723–36

Birdsall, N. J. M. and Hulme, E. C. (1976). Biochemical studies on muscarinic acetylcholine receptors. J. Neurochem., 27, 7–16

Birdsall, N. J. M., Hulme, E. C. and Burgen, D. S. V. (1980). The character of the muscarinic receptors in different regions of the rat brain. Proc. R. Soc. Lond.(Biol.), 207, 1–12

Calne, D., Chase, T. W. and Barbeau, A. (1975). Dopaminergic Mechanism, Raven Press, New York

Chase, T. N., Schnur, J. A. and Gordon, E. K. (1970). Cerebrospinal fluid monoamine catabolites in drug-induced extrapyramidal disorders. Neuropharmacology, 9, 265–8

Creese, I., Burt, D. R. and Snyder, S. H. (1976). Dopamine receptor binding predicts clinical and pharmacological potencies of antiparkinsonian drugs. Science, 192, 481–3

Creese, I. and Snyder, S. H. (1977). A simple and sensitive radio-receptor assay for antischizophrenic drugs in blood. Nature, 270, 261–3

Davis, J. M. (1976). Comparative doses and costs of antipsychotic
    medications. Arch. Gen. Psychiatry, 33, 858-63
DiMascio, A. (1971). Towards a more rational use of antiparkin-
    sonian drugs in psychiatry. Drug Ther., 1, 23-37
Donlon, P. T. and Stenson, R. L. (1976). Neuroleptic-induced
    extrapyramidal symptoms. Dis. Nerv. Syst., 37, 629-35
Drachman, D. A. (1971). Memory and cholinergic systems. In
    Neurotransmitter Function (ed. W. S. Felds), Yearbook Publ.,
    New York, pp. 353-62
Eadie, M. J. and Tyrer, J. H. (1974). Anticonvulsant Therapy:
    Pharmacological Basis and Practice, Churchill Livingstone,
    London, pp 35-78
Ferkany, J. W. and Enna, S. J. (1982). Radioreceptor assays. In
    Analysis of Biogenic Amines (ed. G. B. Baker and R. T.
    Coults), Elsevier/North-Holland, Amsterdam, in press
Folstein, M., Folstein, S. and McHugh, P. R. (1975). Minimental
    state. A practical method for grading the cognitive state of
    patients for the clinician. J. Psychiat. Res., 12, 289-98
Johnston, M. V., McKinney, M. and Coyle, J. T. (1981).
    Neocortical cholinergic innervation: a description of ex-
    trinsic and intrinsic components in the rat. Exp. Brain
    Res., 43, 159-72
Kebabian, J. W. and Calne, D. B. (1979). Multiple receptors for
    dopamine. Nature, 277, 93-6
Longo, V. G. (1966). Behavioral and electroencephalographic
    effects of atropine and related compounds. Pharmacol. Rev.,
    18, 965-89
Olton, D. S. and Feustle, W. A. (1981). Hippocampal function
    required for nonspatial working memory. Exp. Brain Res., 41,
    380-9
Racagni, G., Cheney, D. L., Trabuchi, M. and Costa, E. (1976). In
    vivo actions of clozapine and haloperidol on the turnover
    rate of acetylcholine in rat striatum. J. Pharmacol. Exp.
    Ther., 96, 323-32
Richelson, E. and Divinitz-Romero, S. (1977). Blockade by
    psychotropic drugs of the muscarinic acetylcholine receptor
    in cultured nerve cells. Biol. Psychiat., 12, 771-82
Rish, S. C., Hicey, L. Y. and Janowsky, D. S. (1979). Plasma
    levels of tricyclic antidepressants and clinical efficacy.
    Review of the literature. J. Clin. Psychiat., 40, 4-116
Spitzer, R. L., Endicott, J. and Robins, E. (1975). Research
    Diagnostic Criteria., New York State Psychiatric Institute,
    New York, Biometrics Research, 2nd edn
Tune, L. E. and Coyle, J. T. (1980). Serum levels of anti-
    cholinergic drugs in treatment of acute extrapyramidal side
    effects. Arch. Gen. Psychiatry, 37, 293-7
Tune, L. E. and Coyle, J. T. (1981). Acute extrapyramidal side
    effects: serum levels of neuroleptics and anticholinergics.
    Psychopharmacology, 75, 9-15

Tune, L. E., Creese, I., Coyle, J. T., Pearlson, G. and Snyder, S. H. (1979). Low neuroleptic serum levels in patients receiving fluphenazine decanoate. Am. J. Psychiatry, 137, 80-2

Tune, L. E., Holland, A., Folstein, M., Damlouji, N. F., Gardner, T. J. and Coyle, J. T. (1981). Association of post-operative delirium with raised serum levels of anticholinergic drugs. Lancet, ii, 651-3

Tune, L. E., Strauss, M. E., Lew, M. F., Breitlinger, E. and Coyle, J. T. (1982). Serum levels of anticholinergic drugs and impaired recent memory in chronic schizophrenic patients. Am.J.Psychiatry, 139, 1460-2

Van Putten, T. (1974). Why do schizophrenic patients refuse to take their drug? Arch. Gen. Psychiatry, 31, 67-72

Whitehouse, P. J., Price, D. L., Struble, R. G., Clark, A. W., Coyle, J. T. and DeLong, M. (1982). Alzheimer's disease and senile dementia: loss of neurons in the basal forebrain. Science, 215, 1237-9

Wing, J. K., Cooper, J. E. and Sartorius, N. (1974). Measurement and Classification of Psychiatric Symptoms, Cambridge University Press, Cambridge

Yamamura, H. I. and Snyder, S. H. (1974). Muscarinic cholinergic receptor binding in the longitudinal muscle of guinea pig ileum with [^{3}H]-quinuclidinyl benzilate. Mol. Pharmacol., 10, 861-7

Clinical effects related to the serum concentrations of thioridazine and its metabolites

Rolf Axelsson[1] and Erik Mårtensson[1]

INTRODUCTION

Neuroleptic drugs have vastly improved the treatment of psychotic disorders and increased our capacity to ameliorate severe symptoms and to rehabilitate patients. The first substance used, chlorpromazine, has been followed by a variety of others, mostly without major differences in antipsychotic activity. These drugs do, however, differ in respect to type and frequency of induced side-effects. Since some side-effects are concentration-dependent, it is important to keep both acute and maintenance doses minimal without loss of therapeutic effect. With the aid of routine serum determinations, we have therefore sought to optimize the treatment with a commonly used neuroleptic drug, thioridazine. Earlier studies of the metabolism (Mårtensson *et al.*, 1975), protein binding (Nyberg *et al.*, 1978) and metabolite characteristics (Axelsson and Mårtensson, 1977) of this drug have provided the basis for the present study, in which our aim has been to explore any correlations between the serum concentrations of thioridazine and its metabolites on the one hand, and clinical effects, including side-effects, on the other.

METHODS

Patients

Patients with acute paranoid psychosis were screened for inclusion in the study on admission to Psychiatric Department III, Lillhagen Hospital. Those with affective disorders or dementia were excluded. Extensive examinations, including laboratory tests and ECG recordings, showed good physical health without abuse of alcohol and narcotics in the 65 patients, 29 men and 36 women, who

---

[1]Psychiatric Department III, University of Göteborg, Sweden.

were accepted. With no age restriction used, their ages ranged from 16 to 78 (mean 50) years.

During the observation period of 20-50 days from admission to discharge from hospital, thioridazine was the only drug given. With variable dose schedules determined by the attending psychiatrist, the mean daily dose ranged between 123 and 1007 mg and the maximum between 200 and 1200 mg. The medication was given in equal amounts at 7 a.m., 12 noon, 4 p.m. and 8 p.m. After a week constant medication (steady-state level), blood samples were obtained before the first dose of the day. The sampling procedure was repeated once a week, before any change in dosage and in connection with discharge from hospital. The total serum concentrations of thioridazine and its main metabolites, side-chain sulfoxide, side-chain sulfone and ring sulfoxide, were determined by use of gas chromatography (Mårtensson *et al.*, 1975).

Rating of Therapeutic Effect

Before the start of treatment and at the end of the observation period, the psychiatric symptoms were rated according to the Comprehensive Psychopathological Rating Scale (CPRS) (Asberg *et al.*, 1978). An independent psychiatrist performed the ratings without knowledge of the doses and serum concentrations involved. Separate registrations were made of the total CPRS score and the score for paranoid symptoms alone. The percentage of the admission score still remaining at the end of the observation period served as a measure of the therapeutic effect.

Comparative analyses were made of patients at or below the age of 40 years ($n=21$) and those above ($n=44$). Patients with a mean total serum concentration of thioridazine between 1 and 2 μmol 1^{-1} were separately studied concerning the influence of dose and concentration of metabolites on the clinical outcome.

Evaluation of Side-Effects

Side-effects were especially studied in 38 patients, 14 men and 24 women between the ages of 16 and 78 (mean 59) years. Both objective signs and subjective reports of the side-effects most commonly seen during treatment with neuroleptics (table 1) were rated according to frequency and intensity (Axelsson and Mårtensson, 1980). A slight degree of a reported or observed side-effect was given the score 1, a moderate degree the score 2 and a severe degree the score 3. The tremor rating, based on objective findings only, was given the score 1 for finger tremor with extended hands, 2 for finger and hand tremor with extended hands and 3 for continuously observable hand tremor.

Body weight and cardiovascular parameters were registered on admission, during treatment, in connection with blood sampling and

Table 1. Rated side-effects

Drowsiness	Sweating
Headache	Blurred vision
Sensibility disturbance	Palpitation
Paresthesia	Vertigo
Tremor	Postural hypotension
Rigidity	Nausea/vomiting
Hyperkinesia	Constipation
Hypokinesia	Diarrhea
Dyskinesia	Itching
Acute dystonia	Dermatological reactions
Akathisia	Menstrual disturbances
Inhibition of micturition	Gynecomastia
Dry mouth	Galactorrhea
Salivation	Altered libido
Nasal congestion	Inhibition of ejaculation

at discharge. Owing to poor cooperation, some patients could not be included on every occasion. Systolic and diastolic blood pressures and heart rates (erect and recumbent) were recorded, and the orthostatic blood pressure change was calculated from these values. ECG recordings (XII leads) were performed at the Medical Centre of Lillhagen Hospital throughout the observation period. An independent physician made the ECG analyses, which included measures of Q-S and P-Q time and heart rate. With the aid of a new classification system (Axelsson and Aspenström, 1982), two types of T-wave changes were distinguished: type I with rounded (grade 1), plateau-shaped (grade 2) or bifid (grade 3) T-waves; and type II with diphasic or inverted T-waves.

Only the most prevalent side-effects, seen in a significant number of patients, are presented in this study.

Statistics

Non-parametric correlation analyses were performed by use of Pitman's test (Bradley, 1968). The technique suggested by Mantel was used to test the partial correlation between two variables and eliminate the influence of a third (Mantel, 1963). Quadratic regression analysis was applied to the calculations of non-linear relationships. In comparisons between groups of patients, Wilcoxon's test for two samples was used.

The mean dose was defined as accumulated dose divided by number of days of the observation period. The mean serum concentration was calculated from the area under the time-concentration curve.

RESULTS

Serum Concentrations

The total serum concentrations of thioridazine, side-chain sulfoxide, side-chain sulfone and ring sulfoxide were in the ranges
0.35-6.44, 0.32-4.53, 0.11-1.63 and 0.81-12.19 μmol l^{-1}, respectively.

Therapeutic Effect

The total CPRS score remaining at the end of the observation
period was, in mean, 37% (range 0-121%). In 50 of the 65 patients,
there was a reduction of at least 50%.

On average 22% (range 0-100%) of the paranoid score on admission was still present at the time of discharge. Absence of
paranoid symptoms was noted in 37 out of 65 patients, and in 57
the paranoid score was reduced by 50% or more.

Correlations between therapeutic effect, dose and age

Positive correlations were seen in all patients between mean daily
dose and therapeutic effect as reflected by both the total CPRS
score ($p<0.01$) and the paranoid score ($p<0.05$). A negative correlation was found between age and dose. With age taken into consideration, linear and quadratic regression analyses showed no
correlation of significance between dose and therapeutic effect.

Correlations between therapeutic effect and total serum concentration of thioridazine

Positive correlations were found between therapeutic effect and
serum concentration of thioridazine in patients aged 40 or less,
but not in those above 40 years (table 2). The correlation between
serum concentration and total remaining CPRS score satisfied best
a non-linear relation as verified by the difference between the
correlation coefficients of the quadratic and linear regression
analyses, which were 0.58 ($p<0.02$) and 0.46 ($p<0.05$), respectively. The corresponding figures for the paranoid score were 0.63
($p<0.01$, quadratic) and 0.45 ($p<0.05$, linear).

Comparisons were made between groups of patients at a given
total serum concentration of thioridazine in order to explore the
possibility of an optimal serum concentration interval, indicated
by the quadratic regression analysis. The patients aged 40 or
less were classified according to serum concentration of thioridazine, which was below 1.0 μmol l^{-1} in six patients, between 1.0
and 2.0 μmol l^{-1} in 10 and above 2 μmol l^{-1} in five. The classifi-

Table 2. Therapeutic effect at different serum concentration
intervals of total thioridazine in patients aged 40 years or less,
and in those above the age of 40

Age range	Concentration interval ($\mu mol\ l^{-1}$)	Remaining total CPRS score (%)	
		Mean	Range
40 years or less	<1.0	45	23–84
	1.0–2.0	22	4–61
	>2.0	14	8–20
Above 40 years	<0.7	63	52–76
	0.7–2.0	37	4–104
	>2.0	45	0–121

cation of the patients above 40 years of age gave four patients
with serum concentrations of thioridazine below 0.7 $\mu mol\ l^{-1}$, 27
in the interval between 0.7 and 2.0 $\mu mol\ l^{-1}$ and 13 above 2.0 μmol
l^{-1}.

Among the patients at or below the age of 40, the therapeutic
response was clearly better in those with serum concentrations
above 2.0 $\mu mol\ l^{-1}$ than in those below 1.0 $\mu mol\ l^{-1}$ ($p<0.01$). The
patients in the interval between 1.0 and 2.0 $\mu mol\ l^{-1}$ tended to
respond better to treatment than those below 1.0 $\mu mol\ l^{-1}$
($p<0.10$), but differed little from those above 2.0 $\mu mol\ l^{-1}$. In
the patients above 40 years, the therapeutic effects were distinctly more pronounced in patients with serum concentrations
between 0.7 and 2.0 $\mu mol\ l^{-1}$ than in those below 0.7 $\mu mol\ l^{-1}$
($p<0.02$). No other differences in therapeutic response were
found between the groups of older patients. Table 2 shows the mean
and range of the remaining total CPRS scores at the various concentration intervals of thioridazine.

*Influence of dose and metabolite concentrations on therapeutic
effect at a given concentration of total thioridazine*

Since positive correlations were found between the thioridazine
concentration and dose, between the thioridazine concentration and
therapeutic effect and between dose and therapeutic effect, the
serum concentration of thioridazine was used as background variable in the correlation analysis of dose and therapeutic effect.
The serum concentrations of thioridazine and metabolites and the
therapeutic effect were also intercorrelated. The 31 patients
with serum concentrations between 1.0 and 2.0 $\mu mol\ l^{-1}$ were therefore especially studied. In this group of patients between the

ages of 16 and 78 (mean 50) years, the serum concentration of thioridazine was, in mean, 1.50 (range 1.02-1.99) μmol 1^{-1}, equally distributed over the dose intervals. The mean dose ranged between 154 and 1007 (mean 502) mg.

Patients with a dose above 600 mg of thioridazine showed a better therapeutic effect than those with a dose below 400 mg ($p<0.01$). For further exploration of this finding, the serum concentration/dose ratio was calculated in each case. Patients with low concentration/dose ratios, below 3×10^{-3} μM mg^{-1} ($n=15$), showed better therapeutic effect, reflected by the percent remaining total CPRS score of, in mean, 25 (range 4-61), than patients with concentration/dose ratios above 3×10^{-3} μM mg^{-1} ($n=16$), where the score was, in mean, 43 (range 5-104) ($p<0.03$).

The ratio between the metabolite/thioridazine concentrations was also calculated in each of the 31 patients involved in this part of the study. The following values were obtained: side-chain sulfoxide, mean 1.04, range 0.37-2.0; side-chain sulfone, mean 0.33, range 0.08-0.62; ring sulfoxide, mean 2.91, range 1.14-7.73. When patients with high and low ratios, determined according to the median values (side-chain sulfoxide 0.95, side-chain sulfone 0.33 and ring sulfoxide 2.70), were compared regarding therapeutic effect, no significant difference was revealed. There was, however, a tendency toward difference in the case of side-chain sulfoxide, reflected by the total remaining CPRS score, which in patients with low side-chain sulfoxide/thioridazine ratios was, in mean, 39 (range 4-104), while it was 29 (range 4-87) in patients with high ratios. Comparison of patients with side-chain sulfoxide/thioridazine ratios above and below 1.0 at serum concentrations of thioridazine between 1.0 and 2.0 μmol 1^{-1} showed marked differences. The patients with a ratio above 1.0 had a total remaining CPRS score of, in mean, 20 (range 4-46) ($n=12$); those with a ratio below 1.0 had a corresponding score of 43 ($n=19$) ($p<0.01$).

Side-Effects

Type

The side-effects found to be most frequent were dry mouth, tremor, drowsiness, nasal congestion, increase in body weight, decrease in blood pressures, increase in diastolic orthostatic blood pressure, decrease in heart rate and ECG T-wave changes of type I. These symptoms were seen in about three-fourths of the patients and were most often of a slight degree (score 1). The increase in body weight during the observation period was, in mean, 3.7 (range 1-8) kg, or 6% (range 1-18%) more than the weight recorded on admission. The systolic and diastolic blood pressures and the heart rate decreased by, in mean, 11% (range 6-14%). All patients but one showed ECG T-wave changes of type I.

Variation with time

The side-effects differed regarding variation in intensity during the course of treatment. Dry mouth, drowsiness and nasal congestion reached their maximum intensity after 10–19 days of medication, after which time they decreased. The orthostatic blood pressure change followed a similar pattern with a peak value after about 7 days of treatment and returned to pre-treatment level toward the end of the observation period. The onset of tremor, decrease in blood pressures and ECG T-wave changes of type I did, however, occur immediately after the start of treatment and remained constant throughout the observation period. The changes in body weight and heart rate followed a pattern of successive accentuation during treatment.

Intercorrelations and correlations to other variables

Tremor was more often observed in women than in men ($p<0.05$), and the same variation with sex was indicated by the dry mouth score. Women below the age of 50 showed a greater increase in body weight than older women ($p<0.02$), and tended to increase more in weight than men below the age of 50 ($p<0.10$). Significant intercorrelations were found between the mean scores for dry mouth, drowsiness and nasal congestion, none of which were correlated to increase in body weight. The weight increase was, however, correlated to therapeutic effect reflected by the total CPRS score, which more often was reduced by 50% in patients with increase in body weight (18 out of 22) than in those without weight gain (2 out of 9) ($p<0.01$, fourfold table test). The diastolic blood pressure in the erect position was more often decreased in women (18 out of 22) than in men (3 out of 6) ($p<0.04$).

Concentration dependence

Inter-individual correlation analysis showed that patients with dry mouth had higher serum concentrations of side-chain sulfoxide ($p<0.02$) and side-chain sulfone ($p<0.01$) than patients without this side-effect. The serum concentration of side-chain sulfone was also higher in patients with tremor than in those without ($p<0.05$).

Positive correlations were found between changes in systolic and diastolic blood pressures (values on admission minus values at the end of the observation period) on the one hand, and the serum concentration of ring sulfoxide on the other ($p<0.05$ and $p<0.003$, respectively).

No significant intercorrelations were found between the other variables investigated, or between patients with and without other types of side-effects.

Table 3. Values of p for the correlation analysis between drug concentrations and side-effects

Variable	Serum concentrations			
	Thioridazine	Thioridazine side-chain sulfoxide	Thioridazine side-chain sulfone	Thioridazine ring sulfoxide
Dry mouth	n.s.	n.s.	n.s.	n.s.
Tremor	n.s.	$p<0.03$	n.s.	$p<0.01$
Drowsiness	n.s.	n.s.	n.s.	n.s.
Nasal congestion	n.s.	n.s.	n.s.	n.s.
Body weight	n.s.	n.s.	n.s.	n.s.
Heart rates (erect, recumbent)	$p<0.002$	$p<0.02$	$p<0.02$	$p<0.002$
Blood pressures (systolic, diastolic, erect, recumbent)	$p<0.002$	$p<0.002$	$p<0.002$	$p<0.002$
Orthostatic blood pressure (diastolic)	$p<0.01$	$p<0.002$	$p<0.006$	$p<0.005$
ECG T-wave changes of type I	$p<0.001$	$p<0.01$	$p<0.001$	$p<0.0001$

n.s. = non-significant

The results of the intra-individual correlation analysis are given in table 3. All cardiovascular parameters showed strong, positive correlations at all drug concentrations. The tremor score was positively correlated to the sulfoxide metabolites. Dry mouth, drowsiness, nasal congestion and body weight showed no significant correlations.

CONCLUDING REMARKS

The following conclusions summarize our findings of direct interest to the clinician during acute treatment of paranoid psychosis with thioridazine alone.

Therapeutic Effect

For optimal antipsychotic effect, patients aged 40 years or less should have a serum concentration of total thioridazine above 2.0 μmol 1^{-1}. This level is usually reached with a daily dose of 800 mg.

Patients aged 40 years or less may respond favorably within the concentration interval 1.0-2.0 μmol 1^{-1}, provided that this level is reached with a high dosage (concentration/dose ratio below 0.3) or with a side-chain sulfoxide/thioridazine ratio exceeding 1.0.

Patients above the age of 40 should have a serum concentration of total thioridazine between 0.7 and 2.0 μmol 1^{-1} for optimal therapeutic effect. At concentrations above or below this level, the response to the drug is generally unsatisfactory.

Side-Effects

The most pronounced side-effects during acute treatment with thioridazine are dry mouth, tremor, drowsiness, nasal congestion, increase in body weight, decrease in blood pressures, decrease in heart rates and ECG T-wave changes of type I.

Drowsiness, dry mouth, nasal congestion and decrease in diastolic/orthostatic blood pressure are temporary at constant serum concentrations of thioridazine and its metabolites.

Women are more prone to develop side-effects than are men.

Increase in body weight is a favorable prognostic sign.

Tremor is significantly correlated to the concentrations of side-chain sulfoxide, side-chain sulfone and ring sulfoxide, but not to thioridazine.

The cardiovascular side-effects are strongly correlated to the serum concentrations of thioridazine and its main metabolites.

Acknowledgements

The study was supported by the Swedish Medical Research Council
(Grants no. 5998-01 and 5998-02). Agneta Andersson is gratefully
acknowledged for valuable aid in the preparation of the manuscript.

REFERENCES

Asberg, M., Montgomery, S.A., Perris, C., Schalling, D. and
    Sedvall, G. (1978). A comprehensive psychopathological
    rating scale. Acta Psychiatr. Scand., Suppl. 271
Axelsson, R. and Aspenström, G. (1982). Electrocardiographic
    changes and serum concentrations in thioridazine-treated
    patients. J. Clin. Psychiatry, 43, 332-5
Axelsson, R. and Mårtensson, E. (1977). The concentration pattern
    of nonconjugated thioridazine metabolites in serum by thio-
    ridazine treatment and its relationship to physiological and
    clinical variables. Curr. Ther. Res., 21, 561-86
Axelsson, R. and Mårtensson, E. (1980). Side effects of
    thioridazine and their relationship with the serum concen-
    trations of the drug and its main metabolites. Curr. Ther.
    Res., 28, 463-89
Bradley, J.V.(1968). Distribution-Free Statistical Tests,
    Prentice-Hall, London
Mantel, N. (1963). Chi-square tests with one degree of freedom;
    extensions of the Mantel-Haenszel procedure. J. Am. Stat.
    Assoc., 58, 690-700
Mårtensson, E., Nyberg, G., Axelsson, R. and Serck-Hansen, C.
    (1975). Quantitative determination of thioridazine and
    nonconjugated thioridazine metabolites in serum and urine of
    psychiatric patients. Curr. Ther. Res., 18, 687-700
Nyberg, G., Axelsson, R. and Mårtensson, E. (1978). Binding of
    thioridazine and thioridazine metabolites to serum proteins
    in psychiatric patients. Eur. J. Clin. Pharmacol., 14,
    341-50

Plasma levels of perphenazine related to clinical effect and extrapyramidal side-effects

Lars Bolvig Hansen[1] and Niels-Erik Larsen[2]

INTRODUCTION

Many investigators have attempted to evaluate a correlation between the therapeutic effect and the plasma concentration of
neuroleptic drugs (Buyze *et al.*, 1973; Davis *et al.*, 1974;
Mjørndal and Oreland, 1971; Wiles and Franklin, 1978). Unfortunately, simultaneous registration of the degree of side-effects is
often lacking. However, clinical experience shows that development of side-effects of neuroleptic drugs, especially extrapyramidal reactions, may have such substantial negative influence
on the effort of resocialization that the total situation remains
unsatisfactory in spite of amelioration of the psychotic symptoms
(Bolvig Hansen *et al.*, 1981). Therefore, it is of the utmost
importance to handle neuroleptics in a way which gives maximal
therapeutic effect with a minimum of side-effects.

MATERIAL AND METHODS

In light of the above-mentioned problems, we have done three
clinical pharmacological studies involving acute psychotic inpatients, who have not received neuroleptic treatment within the
last four months prior to the studies. Patients with signs of
affective disorders, disturbed consciousness and alcohol or drug
abuse were excluded. Informed consent was obtained from all the
patients in accordance with Helsinki Declaration II.

As a first step we investigated 26 patients (16 males and 10
females) during a four-week period of treatment to evaluate the
correlation between plasma levels of perphenazine and the degree

[1] Department B, Sct. Hans Mental Hospital, DK-4000 Roskilde, Denmark.
[2] Clinical Pharmacological Laboratory, Department of Clinical Chemistry, Glostrup
University Hospital, DK-2600 Glostrup, Denmark.

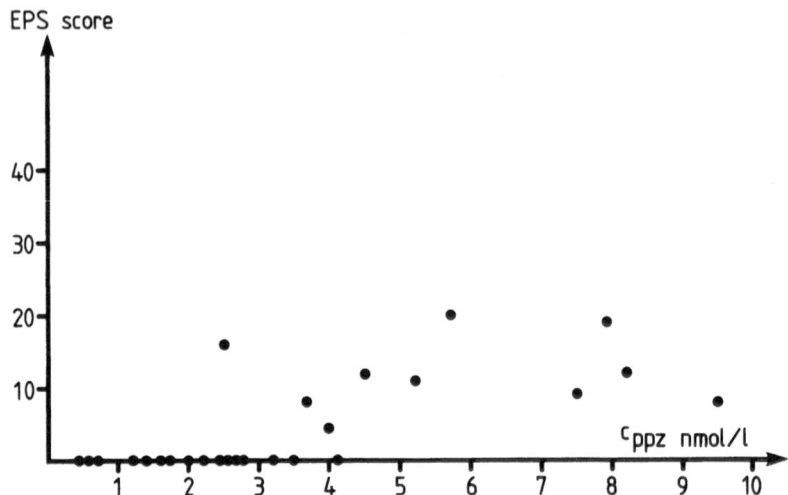

Figure 1. A single plasma concentration value of perphenazine from
          each of 26 patients plotted versus the degree of total
          extrapyramidal side-effects (EPS), which are expressed
          as the sum of scale points from Simpson and Angus Rating
          Scale plus the degree of akathisia and dystonia quan-
          titated by means of a four-point scale. Plasma concen-
          trations eliciting side-effects differ significantly
          from those not provoking side-effects ($p < 0.02$), using
          the Mann-Whitney test.

of total extrapyramidal side-effects. All patients were given
oral perphenazine treatment continuously with the dosage individu-
ally determined on the basis of body weight. The dosage was kept
at a constant level during the entire investigation period. The
medication was given t.i.d. in equal doses with constant intervals
(8 h). Blood samples to determine the perphenazine concentration
were drawn at the end of a dose interval (minimum values). No
other medication was allowed except occasionally for nitrazepam.
The psychiatrist and the chemist were kept blind to each other's
results.

Secondly, we investigated another 26 patients (17 males and 9
females) during a five-week period with the aim of evaluating the
correlation between plasma levels and the degree of antipsychotic
effect. All patients were given oral perphenazine treatment
continuously and the medication was likewise given in equal doses
with constant intervals (8 h), with blood samples drawn at the end
of a dose interval. Based on the perphenazine concentration
determined after three days of treatment, the doses were adjusted
to give concentrations of either below 3 nmol 1^{-1} or between 5 and

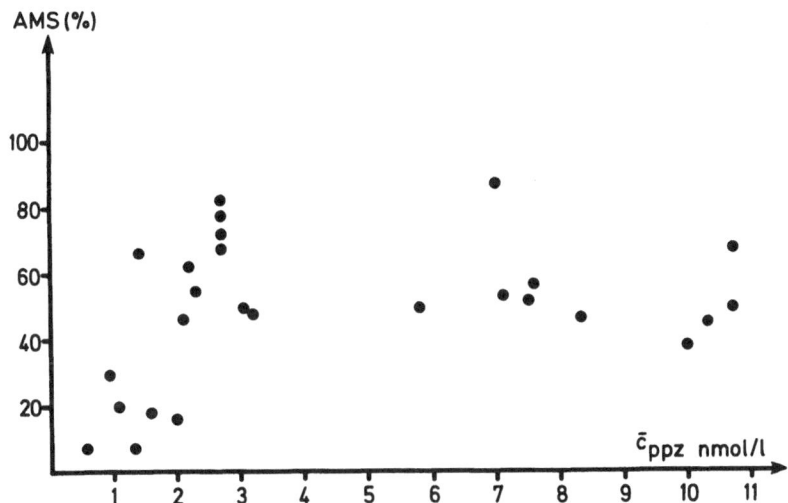

Figure 2. Average plasma concentrations of perphenazine for each
of 26 patients plotted versus the degree of antipsychotic effect (AMS), which is the amelioration expressed in percent of the initial value, as judged from
the Brief Psychiatric Rating Scale. Plasma concentrations above 2 nmol l^{-1} induce a significantly better
therapeutic outcome than do concentrations below this
value ($p<0.005$), using the Mann-Whitney test.

10 nmol l^{-1}. To camouflage the allocation from the psychiatrist,
all patients received from the beginning biperidine, 2 mg t.i.d.
The only additional medication allowed was occasional use of
nitrazepam. The psychiatrist and the chemist were kept blind to
each other's results.

Finally, we investigated 23 patients (15 males and 8 females)
selected using the above-mentioned criteria in order to evaluate
the differences in clinical effects between depot preparations of
perphenazine-enanthate and the new perphenazine-decanoate. Injections were given either fortnightly or weekly. The only additional
medication allowed was, occasionally, nitrazepam. The psychiatrist
and the chemist were kept blind to each other's results.

RESULTS

In figure 1, the plasma level of perphenazine for each of the 26
patients is plotted versus the degree of total extrapyramidal
side-effects. Dividing the patients into two clinical groups

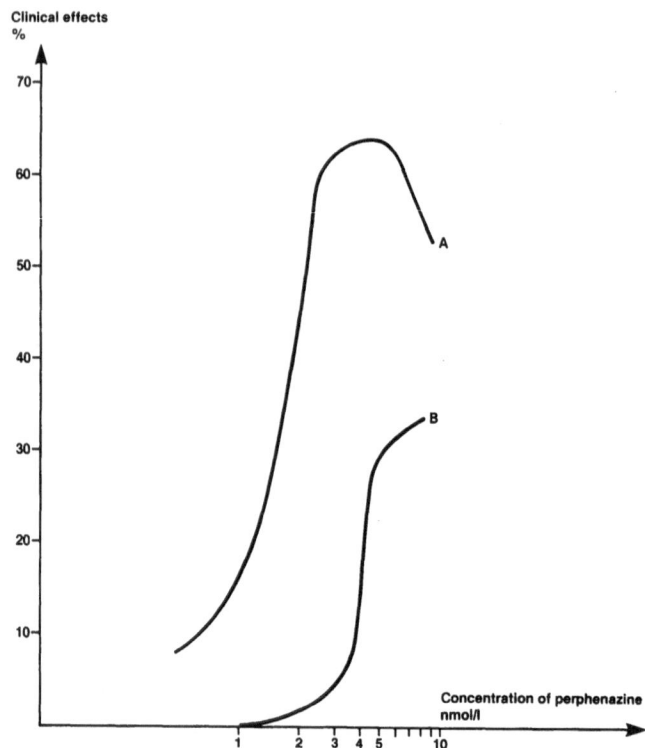

Figure 3. Clinical effects versus logarithmic plasma concentration
scale.   Curve A gives the amelioration expressed in
percent of the initial values as judged from the Brief
Psychiatric Rating Scale (data from figure 2).   Curve B
gives the total extrapyramidal side-effect scores expressed in percent of the maximal obtainable value (48
points) (data from figure 1).

(showing or not showing side-effects, respectively), a significant
difference in plasma levels between the groups was found ($p<0.02$),
using the Mann-Whitney test.   However, a rather poor correlation
($R=0.64$) between the perphenazine plasma concentration and the
intensity of the total extrapyramidal side-effects was found.
   Figure 2 illustrates the relation between therapeutic outcome
and the plasma levels of perphenazine for each of the other 26
patients.   Patients with low levels (<2 nmol 1^{-1}) generally
achieved a substantially poorer clinical response compared to
those with higher concentrations ($p<0.005$), using the Mann-Whitney
test.   There was also a tendency to a weaker antipsychotic effect
among the patients in the high plasma concentration group (>5

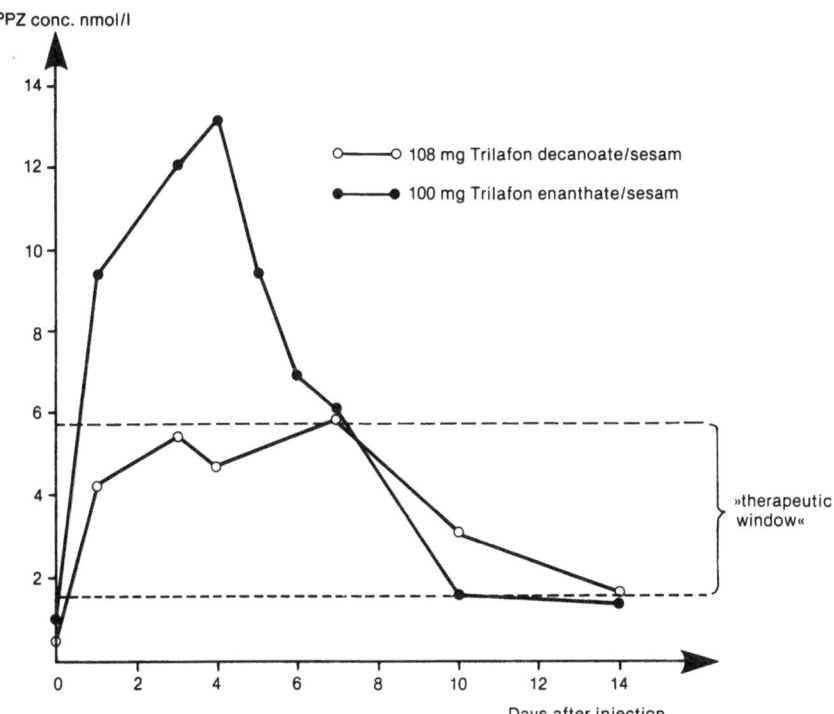

Figure 4. Plasma concentrations of perphenazine in a single
patient after injection of 100 mg perphenazine-enanthate
and 108 mg perphenazine-decanoate, respectively. The
broken lines give the limits for the optimal plasma
concentration range. During the enanthate period extrapyramidal side-effects appeared. No side-effects were
seen during the decanoate period.

nmol 1^{-1}) than among those with plasma concentrations in the
range 2-3 nmol 1^{-1}. This difference was not statistically significant ($p>0.05$), using the Mann-Whitney test.

The relationship between the antipsychotic effect and the
risk of eliciting extrapyramidal side-effects at different plasma
levels is shown in a 'dose-response' curve (figure 3). It can be
seen that a maximal therapeutic response is achieved before the
incidence of extrapyramidal side-effects increases drastically.

Based on the results from the oral studies one might, therefore, conclude that it is possible to obtain a maximal therapeutic
effect without provoking extrapyramidal side-effects. The optimal
plasma concentration range seems to be between 2 and 3 nmol 1^{-1}
(figure 3).

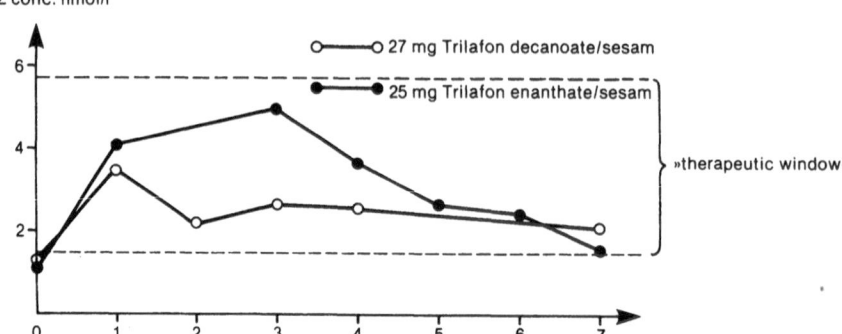

Figure 5. Plasma concentrations of perphenazine in a single
patient after injection of 25 mg perphenazine-enanthate
and 27 mg perphenazine-decanoate, respectively. The
broken lines give the optimal plasma concentration
range. No side-effects were seen in either of the two
depot periods.

Patients treated continuously with oral perphenazine had a
constant ratio of 1.8 between maximum and minimum plasma concentration within an 8 h dose interval (Bolvig Hansen and Larsen,
1977). This means that a minimum concentration of e.g. 3 nmol 1^{-1}
corresponds to a maximum concentration of 5.4 nmol 1^{-1}. Consequently, the operational plasma concentration range for depot
administration should be about 2-6 nmol 1^{-1} for attainment of
maximal therapeutic effect without extrapyramidal side-effects.

Figure 4 shows typical plasma profiles of perphenazine after
injection of a standard dose of perphenazine-enanthate and
perphenazine-decanoate, respectively. As seen, the enanthate
curve far exceeds the upper limit of the optimal concentration
range resulting in appearance of extrapyramidal side-effects. In
order to avoid the rather often seen extrapyramidal side-effects
during perphenazine-enanthate treatment, we lowered the dose and
shortened the injection intervals to one week. In figure 5 typical
plasma concentration profiles of perphenazine after injection of a
low dose of perphenazine-enanthate and perphenazine-decanoate, in
a single patient, are shown. As seen, the enanthate curve now
lies within the optimal therapeutic range. Consequently, no
extrapyramidal phenomena occurred.

CONCLUSION

When treating acute psychotic states with perphenazine, it is in
most cases possible to achieve an excellent therapeutic effect

without provoking extrapyramidal side-effects. During oral treatment given in three equal daily doses with constant intervals, one should guide the plasma level into the range of 2-3 nmol 1^{-1} as measured at the end of the dose interval. Using depot preparations of perphenazine, the plasma concentrations should lie within the limits of 2 and 6 nmol 1^{-1}.

REFERENCES

Bolvig Hansen, L. and Larsen, N.-E. (1977). Plasma concentrations of perphenazine and its sulphoxide metabolite during continuous oral treatment. Psychopharmacology, 53, 127-30

Bolvig Hansen, L., Larsen, N.-E. and Vestergård, P. (1981). Plasma levels of perphenazine related to development of extrapyramidal side effects. Psychopharmacology, 74, 306-9

Buyze, G., Egberts, P.F.C., Muunsze, R.G. and Poslavska, A. (1973). Blood levels of thioridazine and some of its metabolites in psychiatric patients. A preliminary report. Psychiatr. Neurol. Neurochir., 76, 229-39

Davis, J.M., Janowski, D.S., Sekerti, H.J., Manier, D. and El-Youssef, M.K. (1974). The pharmacokinetics of butaperazine in serum. In Phenothiazines and Structurally Related Drugs (ed. I.S. Forrest, C.J. Carr and E. Usdin), Raven Press, New York, pp 433-43

Mjørndal, T. and Oreland, L. (1971). Determination of thioxanthenes in plasma at therapeutic concentrations. Acta Pharmacol. Toxicol., 29, 295-302

Wiles, D.H. and Franklin, M. (1978). Radioimmunoassay for fluphenazine in human plasma. Br. J. Clin. Pharmacol., 5, 265-8

Saliva haloperidol concentrations in schizophrenic patients: relation to serum haloperidol and prolactin concentrations

Russell E. Poland[1], Robert T. Rubin[1], Claude T. H. Friedmann[2]
and Barbara Kaston[2]

INTRODUCTION

Measurement of drugs in saliva has been proposed as a non-invasive means by which serum drug concentrations can be assessed (Horning *et al.*, 1977). The concentrations of many drugs in saliva are equal to or less than the concentrations of free (non-protein-bound) drug in plasma or serum (Horning *et al.*, 1977; Stephen *et al.*, 1980). However, recent studies have shown that neuroleptics such as chlorpromazine (May *et al.*, 1981) and haloperidol (Yamazumi and Miura, 1981) are present in saliva in concentrations exceeding the total plasma concentration of drug.

Some of the variables which can affect saliva drug concentrations include: (1) the amount of drug bound to blood proteins or lipids; (2) the physio-chemical properties of the drug including its pK_a and its lipophilicity; (3) the extent to which the drug is actively transported from serum into saliva; (4) the flow dependence of the drug from serum into saliva; and (5) the pH difference between blood and saliva (Horning *et al.*, 1977; Stephen *et al.*, 1980). Which, if any, of the above variables account for high saliva versus serum neuroleptic concentrations is unknown.

One of the benefits of measuring drugs and other compounds in saliva is the ease with which samples can be collected (Poland and Rubin, 1982). More importantly, however, is the possibility that saliva drug concentrations may be pharmacologically more relevant than serum or plasma concentrations. In fact, May *et al.* (1981) reported that saliva chlorpromazine concentrations 24 h after the first dose related more strongly to clinical outcome than did plasma concentrations. Previous studies have shown a strong positive association between serum haloperidol and serum prolactin

[1]Department of Psychiatry, Harbor-UCLA Medical Center, Torrance, California 90509, USA.
[2]Department of Psychiatry and Human Behavior, University of California at Irvine, School of Medicine, Irvine, California 92668, USA.

concentrations (Rubin and Hays, 1980; Rubin *et al.*, 1980; Poland and Rubin, 1981). Strong correlations between saliva and serum haloperidol and between saliva haloperidol and serum prolactin would suggest that, under appropriate conditions, saliva haloperidol measurements might prove to be clinically useful. Accordingly, we undertook the present study to determine the relationships among serum and saliva haloperidol concentrations and serum prolactin levels in chronically medicated patients.

MATERIALS AND METHODS

Paired serum and saliva samples were obtained from 27 chronically medicated schizophrenic patients in the morning, approximately 10 h after their last dose of medication. After rinsing his/her mouth with water, each subject was asked to allow saliva to accumulate. One to two milliliters of mixed saliva was collected by expectoration into small polypropylene funnels inserted into 12x75 mm polypropylene tubes. The saliva samples were centrifuged for 30 min at 500g to remove particulate matter, and the supernatant was frozen. Immediately after the saliva was collected, a blood sample was obtained by venipuncture. The blood was allowed to clot overnight at 4°C and centrifuged the next morning at 500g for 30 min. The serum was removed and frozen for subsequent haloperidol and prolactin measurements.

Serum and saliva haloperidol were measured by radioimmunoassay (RIA) as described previously (Poland and Rubin, 1981). This RIA does not cross-react appreciably with any known haloperidol metabolite and only cross-reacts to a limited extent (0.32%) with reduced haloperidol, a metabolite which is present in serum at approximately equal concentrations to that of the parent compound but with only one-tenth the neuroleptic activity of haloperidol (Forsman and Ohman, 1979; Hays *et al.*, 1980). Prolactin was measured by RIA using the hormone kit provided by Dr A.F. Parlow on behalf of the National Pituitary Agency.

To achieve a Gaussian distribution for the haloperidol and prolactin values, the data were log-transformed prior to the calculation of Pearson correlation coefficients (Zivin and Bartko, 1976). The nominal significance levels were corrected for the multiple correlations (Jacobs, 1976).

RESULTS

Table 1 shows the serum and saliva haloperidol concentrations, the saliva-to-serum ratios of haloperidol, and the serum prolactin concentrations of 24 chronically medicated patients during pharmacokinetic steady-state conditions. There was a significant correlation between the serum and saliva haloperidol concentrations

Table 1.   Serum and saliva haloperidol (HAL) concentrations,
saliva-to-serum HAL ratios, and serum prolactin (PRL)
concentrations in 24 chronically medicated patients
during pharmacokinetic steady-state conditions

Subject	Serum HAL (μg l^{-1})	Saliva HAL (μg l^{-1})	Saliva-to-serum ratio	PRL (μg l^{-1})
1	6	3	0.50	25
2	7	2	0.29	24
3	10	4	0.40	103
4	11	102	9.27	63
5	12	26	2.17	296
6	15	58	3.87	62
7	15	22	1.47	7
8	16	110	6.88	59
9	22	131	5.95	57
10	22	4	0.18	166
11	24	53	2.21	55
12	25	67	2.68	36
13	26	61	2.35	51
14	26	55	2.12	18
15	27	56	2.07	37
16	28	36	1.29	70
17	28	60	2.14	23
18	31	23	0.74	39
19	34	109	3.20	137
20	34	111	3.26	59
21	35	86	2.43	28
22	51	448	8.78	32
23	60	472	7.87	240
24	66	40	0.61	97
Range	6–66	2–472	0.2–9.36	7–296

(r = +0.70, p<0.005), but there was no significant correlation
either between serum haloperidol and serum prolactin (r = +0.23)
or between saliva haloperidol and serum prolactin (r = +0.21).

Table 2 shows weekly serum and saliva haloperidol concentrations, saliva-to-serum haloperidol ratios, and serum prolactin
levels in three chronically medicated patients studied repeatedly
during pharmacokinetic steady-state conditions.   For the three
subjects, serum haloperidol concentrations were relatively stable,
but saliva haloperidol concentrations were more variable, particularly for subjects 25 and 27.   The saliva-to-serum haloperidol
ratios also were relatively constant within each subject, except
for sample 6 of subject 25 and sample 2 of subject 27.

Table 2. Weekly serum and saliva haloperidol (HAL)
concentrations, saliva-to-serum HAL ratios, and serum
prolactin (PRL) concentrations in three chronically medicated
patients during pharmacokinetic steady-state conditions

Subject 25 - 10 mg haloperidol per day

Sample	Serum HAL (μg l^{-1})	Saliva HAL (μg l^{-1})	Saliva-to-serum ratio	Serum PRL (μg l^{-1})
1	41	10	0.24	146
2	22	5	0.23	166
3	42	28	0.67	136
4	21	4	0.19	131
5	25	8	0.32	157
6	64	73	1.14	179
7	30	24	0.80	151
8	25	13	0.52	142
Range	21-64	4-73	0.23-1.14	131-179

Subject 26 - 5 mg haloperidol per day

Sample	Serum HAL (μg l^{-1})	Saliva HAL (μg l^{-1})	Saliva-to-serum ratio	Serum PRL (μg l^{-1})
1	7	3	0.43	24
2	4	3	0.75	14
3	12	6	0.50	41
4	5	3	0.60	22
Range	4-12	3-6	0.43-0.75	14-41

Subject 27 - 5 mg haloperidol per day

Sample	Serum HAL (μg l^{-1})	Saliva HAL (μg l^{-1})	Saliva-to-serum ratio	Serum PRL (μg l^{-1})
1	12	26	2.17	17
2	21	500	23.8	24
3	28	142	5.07	37
4	20	50	2.50	15
Range	12-28	26-500	2.17-23.8	15-37

Table 3 shows the within-subject correlations between serum and saliva haloperidol, serum haloperidol and serum prolactin, and saliva haloperidol and serum prolactin for the three subjects of table 2. The within-subjects serum-to-saliva correlations were comparable to the across-subjects correlation of these two measures (r = +0.70). The saliva-to-serum haloperidol ratios for each of the three subjects also were relatively stable. Excluding sample 6 (subject 25) and sample 2 (subject 27), the within-subjects haloperidol ratios were less variable than the across-subjects haloperidol ratios (table 1). In contrast to the saliva-to-serum drug correlations, both the serum and saliva haloperidol-to-prolactin correlations were much higher within subjects than they were across subjects (see above).

Table 3. Within-subject correlations among serum and saliva
          haloperidol (HAL) and serum prolactin (PRL)

Correlations	Subject 25	Subject 26	Subject 27
Serum HAL vs Saliva HAL	r = +0.87	r = +0.88	r = +0.65
Serum HAL vs Serum PRL	r = +0.61	r = +0.98	r = +0.73
Saliva HAL vs Serum PRL	r = +0.41	r = +0.84	r = +0.60

DISCUSSION

The present study confirms and extends the work of Yamazumi and Miura (1981) on saliva haloperidol concentrations. Although the haloperidol RIA used by those investigators probably measured reduced haloperidol as well as haloperidol itself (Rubin and Poland, 1981), the results of their study are similar to ours. They found a positive across-subjects correlation between saliva and serum haloperidol concentrations (r = +0.75) which was similar to that found in our subjects (r = +0.70). In addition, many of their subjects showed saliva-to-serum haloperidol ratios of 5 or more, which also is comparable to the ratios found in some of our subjects.

The presently accepted view is that, for many drugs, the salivary concentration reflects the unbound drug concentration in plasma, which presumably is the fraction of drug in blood that is pharmacologically active. For many drugs the correspondence between saliva and free plasma concentrations has been shown to be close (Horning *et al.*, 1977) and, depending upon the drug, the saliva concentration often is equal to or less than the free drug concentration in plasma, but not greater than the total drug concentration. Thus, drug saliva-to-plasma ratios are usually 1 or less.

However, as indicated by the present study, for most patients the saliva-to-serum haloperidol ratios were greater than 1, and thus the saliva haloperidol concentrations were obviously greater than the amount of free haloperidol in serum, which is approximately 8% of the total (Forsman and Ohman, 1977). Part of the reason for the elevated saliva haloperidol concentrations is due to trapping of haloperidol in its ionic form. Saliva generally is more acidic than plasma, so that a greater percentage of the haloperidol in saliva is positively charged and not able to diffuse back into blood. However, haloperidol has a pK_a of 8.25, so that even at a saliva pH of 6, the trapping effect would not account entirely for the high saliva concentrations in some of the patients. Interestingly, chlorpromazine and desmethylimipramine also are concentrated in saliva. Chlorpromazine sequesters in saliva up to concentrations 100-fold higher than that found in plasma (May *et al.*, 1981), and desmethylimipramine concentrations in saliva can be up to 16 times higher than serum concentrations (Cooper *et al.*, 1981). Again, the free concentrations of both chlorpromazine and desmethylimipramine are 10% or less. The reasons for the high saliva concentrations of these three psychoactive drugs are unknown.

We previously have found a significant correlation between serum haloperidol and serum prolactin levels in chronically medicated patients (Rubin *et al.*, 1980; Rubin and Poland, 1981; Poland and Rubin, 1981). However, in the present study we found no significant across-subjects correlation between serum haloperidol and serum prolactin. The large inter-subject variability in the prolactin response to neuroleptic drug administration may account in part for this finding (Rubin and Hays, 1980). Although only three subjects were studied, the within-subjects correlations between serum haloperidol and serum prolactin were much higher.

Prolactin concentrations were measured to determine if saliva haloperidol correlated better with serum prolactin than did serum haloperidol. If this were so, then saliva levels might in some way have reflected free serum haloperidol concentrations. However, saliva haloperidol correlated less well with serum prolactin than did serum haloperidol, suggesting that saliva haloperidol is not a good measure of pharmacologically relevant haloperidol concentrations. More specifically, subject 27 had a saliva haloperidol concentration which fell from 500 μg 1^{-1} in sample 2 to 142 μg 1^{-1} in sample 3, while serum haloperidol concentrations increased 33% between sample 2 and sample 3 (table 2). The corresponding serum prolactin concentrations also increased between samples 2 and 3, showing a positive relationship with serum haloperidol but a negative relationship with saliva haloperidol. These data also suggest that saliva haloperidol is not a good reflection of serum free haloperidol, but additional studies need to be performed on larger samples of patients before this issue can be settled.

Acknowledgements

This work was supported in part by McNeil Pharmaceutical, Spring House, PA, and NIMH Research Scientist Development Award MH 37363 (to RTR). We thank Mrs Leslie Land and Mrs Bella Forster for excellent technical assistance and Mrs Debbie Hanaya for outstanding editorial assistance.

REFERENCES

Cooper, T.B., Bark, N. and Simpson, G.M. (1981). Prediction of steady state plasma and saliva levels of desmethylimipramine using a single dose, single time point procedure. Psychopharmacology, 74, 115-21

Forsman, A. and Ohman, R. (1977). Studies on serum protein binding of haloperidol. Curr. Ther. Res., 21, 245-55

Forsman, A. and Ohman, R. (1979). Interindividual variation of clinical response to haloperidol. In Biological Psychiatry Today (ed. J. Obiols, C. Ballus, E. Gonzalez Monclus and J. Pujol), Elsevier/North-Holland, Amsterdam, pp. 949-54

Hays, S.E., Poland, R.E. and Rubin, R.T. (1980). Prolactin releasing potencies of antipsychotic and related nonantipsychotic compounds in female rats: relation to clinical potencies. J. Pharmacol. Exp. Ther., 214, 362-7

Horning, M.G., Brown, L., Nowlin, J., Lertratanangkoon, K., Kellaway, P. and Zion T.E. (1977). Use of saliva in therapeutic drug monitoring. Clin. Chem., 23, 157-64

Jacobs, K.W. (1976). A table for the determination of experimentwise error rate (alpha) from independent observations. Ed. Psychol. Measur., 36, 899-903

May, P.R.A., Van Putten, T., Jenden, D.J., Yale, C. and Dixon, W.J. (1981). Chlorpromazine levels and the outcome of treatment in schizophrenic patients. Arch. Gen. Psychiatry, 38, 202-7

Poland, R.E. and Rubin, R.T. (1981). Radioimmunoassay of haloperidol in human serum: correlation of serum haloperidol with serum prolactin. Life Sci., 29, 1837-45

Poland, R.E. and Rubin, R.T. (1982). Saliva cortisol levels following dexamethasone administration in endogenously depressed patients. Life Sci., 30, 177-81

Rubin, R.T., Forsman, A., Heykants, J., Ohman, R., Tower, B. and Michiels, M. (1980). Serum haloperidol determinations in psychiatric patients. Arch. Gen. Psychiatry, 37, 1069-74

Rubin, R.T. and Hays, S.E. (1980). The prolactin secretory response to neuroleptic drugs: mechanisms, applications and limitations. Psychoneuroendocrinology, 5, 121-37

Rubin, R.T. and Poland, R.E. (1981). Serum haloperidol determinations and their contribution to the treatment of schizophrenia. In <u>Clinical Pharmacology in Psychiatry; Neuroleptic and Antidepressant Research</u> (ed. E. Usdin, S.G. Dahl, L.F. Gram and O. Lingjaerde), Macmillan, London, pp. 217-25

Stephen, K.W., McCrossan, J., Mackenzie, D., Macfarlane, C.B. and Speirs, C.F. (1980). Factors determining the passage of drugs from blood into saliva. <u>Br. J. Clin. Pharmacol</u>., 9, 51-5

Yamazumi, S. and Miura, S. (1981). Haloperidol concentrations in saliva and serum: determination by the radioimmunoassay method. <u>Int. Pharmacopsychiat</u>., 16, 174-83

Zivin, J.A. and Bartko, J.J. (1976). Statistics for disinterested scientists. <u>Life Sci</u>., 18, 15-26

Section Four

Clinical Pharmacokinetics of Lithium and Antidepressants

Significance of the serum lithium concentration and the treatment regimen for wanted and unwanted effects of lithium treatment

Mogens Schou[1]

INTRODUCTION

Lithium (Li) treatment was the first psychiatric therapy to be monitored through determination of serum concentrations of the drug. In the beginning this served to guard against overdosage and poisoning, but later it was used to ensure sufficient levels for achievement of effect. When Li started being used for prophylactic purposes, i.e. for prevention or alleviation of manic-depressive recurrences, the monitoring procedure became particularly important, because under these circumstances no symptoms were present, and dosage adjustment could therefore not be based on clinical assessment.

SERUM LITHIUM UNDER STANDARDIZED CONDITIONS

The lithium ion is absorbed readily from the gastrointestinal tract; it is not bound to proteins; it penetrates into tissues with varying rapidities; and its apparent distribution volume corresponds to about 70% of the body. Elimination takes place almost exclusively through the kidneys with an elimination half-life of about 15-30 h.

The Li concentration in blood serum is used for monitoring purposes. The serum concentration is clearly not identical with the Li concentration in those - unknown - brain cells in which the ion exerts its therapeutic and prophylactic actions, but there is reason to suppose that the serum concentration can be used as at least an indicator of that concentration.

Owing to differences in the rates of Li absorption, distribution and elimination, the serum Li concentration fluctuates throughout the day with peak values 2-4 h after each intake, followed by gradual and largely exponential fall until the next

---
[1]The Psychopharmacology Research Unit, Aarhus University Institute of Psychiatry and the Psychiatric Hospital, DK-8240 Risskov, Denmark.

193

intake. Administration with one or two daily intakes is customary.
Studies carried out by Amdisen in our Institute (Amdisen, 1980)
indicate that the serum concentration which is best suited for
monitoring purposes is that obtained in blood samples drawn in the
morning 12 h after the last intake of Li. At this time the serum
concentration is least influenced by individual differences in
gastrointestinal absorption and renal elimination. The samples
should be drawn under steady-state conditions, i.e. about one week
after start of treatment and after dosage changes. When, in the
following, I use the terms 'serum Li' or 'serum Li concentration'
without further qualification, I am referring to the serum concentration determined under these standardized circumstances.

It has been debated whether the Li concentration in erythro-
cytes might reflect the Li concentration in brain cells better
than does the serum Li concentration, and erythrocyte Li levels or
erythrocyte/plasma Li ratios have been suggested as predictors of
response to Li or of Li toxicity. However, the evidence presented
in support of these notions has, in my opinion, not been sufficiently strong to justify the rather elaborate procedure of
erythrocyte Li determinations as a routine procedure.

Determination of the Li concentration in saliva has also been
proposed as an aid in treatment monitoring, especially for remote
parts of developing countries where the drawing of blood samples
might present difficulties. The proposal has in fact been made
many times, but I do not know of any place where the procedure is
in fact used.

SERUM LITHIUM RESPONSE CURVE FOR PROPHYLACTIC EFFECT

Whereas in pharmacology in general it is customary to deal with
dose-response curves, we can, when Li treatment is concerned,
advantageously replace these with serum Li - response curves,
because the renal Li clearance shows such pronounced individual
variation that different patients may require markedly different
Li dosages in order to achieve the same serum Li level. Response
to Li may be either wanted or unwanted. I shall deal first with
wanted response, which in this connection means response to prophylactic Li treatment, i.e. prevention or alleviation of manic
and depressive relapses through Li administration over months and
years.

Figure 1 shows how a serum Li - response curve for prophylactic effect *might* look, but it should be emphasized that what is
shown is a schematic approximation based on uncertain and mostly
retrospective information. It corresponds largely to the graph
published by Baastrup (1980), which shows serum Li concentrations
in 75 patients given successful Li treatment. The curve shown
here takes into account that some patients do not respond to Li.

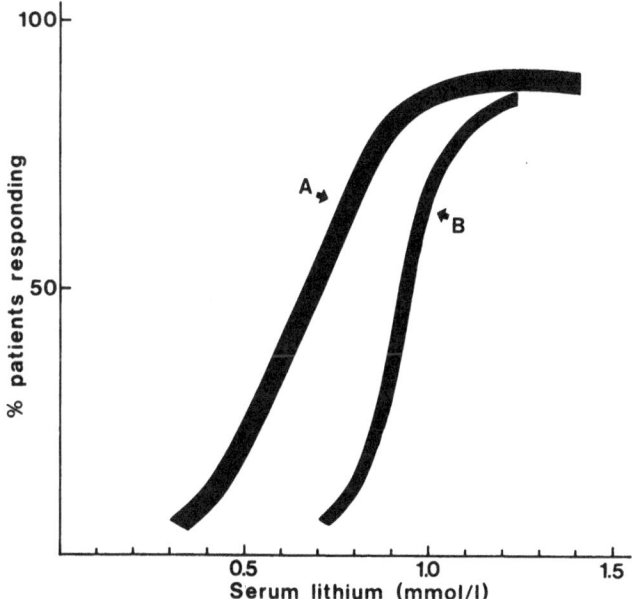

Figure 1. Serum lithium response curve for the prophylactic effect of lithium (curve A) and for lithium-induced polyuria (curve B). The graphs are schematic approximations.

The exact shape and location of a serum Li – response curve can be determined only through prospective studies in which patients are allocated randomly to different serum Li levels over the expected effective concentration range and maintained at these levels for sufficiently long periods to permit calculation of degrees of prophylactic effectiveness. Such studies involve considerable practical difficulties, and their ethical justification seems debatable.

A lower limit for effective serum Li levels of about 0.4 mmol 1^{-1} corresponds to Baastrup's experiences and is also in accordance with data presented by Hullin (1981). His study was prospective and showed that patients maintained at serum Li levels below 0.4 mmol 1^{-1} had a markedly higher frequency of relapse than patients maintained at higher serum Li levels.

An upper limit is more difficult to establish because of the increasing frequency of side-effects with increasing dosage and serum levels, but there is at least no evidence to support the notion of further prophylactic benefit at levels higher than about 1.1-1.3 mmol 1^{-1} nor of a 'therapeutic window' with falling efficiency at higher levels. None of Baastrup's successfully treated patients had serum levels higher than 1.1 mmol 1^{-1} and curve A has accordingly been drawn between the points 0.4 and 1.1 mmol 1^{-1}.

The relationship between serum Li and prophylactic outcome may, in fact, not be quite so simple. Sarantidis and Waters (1981) found that patients with an excellent prophylactic response had a higher average serum Li level (0.74 mmol 1^{-1}) than patients with only a fair prophylactic response (average serum Li 0.63 mmol 1^{-1}), but then they found that patients with a poor response also had a high level (0.79 mmol 1^{-1}), possibly because in these patients the dosage had been 'pushed' in order to achieve effect but without this actually being obtained. Sashidharan *et al.* (1982) studied serum Li levels from 53 patients with varying outcomes of prophylactic Li treatment and found that the levels for both those with poor outcome and those with good outcome spread over the full range between 0.3 and 1.3 mmol 1^{-1}. In fact, those with a favorable outcome spent significantly less time at serum Li levels above 0.9 mmol 1^{-1} than did those with a poor outcome; an interpretation of this finding is made difficult by the retrospective nature of the study.

Curve A in figure 1 is drawn in such a way that it becomes horizontal at a level lower than 100% response. This merely reflects that some patients do not respond to the treatment. The frequency of non-response, partial or total, is difficult to estimate, because it depends so much on the wideness of indications on which Li treatment is started.

SERUM LITHIUM RESPONSE CURVES FOR SIDE-EFFECTS

Serum Li - response curves for side-effects of Li are generally located at a somewhat higher concentration range than that of the serum Li response curve for wanted effects. This is fortunate for the patients.

In figure 1, curve B has been superimposed on curve A. Curve B might, in principle, represent any of the Li-induced side-effects; as shown here it reflects the situation for one of the more frequent side-effects of long-term Li treatment, namely impairment of renal water reabsorption. As before, we are not dealing with a precisely 'titrated' curve but rather with a schematic diagram which reflects the outcome of different studies with different approaches.

Various measures are available of the extent to which Li treatment inhibits the response of the distal tubules and collecting ducts to the action of the antidiuretic hormone. Vestergaard and Amdisen (1981) determined maximum urine osmolality after administration of a vasopressin analog, DDAVP (desmopressin acetate), and introduced this value as the dependent variable in a multiple regression analysis with the following predictor variables: age, sex, serum Li, Li dosage, duration of Li treatment, concomitant treatment with neuroleptic drugs, and concomitant treatment with antidepressant drugs. Data from 147 patients were employed. The renal concentrating ability, as expressed by the maximum urine osmolality, was found to be significantly and positively correlated with the serum Li concentration and with the duration of the Li treatment, but not with any of the other independent variables. The serum Li concentration ranged from 0.4 to 1.1 mmol l^{-1}, average value 0.87 mmol l^{-1}. In another study Vestergaard and Thomsen (1981) employed data from the same patient group for multiple regression analysis but now used as the dependent variable the expression V/CLi, where V is the urine flow and CLi is the renal Li clearance. This expression is a reliable indicator of water handling in the distal parts of the nephron (Thomsen, 1978; Thomsen *et al.*, 1981), and the multiple regression analysis once again showed significant association with the serum Li concentration and the duration of the Li treatment.

A third study indicating that the effect of Li on the distal parts of the nephron is closely associated with the serum Li concentration is that carried out by Penney *et al.* (1981). They demonstrated increased urinary excretion of arginine vasopressin, the antidiuretic hormone in man, and found the logarithm of the urine arginine vasopressin excretion significantly correlated with the serum Li concentration. In this study the serum Li concentration ranged from 0.4 to 1.2 mmol l^{-1} and averaged 0.63 mmol l^{-1}.

Confirmation of the location and of the steepness of the slope of curve B in figure 1 can further be obtained by comparison of polyuria frequencies in different clinics. It has been a striking observation in the Li-kidney studies of recent years that impairment of renal concentrating ability occurs with high frequency in some clinics and with low frequency in others. Vestergaard and Amdisen (1981) found the renal concentrating ability markedly decreased in their patients, treated at the Psychiatric Hospital in Aarhus. Hullin *et al.* (1979) from Leeds found only a moderate lowering of maximum urine osmolality in their Li-treated patients. Treatment duration was approximately the same in the two clinics, but the patients had been maintained at different serum Li levels: in Aarhus, at an average value of 0.85 mmol l^{-1}; in Leeds, at an average value of only 0.59 mmol l^{-1}. It seems likely that this 40% difference in serum level may have played at least a contributory role for the different affection of renal concentrating ability in the two patient groups.

In the Aarhus hospital, we have now taken notice of these findings and within recent years adjusted treatment guidelines so that patients are now maintained at serum levels which are about 25% lower than those employed previously. Rather than aiming at serum levels between 0.8 and 1.0 mmol l^{-1} we now adjust dosages to concentrations within the range 0.6-0.8 mmol l^{-1}, and it is our expectation for the coming years that prophylactic efficacy will remain largely unchanged but that Li-induced polyuria and perhaps other side-effects may become less frequent.

INDIVIDUAL ADJUSTMENT OF LITHIUM DOSAGES AND SERUM LITHIUM LEVELS

The therapeutic range of Li is, as indicated, rather narrow. Doses and serum Li concentrations required for therapeutic and prophylactic effect are not very much lower than concentrations which produce side-effects and there is often overlapping so that some patients can be kept free of relapses only at the cost of suffering side-effects such as tremor, weight gain, thirst and polyuria. It is therefore important that each patient is maintained at the serum Li concentration which is optimum for him or her, i.e. the concentration which produces a maximum of prophylactic protection with a minimum of side-effects. The curves in figure 1 indicate that 0.6-0.8 mmol 1^{-1} is a useful range to aim for initially in the treatment or in groups of patients, but it should be understood that for the individual patient the optimum range may be still narrower, and fine adjustment of dosages and serum Li levels to the individual optimum is a very important task for the physician. Since we are dealing with prophylactic treatment, such adjustment may take a long time, since dosage changes have to be followed by long periods of observation in order to see whether the desired result was obtained.

By 'fine' adjustment I really mean *fine*. Time and again I have been amazed at how much difference it may make for a patient's life quality, if his or her Li dosage is raised by as little as one-half or one Li tablet and the serum concentration correspondingly increased by one-tenth of a millimole per liter. This may take away slight but troublesome manic and depressive mood changes. In other cases a reduction of serum Li by one-tenth of a millimole per liter may effectively remove or reduce troublesome side-effects. It is perhaps difficult for patients and physicians to understand that such seemingly small changes can be so important, and I have sometimes wondered whether it would be didactically preferable if serum Li levels were presented in micromoles per liter rather than in millimoles per liter. A change of serum Li from 700 to 800 µmol 1^{-1} somehow looks more impressive than a change from 0.7 to 0.8 mmol 1^{-1}, and such a change may, as I have indicated, make all the difference for the patient's well-being.

SIGNIFICANCE OF THE TREATMENT REGIMEN

Li is usually administered in one or two, sometimes three, daily doses, and both conventional and slow-release or retard tablets

are in use. The choice of treatment regimen determines the course
of the serum Li concentration over the day. This is illustrated
in figure 2, which shows the mean serum Li concentration around
the clock in a group of patients from the Psychiatric Hospital in
Aarhus and in a group from the Psychiatric Clinic at
Rigshospitalet in Copenhagen. In Aarhus the patients had been
given slow-release tablets twice daily, morning and evening. In
Copenhagen they had been treated with conventional tablets given
once daily, in the evening. It will be noted that fluctuations
were much wider in the Copenhagen group, with the highest
concentrations more than three times the lowest, whereas in Aarhus
the highest value was only 1.4 times the lowest. One may also
note that in Aarhus the maximum value was reached 4-5 h after the
intake of Li, whereas in Copenhagen the peak value was reached
about 2 h after the intake.

Now, which of these two curves is clinically preferable?
This has been the subject of friendly debate between the two
clinics. We in Aarhus felt that the avoidance of high concentration peaks and hence of possible peak-associated side-effects
would offer most advantage. Our colleagues in Copenhagen felt
that the achievement of low concentrations before the next intake
of Li would offer the organism a chance of restitution that might

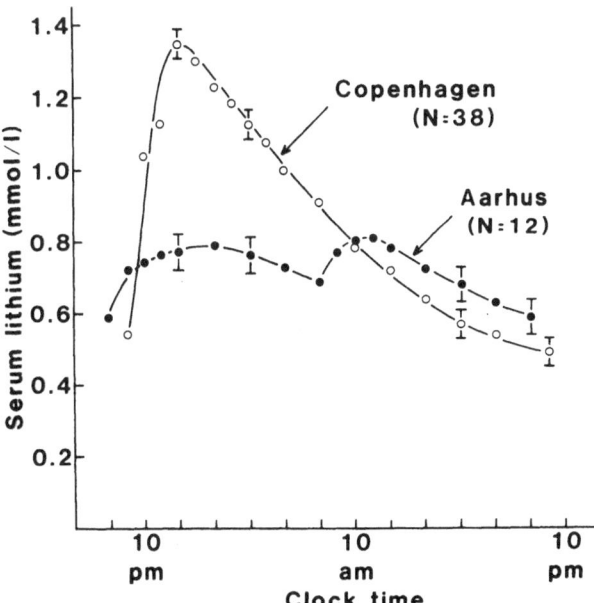

Figure 2. Mean serum lithium concentrations around the clock in
          two groups of patients given different treatment regi-
          mens (see text). Data from Lauritsen *et al.* (1981)

outweigh any disadvantages of the high peaks. Last year we carried out a quantitative comparison with respect to the degree of polyuria in the two groups (Schou et al., 1982). The comparison was based on the assumption, unproven but not unreasonable, that prophylactic efficacy was roughly the same in the two clinics. Since the two groups differed as regards various patient and treatment features, we subjected the data to multiple regression analysis with urine flow as the dependent variable and with age, sex, treatment duration, and serum Li as predictor variables; to this we added the treatment regimen as a further predictor variable, allotting the dummy values of 0 and 1 to each of the two regimens.

I do not mind admitting that the outcome of the study came as a surprise to both clinics (table 1). Each of our groups had expected its own treatment regimen to produce less polyuria than the other regimen. The data showed fairly pronounced polyuria in both groups, median urine flows being between 2 and 3 l per 24 h. Our patients in Aarhus in fact had more polyuria than the patients in Copenhagen, but the difference was not large and only marginally significant. A significant difference appeared when we compared values for the more specific indicator of distal water handling, V/CLi (Thomsen, 1978), and only with this expression as the dependent variable did the treatment regimen add significantly to the explained variation in the multiple regression analysis.

These results have shaken my belief in the superiority of the Aarhus regimen, at least as far as polyuria is concerned, but it has perhaps not quite convinced me that the Copenhagen regimen is

Table 1. Patient and treatment features, urine flow and distal water handling (mean values) in two groups of patients given different lithium treatment regimens (data from Schou et al., 1982)

	Aarhus	Copenhagen
Treatment regimen	Slow-release, twice daily	Conventional, once daily
Number of patients	95	28
F/M	45/50	21/7
Age (years)	43	51
Body weight (kg)	74	70
Duration of treatment (years)	6.5	8.0
12h-SLi (mmol l^{-1})	0.82	0.87
Creatinine clearance (ml min^{-1})	99	90
Urine flow (l/24 h)	2.83	2.38*
V/CLi	0.099	0.076**

*$p = 0.05$; **$p < 0.05$.

better. Definitive conclusions in this respect must await within-clinic trials with random allocation of treatment regimens and with assessment of not only side-effects but also therapeutic and prophylactic effects of the treatment. Perhaps in the future we shall see much less polyuria and polydipsia in our Li-treated patients in Aarhus as we reduce the Li doses and serum levels by about 25%.

EPILOGUE

Determination of serum Li concentrations is a useful aid for monitoring and guidance of Li treatment, but the values reported by the laboratory should not be accorded magical significance. The patient's mental and physical well-being is more important for the choice of dosage level than is the location of the serum Li concentration at one or the other end of the recommended range. Individual adjustment of the dosage to the optimum level is the essential feature; maintenance of this level can then be supported through serum Li determinations.

REFERENCES

Amdisen, A. (1980). Monitoring lithium dose levels: clinical aspects of serum lithium estimation. In Handbook of Lithium Therapy (ed. F.N. Johnson), MTP Press, Lancaster, pp. 196-9

Baastrup, P.C. (1980). Lithium in the prophylactic treatment of recurrent affective disorders. In Handbook of Lithium Therapy (ed. F.N. Johnson), MTP Press, Lancaster, pp. 26-38

Hullin, R.P. (1981). Relationships between plasma lithium levels and clinical and biological responses. In Recent Advances in Neuropsychopharmacology (ed. B. Angrist *et al.*), Pergamon, New York, pp. 373-82

Hullin, R.P., Coley, V.P., Birch, N.J., Thomas, T.H. and Morgan, D.B. (1979). Renal function after long-term treatment with lithium. Br. Med. J., 2, 1457-9

Lauritsen, B.J., Mellerup, E.T., Plenge, P., Rasmussen, S., Vestergaard, P. and Schou, M. (1981). Serum lithium concentrations around the clock with different treatment regimens and the diurnal variation of the renal lithium clearance. Acta Psychiat. Scand., 64, 314-19

Penney, M.D., Hullin, R.P., Srinivasan, D.P. and Morgan, D.B. (1981). The relationship between plasma lithium and the renal responsiveness to arginine vasopressin in man. Clin. Sci., 61, 793-5

Sarantidis, D. and Waters, B. (1981). Predictors of lithium prophylaxis effectiveness. Progr. Neuro-Psychopharmacol., 5, 507-11

Sashidharan, S.P., McGuire, R.J. and Glen, A.I.M. (1982). Plasma
    lithium levels and therapeutic outcome in the prophylaxis of
    affective disorders: a retrospective study. Br. J.
    Psychiatry, 140, 619-22
Schou, M., Amdisen, A., Thomsen, K., Vestergaard, P., Hetmar, O.,
    Mellerup, E.T., Plenge, P. and Rafaelsen, O.J. (1982).
    Lithium treatment regimen and renal water handling: the
    significance of dosage pattern and tablet type examined
    through comparison of results from two clinics with different
    treatment regimens. Psychopharmacology, 77, 387-90
Thomsen, K. (1978). Renal handling of lithium at non-toxic and
    toxic serum lithium levels: a review. Dan. Med. Bull., 25,
    106-15
Thomsen, K., Holstein-Rathlou, N.-H. and Leyssac, P.O. (1981).
    Comparison of three measures of proximal tubular reabsorp-
    tion: lithium clearance, occlusion time, and micropuncture.
    Am. J. Physiol., 241, F348-55
Vestergaard, P. and Amdisen, A. (1981). Lithium treatment and
    kidney function: a follow-up study of 237 patients in long-
    term treatment. Acta Psychiat. Scand., 63, 333-45
Vestergaard, P. and Thomsen, K. (1981). Renal side effects of
    lithium: the importance of the serum lithium level. Psycho-
    pharmacology, 72, 203-4

Hydroxy metabolite concentrations: role of renal clearance

William Z.Potter[1], Elizabeth A.Lane[1] and
Matthew V.Rudorfer[1]

INTRODUCTION

It is generally emphasized that basic lipophilic psychoactive drugs are cleared primarily through metabolism, not renal clearance (Potter *et al.*, 1981). Kidney disease or other sources of alterations of renal clearance are not reported to affect plasma concentrations of drugs such as the tricyclic antidepressants, although the clearance of unmetabolized drugs such as lithium will clearly be affected (Amdisen, 1977). From any but an academic point of view this would be the limit of interest in renal clearance if extensively metabolized parent drugs were the only biologically active forms.

We have known for years however (reviewed in Garattini *et al.*, 1975) that many psychoactive drugs are metabolized to biologically active compounds. More recently it has become established that hydroxylated but unconjugated biologically active metabolites exist in significant steady-state concentrations both in plasma and brain (for review, see Potter and Calil, 1981). The majority of evidence supporting a pharmacodynamic role of hydroxy metabolites, both in terms of therapeutic and side- or toxic effects, stems from investigations with the tricyclic antidepressants (TCAs), although a study of direct clinical efficacy has only been obtained for a hydroxyphenothiazine (Kleinman *et al.*, 1978). This paper focuses primarily on the TCAs but will consider relevant data from studies with another class of basic lipophilic drugs, the beta-adrenergic antagonists.

It was shown over a decade ago that in man the majority of a dose of TCA was metabolized to hydroxy metabolites which were excreted in the urine (Crammer *et al.*, 1969). A few years later,

[1]Clinical Psychobiology Branch, National Institute of Mental Health, and
Pharmacological Sciences Program, National Institute of General Medical Sciences,
Bethesda, Maryland 20205, USA.

203

Alexanderson and Borgå (1973), as part of a remarkably comprehensive series of studies on nortriptyline pharmacokinetics at the Karolinska Institute, showed that there was a high renal clearance of unconjugated as well as conjugated 10-hydroxynortriptyline. Subsequent studies carried out through the same laboratory have replicated and extended this finding (Kragh-Sørensen *et al.*, 1977; Mellström *et al.*, 1981).

More recently, numerous laboratories almost concurrently demonstrated that unconjugated hydroxy metabolites of TCAs might have clinical relevance in light of their preclinical biological activity and the documentation of significant steady-state concentrations in man (reviewed in Potter and Calil, 1981). Table 1 shows relative steady-state concentrations of biologically active hydroxy metabolites following a variety of TCAs. In order to carry out mechanistic pharmacodynamic investigations with TCAs, it is necessary to understand better the determinants of the steady-state concentrations of their hydroxy metabolites. Our special emphasis here is on the renal clearance of these compounds. This, however, can only be understood in terms of an overall pharmacokinetic model which is presented below.

Table 1. Average steady-state concentrations of tricyclic antidepressants and active metabolites. Concentrations are corrected to a 100 mg daily dose

Administered drug	Average concentration for 100 mg/day dose			Reference
	AT	NT	OH–NT	
Amitriptyline (AT)	58	62	–	Potter *et al.* (1981)
Nortriptyline (NT)	–	110	–	Potter *et al.* (1981)
		131	172	Kragh-Sørensen *et al.* (1977)
	IMI	DMI	OH–DMI	
Imipramine (IMI)	45	92	35*	Potter *et al.* (1982)
Desipramine (DMI)	39	55		Potter *et al.* (1981)
	CI	DCI	OH–DCI	
Chlorimipramine (CI)	61	128	63	Linnoila *et al.* (1982)
	42	99	–	Träskmann *et al.* (1979)

OH–NT = 10-hydroxynortriptyline   * Concentrations in children
OH–DMI = 2-hydroxydesipramine
OH–DCI = 8-hydroxychlordesipramine
DCI = desmethylchlorimipramine

THE DETERMINANTS OF METABOLITE CONCENTRATION

In a number of recent studies, the variability in clearance of a drug to a particular metabolite (Mellström *et al.*, 1981) or the elimination clearance of a metabolite (Kitanaka *et al.*, 1982) have been studied with a view to making generalized statements about variability in metabolite concentration. None of these clearances, alone, determines the variability in metabolite concentration. Rather, all of them must be integrated into an overall relationship with all of the clearances that affect metabolite concentration:

$$C_m = \frac{fm_{p \to m} \times (\text{dose rate})_p}{Cl_m} \qquad (1)$$

$$= \frac{Cl_{p \to m} \times (\text{dose rate})_p}{(Cl_{p \to m} + Cl_{p \to \text{other}}) \, Cl_m} \qquad (2)$$

where C_m = steady-state concentration of metabolite, $fm_{p \to m}$ = fraction of parent drug (p) metabolized to the metabolite of interest (m), (dose rate)$_p$ = constant dose rate of parent drug, Cl_m = elimination clearance of metabolite, $Cl_{p \to m}$ = clearance of parent drug to metabolite (m), and $Cl_{p \to \text{other}}$ = clearance of parent drug to other metabolites.

First, variability in the clearance of parent drug to metabolite causes variability in metabolite concentration in the same way that it causes variability in fraction metabolized to that metabolite. Assuming that the clearances of parent drug to this metabolite and to other metabolites vary independently, the fraction metabolized varies directly with clearance of parent drug to metabolite, but in a non-linear manner. That is, higher values of this clearance result in a higher value of the numerator and the denominator as seen by inspection of equation (2). The impact of high values of clearance of parent drug to metabolite upon fraction metabolized, and therefore upon metabolite concentration, depends upon the *absolute value* of fraction metabolized. This relationship is also crucial to understanding the effect of wide variations in rate of clearance to concentrations of metabolite. Although the clearance of parent drug to metabolite can have any value, the fraction metabolized is limited to values between 0 and 1. Furthermore, if one begins with high absolute values of fraction metabolized, large variability in clearance of parent drug to the metabolite causes much less variability in fraction metabolized (figure 1). For example, if the ultimate fraction metabolized is approximately 0.9, a two-times range in rate of clear-

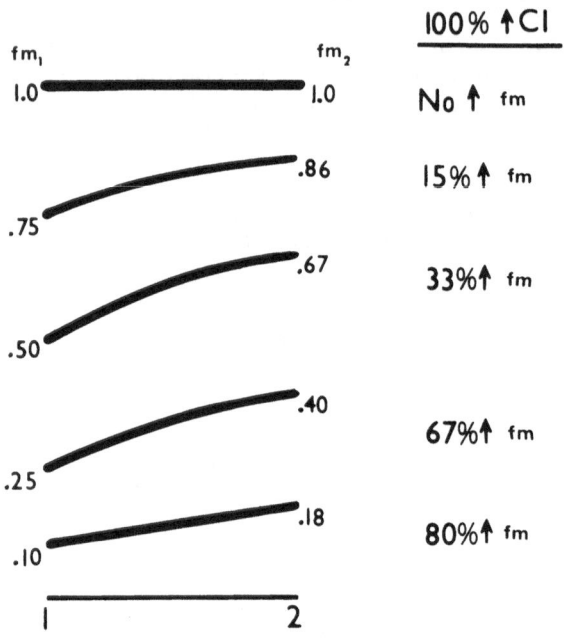

RELATIVE HYDROXYLATION CLEARANCE

Figure 1. The range of fraction of parent drug metabolized to
         hydroxy metabolite for a twofold range in clearance of
         parent drug to hydroxy metabolite. Note that at larger
         values of *fm* a 100% higher hydroxylation clearance
         corresponds to a smaller percentage increase in *fm*.

ance of parent drug to the metabolite will produce very little
variability in fraction metabolized (i.e. 0.90 to 0.95). On the
other hand, if the usual fraction metabolized to a specific metabolite is in the range of 0.10, a two-times range in the rate of
clearance of parent drug to the metabolite will correspond to an
almost twofold range in fraction metabolized (0.10 to 0.18).

Secondly, variability in the elimination clearance of the
metabolite affects metabolite concentration in an inverse manner
(equations (1) and (2)). If the metabolite is eliminated by a
renal and a metabolic route and it is appropriate to sum the
respective clearances, the metabolite concentration becomes:

$$C_m = \frac{fm_{p \to m} \times (\text{dose rate})_p}{Cl_{m, \text{renal}} + Cl_{m, \text{metabolic}}} \qquad (3)$$

For instance, age-dependent decreases in renal function usually result in similar decreases in the renal clearances of metabolites. The impact of a decrease in renal clearance of a metabolite upon the metabolite concentration depends upon the relative values of metabolite renal clearance ($Cl_{m,renal}$) and metabolite clearance by metabolism ($Cl_{m,metabolic}$); that is, upon the fraction of the metabolite excreted unchanged. The denominator of equation (3) may thus be considered as being composed of fractional pathways of metabolite clearance which must add up to 1.0. Hence, if 50% of the metabolite is usually excreted unchanged (i.e. 50% via $Cl_{m,renal}$) then 50% will be metabolized. A comparison population in which renal function is reduced to 10% of normal, such as the aged, could proportionately reduce the fraction excreted unchanged in urine in this case from 50% to 5%. The proportional value of the denominator would now be 0.05 + 0.50 or 0.55. The reciprocal of this is 1.82; thus, a 10-fold reduction in fraction excreted in the urine would increase the metabolite concentration by 82% (equation (3)). If only 10% of the metabolite were excreted unchanged and renal clearance were decreased to 10% of normal, the metabolite concentration would, however, only be about 10% higher (reciprocal of [(0.10 x 0.10)+ 0.90]).

To summarize, the metabolite concentration

(a) varies directly, but non-linearly, with clearance of parent drug to the metabolite;
(b) is more sensitive to variability in clearance of parent drug to the metabolite when the fraction of parent drug metabolized via that pathway is small;
(c) varies inversely with renal clearance of metabolite;
(d) is most sensitive to variability in renal clearance when the fraction of metabolite excreted unchanged is large.

APPLICATION TO ACTIVE METABOLITES OF TRICYCLIC ANTIDEPRESSANTS

Nortriptyline

The hydroxylation of nortriptyline has been shown to range over 10-fold when poor and efficient hydroxylators were compared (Mellström *et al.*, 1981). The fraction of nortriptyline metabolized to hydroxynortriptyline was also reported to be higher in the efficient hydroxylators (60-75%) than in the poor hydroxylators (24-49%). The 10-fold range in hydroxylation clearance, therefore, corresponded to a threefold range in fraction metabolized. These figures are consistent with the clearance of parent drug by other pathways being constant between subjects (figure 1). On the basis of equation (1) one might expect this three-times variability in fraction metabolized to be reflected in a three-times variability in steady-state metabolite concentration (or in area under the curve (AUC) of metabolite after a single dose). However, no such relationship between metabolite concentration and hydroxylation clearance was observed (Mellström et al., 1981). One must conclude that the metabolite AUC was not correlated with hydroxylation clearance (CL_m) because of the independent way in which the elimination clearance of hydroxynortriptyline varied.

In the same set of data, we see that 30-60% of hydroxy-nortriptyline formed from nortriptyline was excreted unchanged. Therefore, age-dependent decreases in renal function in such a group would be expected to result in a maximum 40-200% increase in metabolite concentration as can be calculated from equation (3) according to the examples provided above. Such predicted increases are consistent with the relative elevation of the ratio of hydroxynortriptyline to nortriptyline reported by Bertilsson et al. (1979) in older subjects.

Desipramine

In an initial series of studies of concentrations of active forms of tricyclic antidepressant following drug treatment with desipramine (Kitanaka et al., 1982), we found elevated plasma concentrations of the 2-hydroxy metabolite of desipramine in a group of elderly depressed women as compared to younger patients and healthy volunteers. We also observed a marked increase in the ratio of hydroxydesipramine to desipramine in the elderly as reported for the hydroxynortriptyline-to-nortriptyline ratio. This finding was associated with a markedly diminished renal clearance of hydroxydesipramine in the older patients (figure 2). In this study, the fraction of hydroxydesipramine excreted unchanged was not calculated so that it is not possible to use equation (3) to calculate the predicted increase in the plasma concentration of hydroxydesipramine given the observed decrease in renal clearance.

Recently, we have explored the issue of the renal clearance of 2-hydroxydesipramine more fully in a prospective study. The preliminary results from this study are summarized here.

There were 27 subjects of whom 14 were female ranging in age from 20 to 58 years (mean of 36.4 ± 13.3 years). All but two were pre-menopausal. The remaining 13 male subjects ranged in age from 29 to 55 years, with a mean of 42.3 ± 8.4 years. Subjects revealed no medical or psychiatric abnormalities by history, physical examination or blood tests (including liver chemistry), and took no routine medication. None used alcohol on a daily basis. Two males were smokers, one smoking a pipe and the other smoking cigars.

A five-day protocol was conducted on an outpatient basis. On the first day, each subject took an oral dose of 100 mg desipra-mine after an overnight fast. Venous blood samples for desipramine

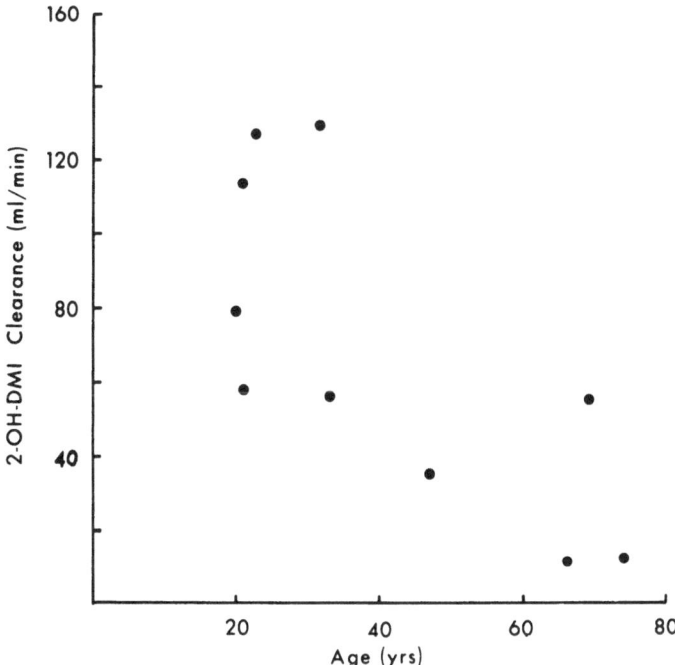

Figure 2.   Decreased renal clearance of 2-hydroxydesipramine with
age ($r = -0.73$, $p < 0.05$) for young normal volunteers
and young and old depressed patients (from Kitanaka *et
al.*, 1982).

and 2-hydroxydesipramine concentration were drawn just before and
at intervals up to 96 h after the dose.   Disposable plastic
syringes and heparinized polypropylene tubes were used instead of
Vacutainers®.   Serial 24 h urine collections were performed by all
subjects for five days beginning with the time of dosage.

Plasma and urinary concentrations of desipramine and 2-
hydroxydesipramine were determined by the high-performance liquid
chromatography assay of Sutfin and Jusko (1979) with previously
described modifications (Kitanaka *et al.*, 1982).   Urine samples
were assayed both before and after overnight incubation with
glucuronidase (pH 4.5) at 37°C.

Renal clearance of hydroxydesipramine was calculated as the
total amount of this metabolite excreted unchanged in urine divided by the total AUC hydroxydesipramine in plasma.   For the first
27 subjects studied, mean clearance was 3.92 ± 1.14 ml min^{-1} kg^{-1}
with a range of 1.68 to 6.49 ml min^{-1} kg^{-1}.   There was a significant negative correlation ($r = -0.56$, $p < 0.005$) between age and
hydroxydesipramine renal clearance for the group as a whole, with

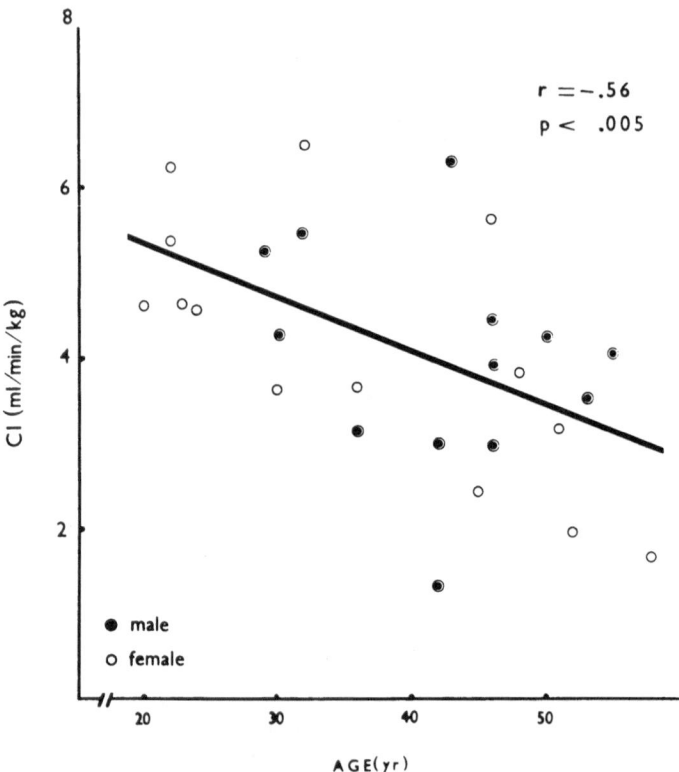

Figure 3. Decreased renal clearance with age for a group of 27
normal volunteers.   Open symbols = women; solid symbols
= men (r = –0.56, p < 0.005).

a pronounced sex difference (figure 3).   The 14 female subjects,
ranging in age from 20 to 58 years, showed a more marked correlation (r = –0.69, p < 0.01) than did the 13 males (29 to 55 years
of age) whose age-clearance association failed to reach significance (r = –0.30).
        Assuming that hydroxydesipramine is eliminated in urine only
in the unchanged form or conjugated to glucuronide, the fraction
of hydroxydesipramine eliminated unchanged in urine may be taken
as the amount of hydroxydesipramine excreted unchanged divided by
the   sum   of   unchanged   plus   glucuronidated   hydroxydesipramine
assayed in urine.   By this method, the fraction of hydroxy metabolite of desipramine excreted unchanged is 0.32 ± 0.09 in 21
subjects, slightly lower than has been reported for the 10-hydroxy
metabolite   of   nortriptyline   (Alexanderson   and   Borgå,   1973;
Mellström *et al.*, 1981) (table 2).   Given this range of the frac-

Table 2. Fraction of hydroxy metabolite excreted unconjugated
(single dose)

			Reference
10-OH-NT	0.47 ± 0.07	(N = 6)	Alexanderson and Borgå (1973)
	0.42 ± 0.12	(N = 8)	Mellström *et al.*(1981)
2-OH-DMI	0.32 ± 0.09	(N = 21)	This work

tion of hydroxydesipramine which is excreted unchanged (up to 50%), a one-half decrease in the average renal clearance of hydroxydesipramine over the 20-58 years age range should correspond to a 12-35% increase in the single dose or steady-state AUC of hydroxydesipramine.

In these subjects, the AUC of hydroxydesipramine did tend to increase with age. Significantly more of the subjects aged 42-58 years had a metabolite AUC greater than 600 ng ml^{-1} h compared with the subjects aged 20-32 years (χ^2, $p < 0.05$). The median hydroxydesipramine AUC for the older group was 768 ng ml^{-1} h (range 438 to 1634) and for the younger group was 565 ng ml^{-1} h (range 408 to 909), representing an average increase of 36% which is at the upper end of our prediction based on an average 50% reduction in hydroxydesipramine renal clearance.

The fraction of desipramine metabolized to hydroxydesipramine (fm) was obtained by summing the total amounts of unbound plus conjugated hydroxydesipramine excreted in the urine and dividing by the dose of desipramine. In 25 individuals, the mean fm was 0.38 ± 0.09, similar to that reported for nortriptyline (Alexanderson and Borgå, 1973; Mellström *et al.*, 1981) (table 3).

Therefore, the fraction of desipramine metabolized to hydroxydesipramine and, thereby, the hydroxydesipramine AUC is also sensitive to variability in the hydroxylation clearance of desipramine. Nevertheless, for this group of subjects, the fraction metabolized was apparently independent of hydroxylation

Table 3. Fraction of drug metabolized to hydroxy metabolite
(single dose)

				Reference
NT	10-OH-NT	0.49 ± 0.03	(N = 6)	Alexanderson and Borgå (1973)
		0.43 ± 0.18	(N = 8)	Mellström *et al.*(1981)
DMI	2-OH-DMI	0.38 ± 0.09	(N = 25)	This work

clearance, despite an eightfold range of hydroxylation clearance. This apparent independence is similar to that seen by Mellström *et al*. (1981) for the AUC of hydroxynortriptyline after nortriptyline.

Our findings that a large amount of unconjugated hydroxydesipramine is excreted unchanged and that there is substantial renal clearance of hydroxydesipramine add to the small, but similar, literature for other antidepressant or cardiovascular compounds. It was originally shown by Alexanderson and Borgå (1973) that the renal clearance of hydroxynortriptyline was over 100 ml min^{-1}. A mean renal clearance of 80.5 ml min^{-1} was reported for the same metabolite by Kragh-Sørensen *et al*. (1977). It was therefore expected (Potter *et al*., 1981) that the renal clearance of these hydroxy metabolites would be affected by processes which alter kidney function such as aging (Vestal, 1978). Thus, as mentioned above, there is a decreased renal clearance of hydroxydesipramine in elderly depressed patients accompanied by an increase in the plasma hydroxydesipramine-to-desipramine ratio at steady state (Kitanaka *et al*., 1982).

This was interpreted to mean that the rate of desipramine hydroxylation was not altered since desipramine concentrations were the same in the elderly as in younger populations. Also, as noted above, preliminary results from our subsequent, more detailed, investigation of single-dose desipramine pharmacokinetics support this interpretation although the age range was more limited. Higher plasma concentrations of the hydroxy metabolite of metoprolol, a beta-receptor antagonist used in cardiovascular disease, have also been reported in elderly versus young volunteers (Lundborg *et al*., 1982), a finding that has likewise been ascribed to the lowering of glomerular filtration rate (GFR) with age.

Little systematic data in this regard have been collected on subjects with other sources of decreased excretory function such as renal disease. Those which are available, however, are consistent with the results seen in healthy aging individuals. Renal clearance of hydroxymetoprolol correlated directly with GFR in four patients with impaired renal function (Hoffmann *et al*., 1980). In an initial study of 20 patients with chronic renal failure who were administered a single dose of nortriptyline, Dawling *et al*. (1981) found no changes in parent drug clearance or half-life in patients as compared to that in controls given the same dose. They did speculate that hydroxy metabolites of nortriptyline might accumulate during renal insufficiency and proceeded to demonstrate subsequently this phenomenon in some of these same patients (Braithwaite and Dawling, 1981). For a given dose of nortriptyline, mean plasma concentrations of unconjugated and, more markedly yet, of conjugated 10-hydroxynortriptyline, were higher in the renal patients than in healthy volunteers.

This finding is consistent with the pharmacokinetic model (equation (3)) since the clearance of conjugated 10-hydroxynortriptyline may be assumed to be dependent on excretion alone and not on further metabolism. Of course, a certain fraction of the conjugate could be excreted via bile as well as urine.

Returning to the plasma pharmacokinetics of biologically active metabolites, there is another detail to be considered and that is related to plasma binding. In the calculation of urinary clearances of hydroxy metabolites as described above, or as reported in the literature by dividing the excretion rate by the mean steady-state concentration of total (bound plus free) drug in plasma (Alexanderson and Borgå, 1973; Kragh-Sørensen *et al.*, 1977; Kitanaka *et al.*, 1982), allowance is not made for the fact that bound drug does not diffuse through the glomerulus. Use of free drug concentrations (at most 20% of total plasma hydroxy metabolite concentration (Potter and Calil, 1981)) in the denominator when computing clearance will yield at least a fivefold increase in calculated renal clearance. The resulting value of greater than 500 ml min^{-1} greatly exceeds GFR, indicating active secretion of unconjugated hydroxy tricyclic metabolite. Thus, factors interfering with active secretion, independent of age or renal failure, might also be expected to increase concentration of OH tricyclics selectively. Such possible specific effects on active secretion have not yet been investigated.

These observations also remind one that changes in the plasma binding of hydroxy metabolites can also affect their renal clearance. As described in the general case by Levy (1980), assuming that renal tubular secretion is a function of the free plasma concentration of compound and that secretion is not limited by the flow rate of plasma perfusing the renal tubules, then the renal clearance of total drug will be linearly and directly related to the free fraction of a compound. Although the free fraction of at least tertiary and secondary amine TCAs does not generally cover more than a twofold range (Potter *et al.*, 1981), there are sometimes extremes. Again, there is no direct evidence that this mechanism plays a significant role in the variability of the renal clearance of hydroxy metabolites of TCAs. One situation that might be expected to produce altered binding of some drugs, uremia, appears to have no effect on that of desipramine (Reidenberg *et al.*, 1971) or the structurally similar tetracyclic antidepressant, maprotiline (Lynn *et al.*, 1981) and may likewise have no effect on the binding of hydroxydesipramine. It will be interesting to see if patients with elevated α_1-acid glycoprotein who show increased binding of parent TCAs (Piafsky *et al.*, 1978) will also have a reduced free fraction of the active hydroxy metabolites. If so, one would predict decreased renal clearance of the hydroxy metabolite and a selective increase in its plasma concentration.

CONCLUSIONS

In summary, there are active hydroxy metabolites of TCAs which are
at least partially dependent on renal excretion for their elimination. Multiple factors can influence the renal clearance of
these active metabolites both at the level of glomerular filtration and active secretion. In real-life situations, however,
the less than 50% fraction of hydroxy TCA metabolites excreted
unchanged in most individuals limits the possible consequences of
major alterations in kidney function. At most, one is likely to
find a doubling of the unconjugated hydroxy TCA metabolite steady-
state concentration secondary to reduced renal clearance. Such an
increase would be likely to have significant pharmacodynamic
effects only for individuals in whom the hydroxy represents a
large proportion of total active compound. One would, therefore,
predict that alterations in urinary clearance might have the
greatest functional significance in patients treated with nortriptyline or amitriptyline since imipramine, desipramine and
chlorimipramine tend to produce relatively low steady-state concentrations of conjugated hydroxy metabolites.

   More generally, this paper has demonstrated how the application of pharmacokinetic theory and relatively simple pharmacokinetic models can produce pharmacodynamically relevant information concerning the expected limits of effects. The clinical
psychopharmacological literature contains many instances of undue
emphasis being placed on factors that might influence pharmacokinetic behavior of parent drug or metabolite. Here, we have not
only identified a number of variables but attempted to assess
their likely relevance to real-life situations by pharmacokineti-
cally appropriate prospective study design and reanalysis of
earlier findings.

REFERENCES

Alexanderson, B. and Borgå, O. (1973). Urinary excretion of nor-
    triptyline and five of its metabolites in man after single
    and multiple doses. Eur. J. Clin. Pharmacol., 5,174-80
Amdisen, A. (1977). Serum level monitoring and clinical pharmaco-
    kinetics of lithium. Clin. Pharmacokin., 2,73-92
Bertilsson, L., Mellström, B. and Sjöqvist, F. (1979). Pronounced
    inhibition of noradrenaline uptake by 10-hydroxy-metabolites
    of nortriptyline. Life Sci., 25,1285-92
Braithwaite, R.A. and Dawling, S. (1981). The pharmacokinetics
    and metabolism of tricyclic antidepressant drugs in patients
    with chronic renal failure. In Clinical Pharmacology in
    Psychiatry; Neuroleptic and Antidepressant Research (ed. E.
    Usdin, S.G. Dahl, L.F. Gram and O. Lingjaerde), Macmillan,
    London, pp. 285-95

Crammer, J.L., Scott, B. and Rolfe, B. (1969). Metabolism of ^{14}C-imipramine. II. Urinary metabolites in man. Psychopharmacologia (Berlin), 15,207-25

Dawling, S., Lynn, K., Rosser, R. and Braithwaite, R. (1981). The pharmacokinetics of nortriptyline in patients with chronic renal failure. Br. J. Clin. Pharmacol., 12, 39-45

Garattini, S., Marcucci, F. and Mussini, E. (1975). Biotransformation of drugs to pharmacologically active metabolites. In Handbook of Experimental Pharmacology, XXVIII/3, Concepts in Biochemical Pharmacology (ed. J.R. Gillette and J.R. Mitchell), Springer-Verlag, Berlin, pp.113-29

Hoffmann, K.-J., Regårdh, C.-G., Aurell, M., Ervik, M. and Jordö, L. (1980). The effect of impaired renal function on the plasma concentration and urinary excretion of metoprolol metabolites. Clin. Pharmacokin., 5, 181-91

Kitanaka, I., Ross, R.J., Cutler, N.R., Zavadil, A.P., III, and Potter, W.Z. (1982). Altered hydroxydesipramine concentrations in elderly depressed patients. Clin. Pharmacol. Ther., 31,51-5

Kleinman, J.E., Nasrallah, H.A., Bigelow, L.B., Rogol, A.D., Zalcman, S., Wyatt, R.J. and Gillin, J.C. (1978). 7-Hydroxychlorpromazine, an active metabolite of chlorpromazine. Presented at American Psychiatric Association Annual Meeting, May 8-12, Atlanta, Georgia, Abstract No. NR29

Kragh-Sørensen, P., Borgå, O., Garle, M., Bolvig Hansen, L., Hansen, C.E., Hvidberg, E.F., Larsen, N.-E. and Sjöqvist, F. (1977). Eur. J. Clin Pharmacol., 11,479-83

Levy, G. (1980). Effect of plasma protein binding on renal clearance of drugs. J. Pharm. Sci., 69,482-3

Linnoila, M., Insel, T., Kilts, C., Potter, W.Z. and Murphy, D.L. (1982). Plasma steady-state concentrations of hydroxylated metabolites of clomipramine. Clin. Pharmacol. Ther., 32, 208-11

Lundborg, P., Regårdh, C.G. and Landahl, S. (1982). The pharmacokinetics of metoprolol in healthy elderly individuals (Abstract). Clin. Pharmacol. Ther., 31,246

Lynn, K., Braithwaite, R., Dawling, S. and Rosser, R. (1981). Comparison of the serum protein binding of maprotiline and phenytoin in uremic patients on haemodialysis. Eur. J. Clin. Pharmacol., 19,73-7

Mellström, B., Bertilsson, L., Säwe, J., Schulz, H.-U. and Sjöqvist, F. (1981). E- and Z-10-hydroxylation of nortriptyline: relationship to polymorphic debrisoquine hydroxylation. Clin. Pharmacol. Ther., 30,189-93

Piafsky, K.M., Borgå, O., Odar-Cederlöf, I., Johansson, C. and Sjöqvist, F. (1978). Increased plasma protein binding of propranolol and chlorpromazine mediated by disease-induced elevation of α_1-acid glycoprotein. New Engl. J. Med., 299, 1435-9

Potter, W.Z., Bertilsson, L. and Sjöqvist, F. (1981). Clinical pharmacokinetics of psychotropic drugs: fundamental and practical aspects. In The Handbook of Biological Psychiatry, (ed. H.M. Van Praag, O. Rafaelsen, M. Lader and A. Sacher) Marcel Dekker, New York, pp. 71–134

Potter, W.Z., and Calil, H.M. (1981). Metabolites of tricyclic antidepressants – biological activity and clinical implications. In Clinical Pharmacology in Psychiatry (ed. E. Usdin), Elsevier/North-Holland, New York, pp. 311–24

Potter, W.Z., Calil, H.M., Sutfin, T., Zavadil, A.P., III, Jusko, W.J., Rapoport, J. and Goodwin, F.K. (1982). Active metabolites of imipramine and desipramine in man. Clin. Pharmacol. Ther., 31,393–401

Reidenberg, M.M., Odar-Cederlöf, I., von Bahr, C., Borgå, O. and Sjöqvist, F. (1971). Protein binding of diphenylhydantoin and desmethylimipramine in plasma from patients with poor renal function. New Engl. J. Med., 285,264–7

Sutfin, T.A., and Jusko, W.J. (1979). High-performance liquid chromatographic assay for imipramine, desipramine, and their 2-hydroxylated metabolites. J. Pharm. Sci., 68,703–5

Träskman, L., Asberg, M., Bertilsson, L., Cronholm, B., Mellström, B., Neckers, L.M., Sjöqvist, F., Thorén, P. and Tybring, G. (1979). Plasma levels of chlorimipramine and its demethyl metabolite during treatment of depression. Clin. Pharmacol. Ther., 26,600–10

Vestal, R.E. (1978). Drug use in the elderly: a review of problems and special considerations. Drugs, 16,358–82

Stereospecific 10-hydroxylation of nortriptyline - genetic aspects and importance for biochemical and clinical effects

Leif Bertilsson[1], Britt Mellström[1], Conny Nordin[2], Bo Siwers[2]
and Folke Sjöqvist[1]

INTRODUCTION

The plasma level of the tricyclic antidepressant nortriptyline is an important determinant for its clinical effects (cf. Sjöqvist *et al.*, 1980). The therapeutic effect is related to the plasma level in a curvilinear manner, with poor outcome both at low and very high plasma concentrations (Asberg *et al.*, 1971). There are two main reasons why nortriptyline has become one of the most thoroughly investigated antidepressants: (a) analytical methods were developed very early for measurement of low plasma levels of this secondary amine, and (b) it was initially thought that nortriptyline had no active metabolites (in contrast to the tertiary amines amitriptyline and imipramine). It was later shown that the major metabolite of nortriptyline, i.e. 10-hydroxy-nortriptyline, is almost as potent as the parent drug in inhibiting the uptake of norepinephrine (NE) in rat brain slices (Bertilsson *et al.*, 1979). The *E*- and *Z*-10-OH-nortriptyline isomers (figure 1) were equipotent in this respect. It was also shown that the plasma levels of 10-OH-nortriptyline often exceeded those of the parent drug during nortriptyline treatment. Levels of 10-OH-nortriptyline and nortriptyline in CSF were comparable, showing that the hydroxy metabolites pass into the central nervous system (*loc. cit*).

We are now reporting on the regulation of the nortriptyline hydroxylation in healthy subjects and in patients treated for depression as well as preliminary observations on the interrelationships between the pharmacokinetics of nortriptyline and 10-OH-nortriptyline, and biochemical and clinical effects.

———————
Departments of [1]Clinical Pharmacology and [2]Psychiatry at the Karolinska Institute, Huddinge Hospital, S-141 86 Huddinge, Sweden.

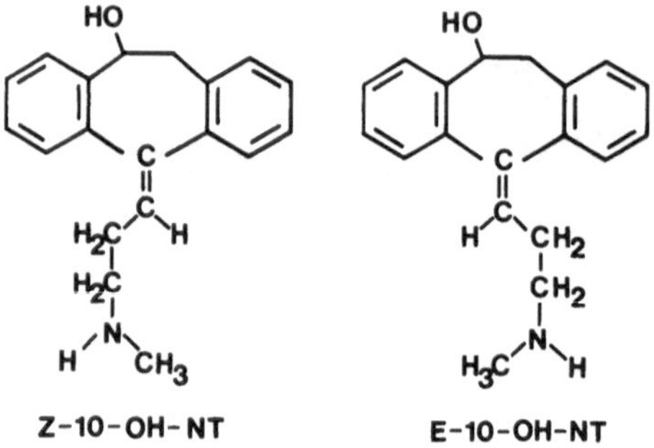

Z-10-OH-NT   E-10-OH-NT

Figure 1. Chemical formulas of the isomeric E- and Z-10-OH-nortriptyline.

GENETIC REGULATION OF THE 10-HYDROXYLATION OF NORTRIPTYLINE

Alexanderson *et al.* (1969) showed that the steady-state plasma levels of nortriptyline were very similar within pairs of mono-zygotic twins. In dizygotic twins and in monozygotic twins treated with some other drugs, e.g. barbiturates, the levels of nortriptyline could be quite different within pairs. As the plasma level of nortriptyline is dependent to a major extent on the rate of 10-hydroxylation (Alexanderson and Borgå, 1973), it can be concluded that this metabolic pathway is genetically controlled, but may be affected by concomitant drug treatment.

During recent years polymorphic 4-hydroxylation of debriso-quine (Mahgoub *et al.*, 1977) and N-oxidation of sparteine (Eichelbaum *et al.*, 1979) have been demonstrated. We later showed that these two polymorphic oxidations are regulated by similar genetic factors and possibly the same subunit of cytochrome P-450 is involved in both metabolic reactions (Eichelbaum *et al.*, 1982). We have also compared the polymorphic oxidation of debrisoquine and sparteine with the metabolism of nortriptyline using crossover studies in healthy volunteers. There was a strong correlation between the debrisoquine metabolic ratio (debrisoquine/4-hydroxy-debrisoquine in urine during 6 h following a single 10 mg dose of debrisoquine) and the total plasma clearance of nortriptyline after a single dose (Spearman rank coefficient of correlation $r_s = -0.83$; $n = 8$; $p = 0.01$) (Bertilsson *et al.*, 1980a). By measuring the excretion of nortriptyline metabolites in urine, it was shown that the metabolic clearance of nortriptyline by hydroxylation in the E-position, but not in the Z-position, correlated even better to the debrisoquine metabolic ratio ($r_s = -0.88$; $p < 0.01$) (Mellström *et al.*, 1981). This implies that common enzymatic mechanisms are involved in the hydroxylation of debrisoquine and in the E-10-hydroxylation of nortriptyline. The strong correlation ($r_s = 0.96$) between the total plasma clearance of nortriptyline and the metabolic clearance by E-10-hydroxylation shows that this metabolic reaction is important for the disposition of the drug (Mellström *et al.*, 1981). The Z-isomer is a minor metabolite compared to E-10-OH-nortriptyline and constitutes only 5-22% of total 10-OH-nortriptyline.

In the clinical study that will be discussed below, patients who had been treated with nortriptyline for depression for at least three weeks were phenotyped with debrisoquine *after* the treatment period. As seen in figure 2 there was a significant correlation (r_S = 0.71; n = 8; $p < 0.05$) between the steady-state plasma level of nortriptyline (per dose unit) and the debrisoquine metabolic ratio. The plasma levels of unconjugated or total (unconjugated plus conjugated) 10-OH-nortriptyline were not significantly related to the debrisoquine metabolic ratio (r_S = -0.36, n = 8; and r_S = - 0.14, n = 7). While plasma levels of nortriptyline are dependent on the rate of hydroxylation, the levels of 10-OH-nortriptyline are determined by its rate of formation, its rate of conjugation and its renal excretion. In a similar study (Bertilsson and Aberg-Wistedt, 1983), it was shown that the steady-state plasma level of desipramine (which is hydroxylated in the aromatic 2-position) and the debrisoquine metabolic ratio correlated significantly (r_S = 0.92; n = 10; $p < 0.01$). These results imply that (a) the hydroxylation of debrisoquine, desipramine and nortriptyline may be mediated by the same isoenzyme of the cytochrome P-450 system and (b) the debrisoquine phenotyping test predicts plasma levels of both desipramine and nortriptyline fairly well. Alexanderson (1972) has previously shown in a crossover study that the metabolism of these two tricyclic antidepressants correlate strongly within individuals.

TREATMENT OF DEPRESSION WITH NORTRIPTYLINE

In an ongoing investigation 16 depressed patients have been treated with 50 mg nortriptyline t.i.d. (25 mg b.i.d. in one old patient) for at least 3 weeks after 4-7 days of placebo treatment. The severity of depression was rated with a subscale of the Comprehensive Psychopathological Rating Scale (CPRS) (Asberg *et al.*, 1978) once a week. Lumbar punctures were performed before and after 3 weeks of nortriptyline treatment. The punctures were performed using a standardized technique (Nordin *et al.*, 1982) early in the morning after at least 8 h of bed rest. Twelve milliliters were drawn with the needle between the fourth and fifth lumbar vertebrae. The levels of 5-HIAA, HVA and MHPG in CSF were determined by mass fragmentography (Bertilsson, 1981). Plasma was drawn once a week and several times during a dosage interval after 3 weeks of treatment. Nortriptyline and 10-OH-nortriptyline in plasma and CSF were analyzed by mass fragmentography (Borgå *et al.*, 1972).

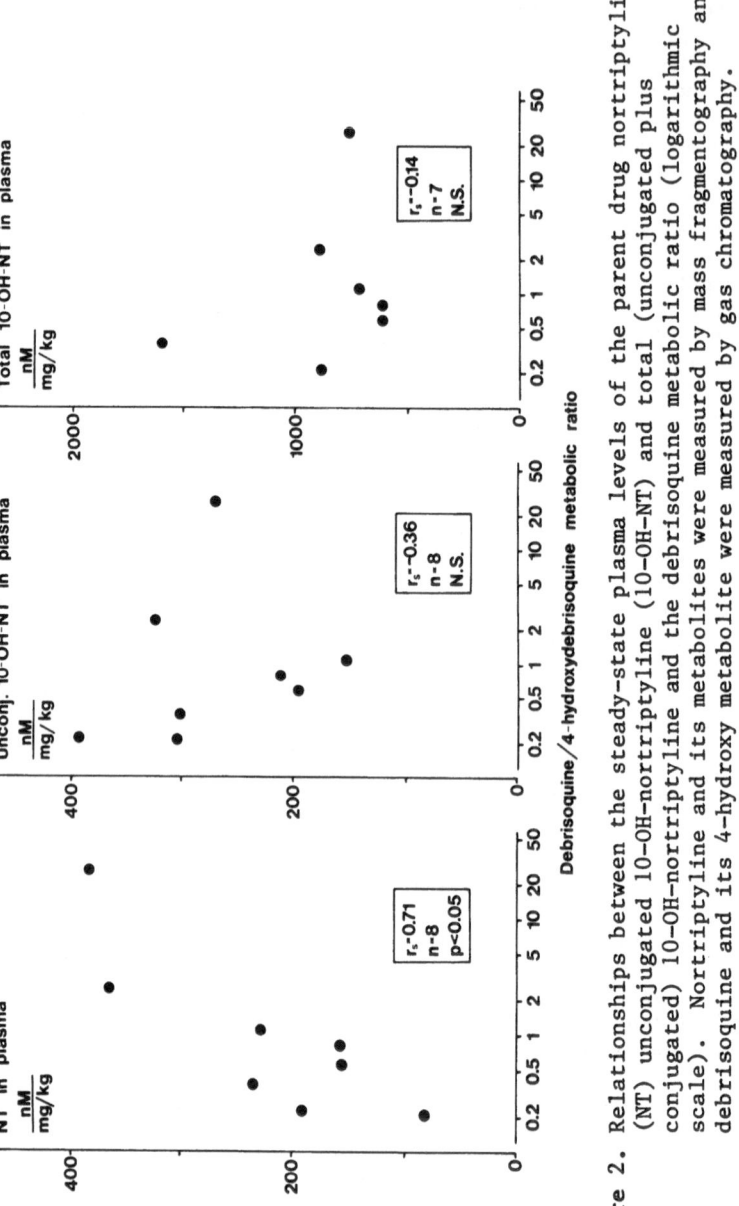

Figure 2. Relationships between the steady-state plasma levels of the parent drug nortriptyline (NT) unconjugated 10–OH–nortriptyline (10–OH–NT) and total (unconjugated plus conjugated) 10–OH–nortriptyline and the debrisoquine metabolic ratio (logarithmic scale). Nortriptyline and its metabolites were measured by mass fragmentography and debrisoquine and its 4–hydroxy metabolite were measured by gas chromatography.

Plasma and CSF Levels of Nortriptyline and 10-OH-Nortriptyline

As previously shown (Bertilsson *et al.*, 1979), the plasma levels
of 10-OH-nortriptyline were high in some patients and low in
others during treatment of depression with nortriptyline. There
was, however, little variation in the plasma levels of both nortriptyline and 10-OH-nortriptyline during a dosage interval as
illustrated in two patients in figure 3. This was true in patients
with both a high (patient 9) and a low (patient 10) ratio of
nortriptyline and 10-OH-nortriptyline (figure 3).

In 15 patients the ratio between the concentrations in CSF
and plasma was similar for nortriptyline ($10.4 \pm 2.0\%$) and
unconjugated 10-OH-nortriptyline ($11.5 \pm 2.4\%$). There was a
strong correlation between the CSF and plasma levels for both
nortriptyline ($r = 0.93$; $p < 0.001$) and 10-OH-nortriptyline ($r =
0.71$; $p < 0.01$) (figure 4). Evidently both plasma and CSF concen-
trations are of a similar order of magnitude for 10-OH-nortripty-
line and nortriptyline. The inter-individual variation in plasma
protein binding for both nortriptyline and 10-OH-nortriptyline is
small and thus the total plasma concentrations should reflect the
concentrations at receptor sites.

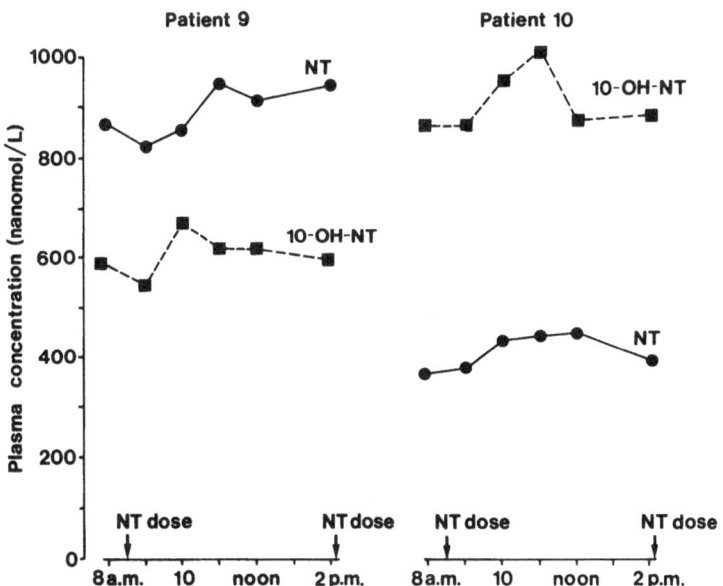

Figure 3. Plasma levels of nortriptyline (NT) and 10-OH-nortripty-
line (10-OH-NT) (unconjugated) during a dosage interval
in two patients treated with 50 mg nortriptyline t.i.d.

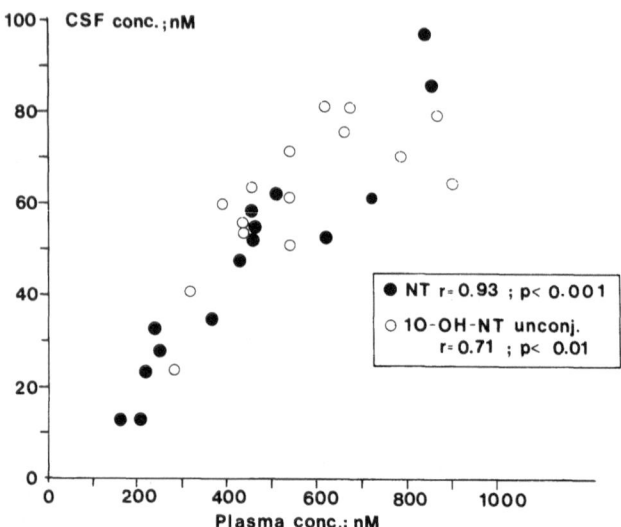

Figure 4. CSF and plasma levels of nortriptyline (NT) and 10-OH-
nortriptyline (10-OH-NT) (unconjugated) in 15 patients
treated with nortriptyline for 3 weeks.

Biochemical and Clinical Effects of Nortriptyline Treatment

Both nortriptyline and 10-OH-nortriptyline are potent inhibitors
of NE uptake with little effect on serotonin (5-HT) uptake
(Bertilsson *et al.*, 1979). After 3 weeks of nortriptyline treatment of 15 depressed patients the CSF level of the NE metabolite
decreased by 36.3% ($p < 0.001$) (table 1). The effect on the 5-HT
metabolite 5-HIAA was less pronounced (-19.7%; $p < 0.01$) and there
was no effect on the dopamine metabolite HVA (table 1). This
confirms the marked effect of nortriptyline treatment on noradrenergic neurons (Bertilsson *et al.*, 1974). Treatment with the
potent inhibitors of 5-HT uptake, chlorimipramine and zimelidine,
have a more pronounced effect on 5-HIAA than on MHPG (Bertilsson
et al., 1974, 1980b).
    In two consecutive studies (Asberg *et al.*, 1973, 1976), it
has been shown that the levels of 5-HIAA in CSF are bimodally
distributed in a group of untreated depressed patients. This
indicates that endogenous depression is biochemically heterogeneous. The relatively selective NE uptake inhibitor nortriptyline seemed to have a more favorable effect in patients with a
pre-treatment 5-HIAA level in CSF above 15 μg 1^{-1} than in patients
with lower CSF 5-HIAA (Asberg *et al.*, 1973). A working hypothesis
was formulated that patients with a low 5-HIAA in CSF have a
disturbance in serotonergic neurons while patients with higher
levels have disturbed noradrenergic functions. Studies with

Table 1. Amine metabolite levels in CSF before and during nortriptyline treatment in 15 patients (mean ± S.D.; nmol 1^{-1})

Amine metabolite	Before treatment	During treatment	Change (%)	Significance
5-HIAA	92.3 ± 42.0	74.1 ± 35.0	-19.7	$p < 0.01$
HVA	201 ± 123	183 ± 125	- 9.0	n.s.
MHPG	49.4 ± 10.6	31.4 ± 5.4	-36.3	$p < 0.001$

chlorimipramine (Träskman *et al.*, 1979), desipramine and zimelidine (Aberg-Wistedt *et al.*, 1982) have given partial support for this hypothesis.

In the present study where 16 depressed patients were treated with nortriptyline, the severity of depression after 3 weeks of treatment was significantly ($p < 0.01$) higher in the patients with a pre-treatment CSF 5-HIAA below 15 µg 1^{-1} (mean CPRS score 11.7 ± S.D. 3.6; $n = 6$) than in patients with a higher pre-treatment 5-HIAA (CPRS score 5.4 ± 3.9; $n = 10$). No definite conclusion should, however, be drawn from this as the former group was more

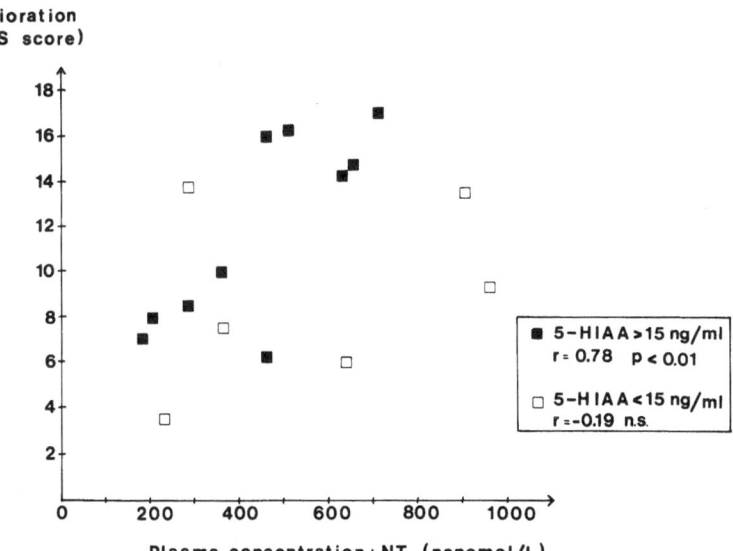

Figure 5. Relationship between the amelioration of depression and plasma concentration of nortriptyline (NT) after 3 weeks of treatment of 16 patients. The patients have been subgrouped according to the pre-treatment CSF level of 5-HIAA.

depressed (CPRS score 20.2 ± 2.1) than the latter group (CPRS score 16.6 ± 2.1) before treatment ($p < 0.01$).

In this relatively small sample of 16 patients there was no linear (or curvilinear) relationship between the amelioration and plasma level of nortriptyline (figure 5). However, among the 10 patients with a pre-treatment 5-HIAA above 15 ng ml^{-1} there was a positive correlation ($r = 0.78$; $p < 0.01$) (figure 5). An even stronger relationship emerged when the amelioration was correlated with the plasma concentration of nortriptyline plus 0.57 x (10-OH-nortriptyline) ($r = 0.84$; $p < 0.01$). The factor 0.57 was the relative potency of 10-OH-nortriptyline and nortriptyline found previously in studies *in vitro* (Bertilsson *et al.*, 1979). The absence of a curvilinear relationship may be due to the fact that none of the patients with a high 5-HIAA had high levels of nortriptyline and/or 10-OH-nortriptyline in plasma. These preliminary results indicate that nortriptyline treatment has a positive effect in patients with high pre-treatment levels of 5-HIAA in CSF and that both nortriptyline and 10-OH-nortriptyline may contribute to this effect.

Acknowledgements

The studies reviewed in this paper were supported by grants from the Swedish Medical Research Council (3902 and 5454) and from the Karolinska Institute.

REFERENCES

Aberg-Wistedt, A., Ross, S.B., Jostell, K.-G. and Sjöqvist, F. (1982). A double-blind study of zimelidine, a serotonin uptake inhibitor, and desipramine, a noradrenaline uptake inhibitor, in endogenous depression: II. Biochemical findings. Acta Psych. Scand., 66, 66-82

Alexanderson, B. (1972). Pharmacokinetics of desmethyl-imipramine and nortriptyline in man after single and multiple doses. A crossover study. Eur. J. Clin. Pharmacol., 5, 1-10

Alexanderson, B. and Borgå, O. (1973). Urinary excretion of nortriptyline and five of its metabolites in man after single and multiple oral doses. Eur. J. Clin. Pharmacol., 5, 174-180

Alexanderson, B., Price Evans, D. A. and Sjöqvist, F. (1969). Steady-state plasma levels of nortriptyline in twins. Influence of genetic factors and drug therapy. Br. Med. J., 2, 764-8

Asberg, M., Bertilsson, L., Tuck, D., Cronholm, B. and Sjöqvist, F. (1973). Indoleamine metabolites in the cerebrospinal fluid of depressed patients before and during treatment with nortriptyline. Clin. Pharmacol. Ther., 14, 277-86

Asberg, M., Cronholm, B., Sjöqvist, F. and Tuck, R. (1971).
Relationship between plasma level of nortriptyline and therapeutic effect. Br. Med. J., 3, 331-4

Asberg, M., Montgomery, S., Perris, C., Schalling, D. and Sedvall,
G. (1978). A comprehensive psychopathological rating scale.
Acta Psychiat. Scand., Suppl. 271, 5-27

Asberg, M., Thorén, P., Träskman, L., Bertilsson, L. and
Ringberger, V. (1976). Serotonin depression - a biochemical
subgroup within the affective disorders? Science, 191, 478-80

Bertilsson, L. (1981). Quantitative mass fragmentography - a
valuable tool in clinical psychopharmacology. In Clinical
Pharmacology in Psychiatry (ed. E. Usdin), Elsevier/North-
Holland, New York, pp. 59-71

Bertilsson, L. and Aberg-Wistedt, A. (1983). The debrisoquine
hydroxylation test predicts steady-state plasma levels of
desipramine. Br. J. Clin. Pharmacol., 15, 388-90

Bertilsson, L., Asberg, M. and Thorén, P. (1974). Differential
effects of chlorimipramine and nortriptyline on metabolites
of serotonin and noradrenaline in the cerebrospinal fluid of
depressed patients. Eur. J. Clin. Pharmacol., 7, 365-8

Bertilsson, L., Eichelbaum, M., Mellström, B., Säwe, J., Schulz,
H.-U. and Sjöqvist, F. (1980a). Nortriptyline and antipyrine
clearance in relation to debrisoquine hydroxylation in man.
Life Sci., 27, 1673-7

Bertilsson, L., Mellström, B. and Sjöqvist, F. (1979). Pronounced
inhibition of noradrenaline uptake by 10-hydroxymetabolites
of nortriptyline. Life Sci., 25, 1285-92

Bertilsson, L., Tuck, J.R. and Siwers, B. (1980b). Biochemical
effects of zimelidine in man. Eur. J. Clin. Pharmacol., 18,
483-7

Borgå, O., Palmér, L., Sjöqvist, F. and Holmstedt, B. (1972).
Mass fragmentography used in quantitative analysis of drugs
and endogenous compounds in biological fluids. In Proc.5th
Int. Congr. on Pharmacology, S. Karger AG, Basel, vol. III,
pp. 56-68

Eichelbaum, M., Bertilsson, L., Säwe, J. and Zekorn, C. (1982).
Polymorphic oxidation of sparteine and debrisoquine: related
pharmacogenetic entities. Clin. Pharmacol. Ther., 31, 184-6

Eichelbaum, M., Spannbrucker, N., Steinecke, B. and Dengler, H.J.
(1979). Defective N-oxidation of sparteine in man: a new
pharmacogenetic defect. Eur. J. Clin. Pharmacol., 16, 183-7

Mahgoub, A., Idle, J.R., Dring, L.G., Lancaster, R. and Smith,
R.L. (1977). The polymorphic hydroxylation of debrisoquine
in man. Lancet, ii, 584-6

Mellström, B., Bertilsson, L., Säwe, J., Schulz, H.-U. and
Sjöqvist, F. (1981). E- and Z-10-hydroxylation of nortripty-
line: relationship to polymorphic debrisoquine hydroxylation.
Clin. Pharmacol. Ther., 30, 189-93

Nordin, C., Siwers, B. and Bertilsson, L. (1982). Site of lumbar puncture influences levels of monoamine metabolites. <u>Arch. Gen. Psychiatry</u>, **39**, 1445

Sjöqvist, F., Bertilsson, L. and Asberg, M. (1980). Monitoring tricyclic antidepressants. <u>Ther. Drug Monit.</u>, **2**, 85-93

Träskman, L., Asberg, M., Bertilsson, L., Cronholm, B., Mellström, B., Neckers, L.M., Sjöqvist, F., Thorén, P. and Tybring, G. (1979). Plasma levels of chlorimipramine and its demethyl metabolite during treatment of depression. <u>Clin. Pharmacol. Ther.</u>, **26**, 600-10

The fate of amitriptyline and its metabolites, taking into account their binding in plasma

P.Baumann[1], D.Tinguely[1], J.Schöpf[1], L.Koeb[1], M.Perey[1], L.Michel[1], A.Balant[2] and B.Dick[3]

INTRODUCTION

At the last meeting in this series, it became clear that the pharmacological activity of the hydroxylated metabolites ought to be considered in future clinical studies on antidepressants (Potter, 1981). Some of the genetic aspects of the metabolism of these antidepressants have been reviewed by Bertilsson et al. (1981).

The penetration of drugs into tissue for metabolism and for pharmacological action partly depends on their binding to plasma proteins and blood cells. Indeed, these blood constituents may act as vehicles and, thus, facilitate elimination by metabolism or through the kidney.

Saliva may be considered to be an ultrafiltrate of blood in those cases where drugs are not actively transported. The analysis of drugs in saliva therefore represents a useful tool for studying their binding to blood constituents.

The present study deals with some of these aspects of the clinical pharmacokinetics of antidepressants.

SALIVA - AND FREE PLASMA CONCENTRATION OF TRICYCLIC ANTIDEPRESSANTS

The analysis of psychotropic drugs in saliva seems not to be a tool of clinical interest. Actually, as demonstrated with lithium,

[1] Clinique Psychiatrique Universitaire de Lausanne, CH-1008 Prilly-Lausanne, Switzerland.
[2] Unité Psychopharmacologie Clinique Extrahospitalière, Centre Médical Universitaire, CH-1211 Geneva, Switzerland.
[3] Department of Clinical Pharmacology, University of Berne, CH-3010 Berne, Switzerland.

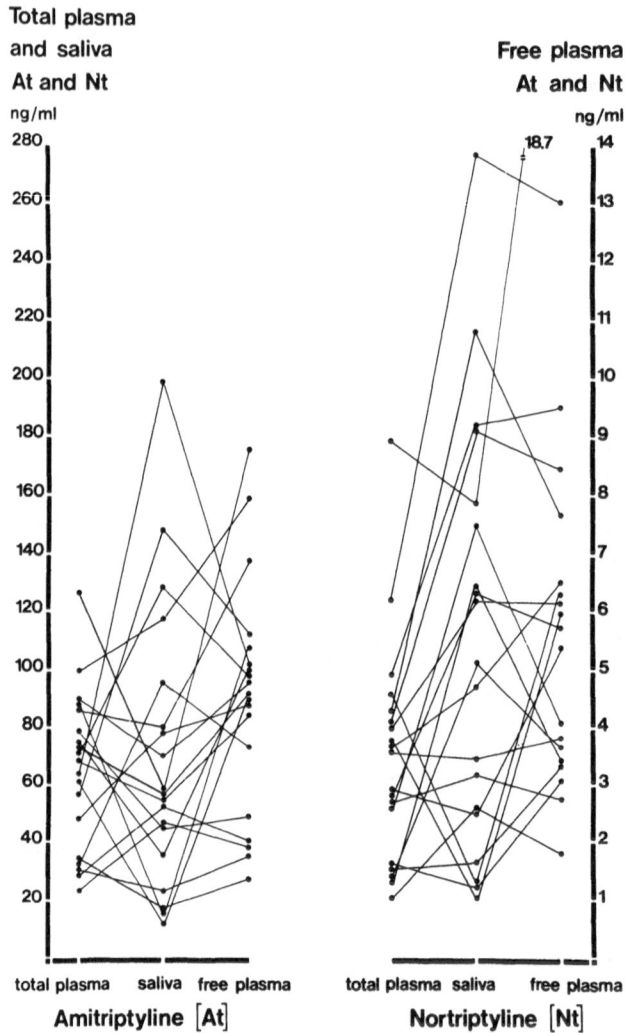

Figure 1.   Distribution of amitriptyline (At) and nortriptyline
(Nt) in total plasma, plasma dialyzate and saliva of 19
patients treated with At (reproduced from Baumann *et*
al. 1982a, with permission of Karger AG, Basel).

patients generally prefer blood samplings to collection of saliva.
Besides, the strong anticholinergic action of some classic tricyclics seriously hinders the collection of saliva for analytical
purposes. Nevertheless, psychotropic drugs such as amitriptyline
and nortriptyline probably reach saliva by diffusion, and measure-

Table 1. Calculation of the coefficients of correlation
(Pearson) between values of amitriptyline (AT) and
nortriptyline (NT), respectively, in plasma
and saliva of 19 patients

Parameters	Coefficient of correlation	Significance
Free AT vs total AT	0.8499	$p \leqslant 0.001$
Free NT vs total NT	0.9451	$p \leqslant 0.001$
Saliva AT vs total AT	0.1124	n.s
Saliva NT vs total NT	0.5121	$p \leqslant 0.05$
Saliva AT vs free AT	0.3813	n.s.
Saliva NT vs free NT	0.6164	$p \leqslant 0.01$
Saliva AT/NT vs total AT/NT	0.8114	$p \leqslant 0.001$
Saliva AT/NT vs free AT/NT	0.8119	$p \leqslant 0.001$
Free AT/NT vs total AT/NT	0.9232	$p \leqslant 0.001$
log(free AT) vs log(saliva AT)	0.4479	n.s.
log(free NT) vs log(saliva NT)	0.5395	$p \leqslant 0.05$

ment of these drugs in this body fluid may give useful information
about the relative importance of plasma protein binding for the
diffusion process of the drugs. Two reports deal with concentration of amitriptyline (Jeffrey and Turner, 1978) and nortriptyline (Kragh-Sørensen and Larsen, 1980) in plasma and saliva, but
neither of these studies takes the free plasma levels into
account. Jeffrey and Turner (1978) found a significant correlation
between the logarithmic drug concentrations of total plasma and
saliva, whereas Kragh-Sørensen and Larsen (1980) found that the
saliva/plasma ratio varied from 2 to 4, intra- and inter-individu-
ally.

Baumann *et al.* (1982a) observed in 19 amitriptyline-treated
patients that in saliva amitriptyline and nortriptyline varied
between 20 and 300% of their respective total plasma levels (figure 1). Free plasma levels were 2–30% of the concentrations
measured in saliva, and salivary levels of amitriptyline and
nortriptyline thus poorly reflect the respective free or total
plasma levels. The calculated coefficients of correlation do not
encourage drug monitoring in saliva for clinical use (table 1).
On the other hand, a highly significant correlation existed between free and total plasma drug levels. The relationships observed for the ratios amitriptyline/nortriptyline between the
different compartments allow us to presume a common mechanism for
the transport of amitriptyline and nortriptyline into saliva.
Indeed, both compounds are weak bases with pK_a values of 9.85 and
10.8 respectively (Maître *et al.*, 1980). As such, their diffusion
into saliva depends on its pH, varying between 5.45 and 7.8
(Mucklow *et al.*, 1978). According to these authors and also

Danhof and Breimer (1978), saliva levels of weak bases depend not only on the pH of saliva, but also on the binding of the drug to plasma proteins:

$$\frac{C_s}{C_p} = \frac{1 + 10^{(pK_a - pH_s)}}{1 + 10^{(pK_a - pH_p)}} \times \frac{f_p}{f_s} \qquad (1)$$

where C_s, C_p = concentration of drug in saliva and in plasma, respectively, pH_s, pH_p = saliva and plasma pH, respectively, f_s, f_p = fraction of drug unbound in saliva and in plasma, respectively, and (free C_p) = unbound concentration of drug in plasma.

As pH_p = 7.4, f_s = 1, f_p = (free C_p)/C_p, $pH_s < 7.8$, $pK_a > 9$, then

$$1 + 10^{(pK_a - pH_s)} \simeq 10^{(pK_a - pH_s)}$$
$$1 + 10^{(pK_a - pH_p)} \simeq 10^{(pK_a - pH_p)}$$

and so

$$C_s = \frac{10^{(pK_a - pH_s)}}{10^{(pK_a - pH_p)}} \times (\text{free } C_p)$$

This equation yields

$$\log C_s = - pH_s + 7.4 + \log(\text{free } C_p)$$

This equation clearly demonstrates that salivary levels of amitriptyline and nortriptyline depend on free plasma levels, and salivary pH. Salivation must be stimulated to get a pH 7.4, at which free plasma level would be equal to that found in saliva. Indeed, most often salivary pH is slightly acidic (5.4-6.8) and thus would lead to an 'extraction' of amitriptyline and nortriptyline from plasma. This mechanism explains why saliva levels are quite similar to total plasma levels (Jeffrey and Turner, 1978). From a theoretical point of view, the increase of saliva pH by one unit reduces the concentration of the drugs in saliva by a factor of 10. When the pH of saliva is calculated from experimental data obtained from amitriptyline and nortriptyline separately, good concordance was found (Baumann *et al.*, 1982a). However, it was not clear whether the calculated pH values reflected the actual pH values. Probably, some other factors which interfere with this model have to be considered: deposit of the drugs on the buccal mucosa or in the salivary ducts and unspecific binding to macromolecules in saliva could thus lead to erroneous results. The salivary flow rate may be a determinant for the accumulation of drug in saliva through an increase in its pH. On the other hand, the question remains open whether differences exist in the secretion of the drugs in saliva of parotic or submandibular origin. It is also important to carry out the collection of samples in the post-absorption phase, when there are no differences in the concentrations of the drugs between venous and arterial blood (Posti, 1982).

These points underline the difficulties encountered in intro-
ducing clinical drug monitoring in saliva for weak bases like
tricyclics or neuroleptics.

The hypothesis that the concentration of drug available for
the active site depends on free rather than total plasma levels
has led to numerous *in vitro* studies concerning the binding of
amitriptyline and nortriptyline to plasma proteins (Borgå *et al.*,
1969; Alexanderson and Borgå, 1972; Brinkschulte and Breyer-Pfaff,
1980; Burch *et al.*, 1981). Using another approach, Baumann *et al.*
(1982a) studied the binding of 'endogenous' amitriptyline and
nortriptyline in patients treated with clinical doses of amitriptyline. Results from these investigations showed an inter-
individual variation in binding with a factor of about 2 in untreated subjects without organic disease. The binding may be
subject to even greater variability under the influence of competing drugs or in physical illness.

The preliminary results of this study, in which 17 patients
already have been studied, show that the mean amitriptyline concentrations in total plasma are slightly higher than the corre-

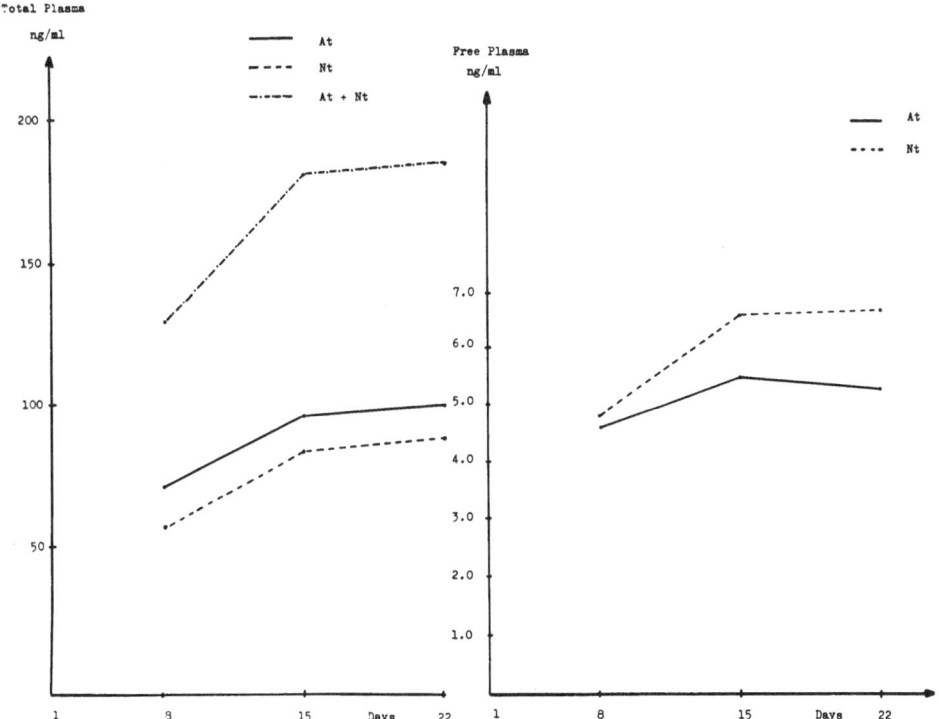

Figure 2. Total and free plasma amitriptyline (At) and
nortriptyline (Nt) in 17 patients.

sponding nortriptyline levels, while the inverse is true for free plasma levels (figure 2). This confirms earlier *in vitro* studies showing that nortriptyline is bound to plasma proteins to a lesser extent than amitriptyline.

STEADY-STATE LEVELS OF HYDROXYLATED METABOLITES

The hydroxylated metabolites of tricyclic antidepressants have gained interest, since it was shown that they exert a central effect in inhibiting the uptake of norepinephrine (Bertilsson *et al.*, 1979), and that the concentration of unconjugated hydroxylated metabolites in plasma may exceed that of the parent compounds (Alvan *et al.*, 1977; Garland *et al.*, 1979; for review, see Potter, 1981). These polar metabolites are probably bound to plasma proteins to a lesser extent than are the parent compounds, and consequently their pharmacological availability in plasma is higher.

Figure 3 presents various concentrations of amitriptyline and its metabolites in a patient treated for three weeks with 150 mg amitriptyline (Laroxyl). The amitriptyline level in plasma exceeded that of hydroxy-amitriptyline by a factor of 3, while the inverse relationship was noticed for nortriptyline and hydroxy-nortriptyline. However, the free plasma concentration of OH-amitriptyline in this case was slightly higher than the free concentration of the parent compound. Very striking is the fact that, on day 22, the free nortriptyline concentration was only 4.5 µg l^{-1}, but that of OH-nortriptyline reached a level of 42 µg l^{-1}. In this patient, free OH-amitriptyline and OH-nortriptyline were 25-40% of their corresponding total plasma concentration. In saliva, the hydroxy metabolite levels were higher than amitriptyline and nortriptyline in plasma, respectively. This finding demonstrates the relevance of free plasma drug levels for diffusional processes.

The phenotype of hydroxylation is one of the principal factors responsible for the inter-individual variation of the metabolism of the drugs in the liver. In the field of antidepressant drugs, its role has been clearly demonstrated for nortriptyline (Bertilsson *et al.*, 1980; Mellström *et al.*, 1981) and recently also for amitriptyline (Balant-Gorgia *et al.*, 1982). The patient presented in figure 3 did not show abnormal hydroxylation.

These preliminary results confirm the necessity of investigations including hydroxylated metabolites and protein binding studies. As already pointed out by Potter (1981), such studies should help to clarify discrepancies in the literature with regard to concentration-response relationships.

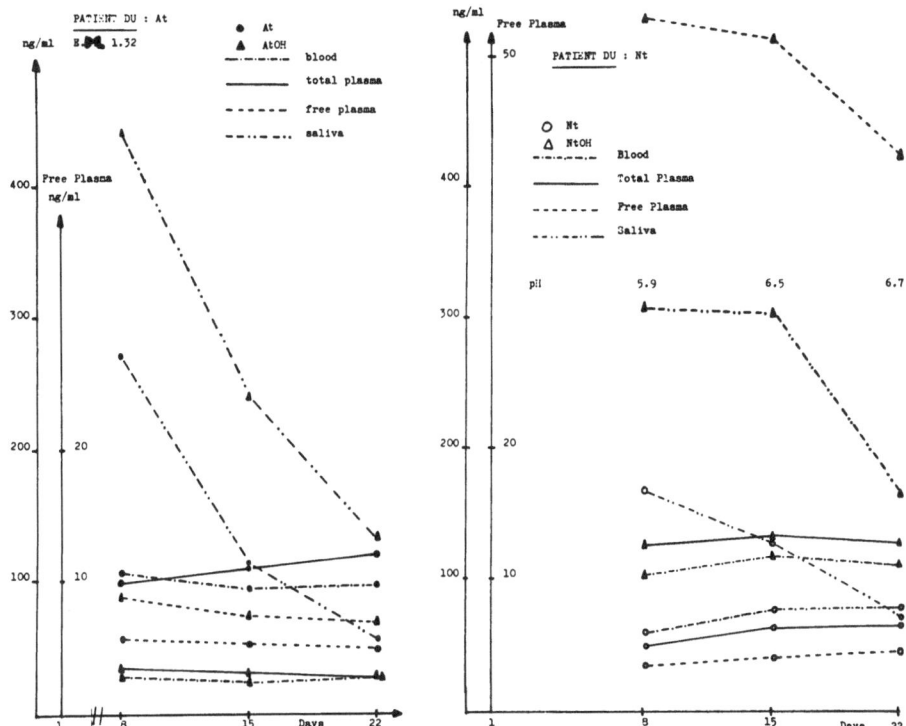

Figure 3. Whole blood, total and free plasma and saliva levels of amitriptyline (At) and its metabolites in a patient treated with 150 mg Laroxyl® daily for three weeks.

THE EFFECT OF AMITRIPTYLINE ON ALPHA$_1$-ACID GLYCOPROTEIN (AAG)

Several blood constituents have been found to be responsible for the plasma protein binding of tricyclic antidepressants. In particular, these basic drugs exhibit high affinity for AAG (Piafsky and Borgå, 1977; Brinkschulte and Breyer-Pfaff, 1980). The clinical significance of the drug binding to this protein has recently been discussed (de Leve and Piafsky, 1981).

Carroll *et al.* (1981) reported an increase of AAG in five depressed women after imipramine treatment. Pre-treatment AAG values were slightly elevated in comparison to controls.

Independently, in a study where AAG was measured by immunodiffusion at the beginning and after three weeks of treatment with 150 mg amitriptyline daily in 16 primary depressive patients without somatic disease, we observed a statistically significant increase ($p < 0.01$) of the AAG levels (Baumann *et al.*, 1982b). The initial and the final mean values remained within the normal

range (50–140 mg per 100 ml) (figure 4). No change in albumin
levels was noticed. For control, the same measurements were
performed in 16 freshly admitted patients with varying diagnoses. Their pharmacological treatment included neuroleptics,
antidepressants (except amitriptyline) and anti-Parkinson agents.
Neither albumin nor AAG concentrations in plasma increased or
decreased significantly during the three weeks in this group
(figure 4). This drug effect seems not to be very specific, as
anti-epileptic drugs also cause an increase in AAG concentration
(Routledge *et al.*, 1981). At the present time, no satisfactory
explanation of this effect can be offered.

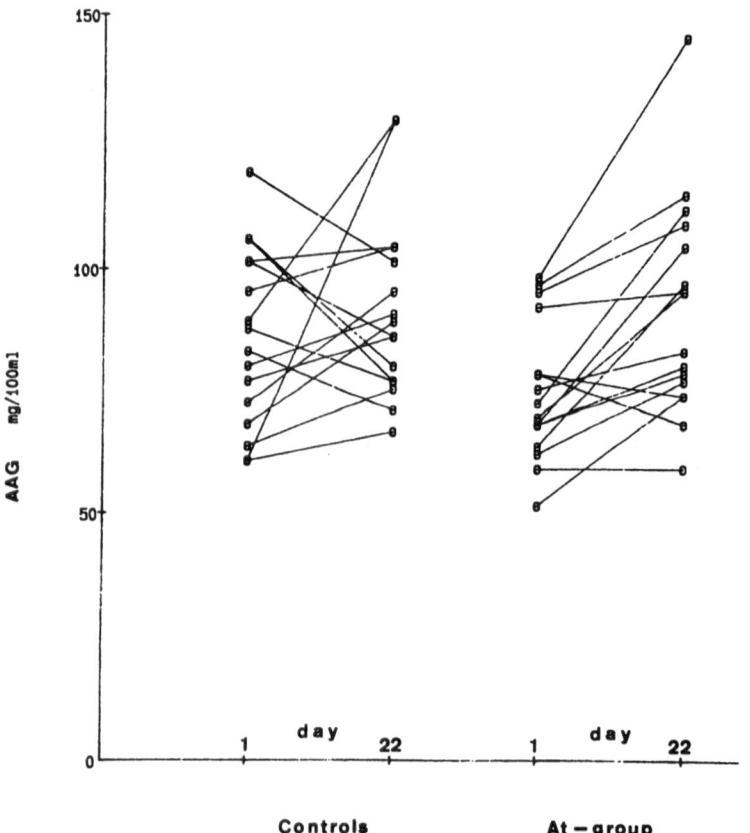

Figure 4. Alpha₁-acid glycoprotein levels in 16 depressive
patients treated for three weeks with 150 mg Laroxyl®
daily and in 16 controls. AAG was measured before (day
1) and during treatment (day 22) in the depressive
patients (from Baumann *et al.*, 1928b).

AAG occurs in three variants and in up to eight polymorphic forms. In 12 depressive patients treated for three weeks with amitriptyline, the number of bands and their relative intensities remained stable within each patient (Tinguely *et al.*, 1982), even if the AAG levels rose. This finding is not quite unexpected, as polymorphism is under genetic control and not markedly influenced by environmental factors.

SUMMARY AND CONCLUSION

Recent investigations have demonstrated the inter-individual differences in plasma protein binding and in the metabolism of tricyclic antidepressants. This means that, in clinical research, the relevance of these variables for blood level monitoring should be examined. The determination of free plasma drug levels still represents a technical problem. The present study shows that saliva level monitoring proves the importance of the unbound fraction of the drug in plasma for diffusional processes. In addition, a detailed case study confirms the need for measuring also the hydroxylated metabolites in the different compartments of the blood. Finally, a treatment with amitriptyline produces an increase in AAG concentration in plasma, which probably is of little relevance for the steady-state levels of the drug, but which encourages further research about the relationship between amitriptyline and glycoproteins.

Acknowledgements

The studies presented were financially supported by the Fonds National de la Recherche Scientifique (No.3.965.78 and 3.864-0.81) and by the Fonds Sandoz. We thank Mrs Chr. Bertschi and J. Bourquin for the preparation of the manuscript.

REFERENCES

Alexanderson, B. and Borgå, O. (1972). Interindividual differences in plasma protein binding of nortriptyline in man - a twin study. Eur. J. Clin. Pharmacol., 4, 196-200

Alvan, C., Borgå, O., Lind, M., Palmer, L. and Siwers, B. (1977). First pass hydroxylation of nortriptyline: concentrations of parent drug and major metabolites in plasma. Eur. J. Clin. Pharmacol., 11, 219-24

Balant-Gorgia, A.E., Schulz, P., Dayer, P., Balant, L., Kubli, A., Gertsch, C. and Garrone, G. (1982). Role of oxidation polymorphism on blood and urine concentration of amitriptyline and its metabolites. Arch. Psychiat. Nervenkr., 232, 215–22

Baumann, P., Tinguely, D., Koeb, L., Schöpf, J. and Le, P.K. (1982a). On the relationship between free plasma and saliva amitriptyline and nortriptyline. Int. Pharmacopsychiat., 17, 136–46

Baumann, P., Tinguely, D. and Schöpf, J. (1982b). Increase of α_1-acid-glycoprotein after treatment with amitriptyline. Br. J. Clin. Pharmacol., 14, 102–3

Bertilsson, L., Alvan, G., von Bahr, C., Lind, M., Mellström, B., Säwe, J., Schulz, H.-U. and Sjöqvist, F. (1981). Active metabolites of antidepressants: novel aspects of hydroxylation and demethylation in man. In Clinical Pharmacology in Psychiatry; Neuroleptic and Antidepressant Research (ed. E. Usdin, S.G. Dahl, L.F. Gram and O. Lingjaerde), Macmillan, London, pp. 161–9

Bertilsson, L., Eichelbaum, M., Mellström, B., Säwe, J., Schulz, H.-U. and Sjöqvist, F. (1980). Nortriptyline and antipyrine clearance in relation to debrisoquine hydroxylation in man. Life Sci., 27, 1673–7

Bertilsson, L., Mellström, B. and Sjöqvist, F. (1979). Pronounced inhibition of noradrenaline uptake by 10-hydroxy-metabolites of nortriptyline. Life Sci., 25, 1285–91

Borgå, O., Azarnoff, D.L., Forshell, G.P. and Sjöqvist, F. (1969). Plasma protein binding of tricyclic anti-depressants in man. Biochem. Pharmacol., 18, 2135–43

Brinkschulte, M. and Breyer-Pfaff, U. (1980). The contribution of α_1-acid glycoprotein, lipoproteins, and albumin to the plasma binding of perazine, amitriptyline, and nortriptyline in healthy man. Naunyn-Schmiedeberg's Arch. Pharmacol., 314,61–6

Burch, J.E., Roberts, S.G., and Raddats, M.A. (1981). Binding of amitriptyline and nortriptyline in plasma determined from their equilibrium distributions between red cells and plasma, and between red cells and buffer solution. Psychopharmacology, 75, 262–72

Carroll, B.J., Mukhopadhyay, S. and Feinberg, M. (1981). Radioimmunoassay of tricyclic antidepressants. In Clinical Pharmacology in Psychiatry; Neuroleptic and Antidepressant Research (ed. E. Usdin, S.G. Dahl, L.F. Gram and O. Lingjaerde), Macmillan, London, pp. 19–25.

Danhof, M. and Breimer, D.D. (1978). Therapeutic drug monitoring in saliva. Clin. Pharmacokin., 3, 39–57

De Leve, L.D. and Piafsky, K.M. (1981). Clinical significance of plasma binding of basic drugs. Trends Pharmacol. Sci., 2, 283–4

Garland, W.A., Muccino, R.R., Min, B.H., Cupano, J. and Fann, W.E. (1979). A method for the determination of amitriptyline and its metabolites nortriptyline, 10-hydroxyamitriptyline, and 10-hydroxynortriptyline in human plasma using stable isotope dilution and gas chromatography-chemical ionization mass spectrometry (GC-CIMS). Clin. Pharmacol. Ther., 25, 844-56

Jeffrey, A.A. and Turner, P. (1978). Relationship between plasma and salivary concentrations of amitriptyline. Br. J. Clin. Pharmacol., 5, 268-9

Kragh-Sørensen, P. and Larsen, N.-E. (1980). Factors influencing nortriptyline steady-state kinetics: plasma and saliva levels. Clin. Pharmacol. Ther., 28, 796-803

Maitre, L., Moser, P., Baumann, P.A. and Waldmeier, P.C. (1980). Amine uptake inhibitors: criteria of selectivity. Acta Psychiat. Scand., 61, Suppl. 280, 97-110

Mellström, B., Bertilsson, L., Säwe, J., Schulz, H.-U. and Sjöqvist, F. (1981). *E*- and *Z*-10-hydroxylation of nortriptyline: relationship to polymorphic debrisoquine hydroxylation. Clin. Pharmacol. Ther., 30, 189-93

Mucklow, J.C., Bending, M.R., Kahn, G.C. and Dollery, C.T. (1978). Drug concentration in saliva. Clin. Pharmacol. Ther., 24, 563-70

Piafsky, K.M. and Borgå, O. (1977). Plasma protein binding of basic drugs. II. Importance of α_1-acid glycoprotein for interindividual variation. Clin. Pharmacol. Ther., 22, 545-9

Posti, J. (1982). Saliva-plasma drug concentration ratios during absorption: theoretical considerations and pharmacokinetic implications. Pharmaceut. Acta Helv., 57, 83-92

Potter, W.Z. (1981). Active metabolites of tricyclic antidepressants. In Clinical Pharmacology in Psychiatry; Neuroleptic and Antidepressant Research (ed. E. Usdin, S.G. Dahl, L.F. Gram and O. Lingjaerde), Macmillan, London, pp.139-53

Routledge, P.A., Stargel, W.W., Finn, A.L., Barchowsky, A. and Shand, D.G. (1981). Lignocaine disposition in blood in epilepsy. Br. J. Clin. Pharmacol., 12, 663-6

Tinguely, D., Baumann, P. and Schöpf, J. (1982). A microprocedure to determine polymorphic forms of acid-α_1-glycoprotein in plasma. Application to depressive patients treated with amitriptyline. J. Chromatogr., 229, 319-25

Protein binding of imipramine and related compounds

C.B.Kristensen[1], L.F.Gram[1] and P.Kragh-Sørensen[2]

INTRODUCTION

Protein binding of drugs is often mentioned as a subject of importance. In relation to psychotropic drugs it is, however, difficult to find works substantiating the importance in relation to either clinical or pharmacokinetic aspects. One of the reasons for this is probably that most works deal with quantitative rather than qualitative binding measurements. Another reason could be that the many different techniques that have been used have led to different results, and difficulties in establishing the possible clinical significance of such measurements.

METHODOLOGICAL PROBLEMS

The most commonly used techniques are equilibrium dialysis (ED), ultrafiltration (UF), and measurement of CSF/plasma ratio. In studies of protein binding of a particular drug, ED generally yields relatively high free fraction measurements whereas UF generally yields relatively low free fractions. CSF/plasma ratio tends to yield results lying between those obtained by ED and UF.

Results from protein binding studies of imipramine and carbamazepine illustrate these tendencies (table 1).

Another problem, probably also primarily related to the techniques, is the difference in inter-individual variation found in different studies. As seen from table 1, the range of inter-individual variation in protein binding of imipramine found in different studies varies from less than twofold to more than fourfold. With carbamazepine the differences seem less dramatic.

Departments of [1]Clinical Pharmacology and [2]Psychiatry, Odense University, DK-5000 Odense C, Denmark.

Table 1. Results from studies on plasma protein binding of imipramine and carbamazepine

Imipramine

Method	*N*	% free		Reference
		Mean	Range	
ED 37°C	26	15	5-23	Glassman *et al.* (1973)
ED 37°C	8	13.7	–	Pruitt and Dayton (1971)
ED 37°C	23	7.9	6.1-11.1	Piafsky and Borgå (1977)
CSF/plasma	12	9.5	4.4-12.9	Muscettola *et al.* (1978)
UF 20°C	5	4.2	–	Borgå *et al.* (1969)

Carbamazepine

Method	*N*	% free		Reference
		Mean	Range	
ED 37°C	8	27.9	26.0-29.8	Rawlins *et al.* (1975)
ED 24°C	12	25.9	–	McAuliffe *et al.* (1977)
CSF/plasma	10	24	19-34	Johannesen *et al.* (1976)
CSF/plasma	11	18.2	13.9-33.3	Meinardi (1972)
CSF/plasma	19	21.0	–	Johannesen and Strandjord (1972)
UF 37°C	24	18.2	10.3-29.7	Hooper *et al.* (1975)
UF 22°C	6	23.9	–	Di Salle *et al.* (1974)
UF 22°C	14	14	19-34	Johannesen *et al.* (1976)

As it must be assumed that the inter-individual variation in protein binding is more important in clinical practice than the absolute degree of binding, it seems reasonable to focus on this problem.

The various problems related to the use of ED have been discussed in detail elsewhere (Kristensen and Gram, 1982).

It seems worth while to mention the important factors to be controlled when using this technique. Probably the most important factors are pH and dilution. To obtain reproducible results, the variation in pH must be less than 0.1 pH unit during dialysis (Henry *et al.*, 1981; Brinkschulte and Breyer-Pfaff, 1979). Calculation of free fraction implies dividing concentration of drug on the buffer side by the concentration on the serum side of the membrane, and it is therefore necessary to correct for the increased volume at the serum side caused by the colloidal osmotic pressure. This, of course, is more important the longer the dialysis lasts. When dilution of serum becomes more than about 5%, corrections should be made, otherwise a too low degree of protein binding will be found. In specific studies precise information on other factors such as temperature, membrane qualities, radiochemicals, buffer, concentration of drugs, storage of samples and the use of serum or plasma should be listed in order to evaluate the results properly.

MEASUREMENT IN DILUTED SERUM

For large-scale studies, it may be possible to use diluted serum for ED. By diluting serum and drug to the same degree, the ratio between drug and proteins remains constant. Then it can be derived from the law of mass action that free fraction of the drug (α) in different dilutions of serum and drug can be calculated from measurement of free fraction at only one concentration (dilution) of drug and protein. The equation to be used is

$$\alpha_1 = \frac{\alpha}{\alpha + y - \alpha y} \tag{1}$$

where α is the free fraction in undiluted serum and α_1 is the free fraction at a particular dilution of drug and protein, and y is the relative concentration after dilution. For example, with imipramine: $\alpha = 0.109$ in undiluted serum ($y = 1$), and α_1 in a 10-times diluted medium can be calculated:

$$\alpha_1 = \frac{0.109}{0.109 + 0.10 - 1.09 \times 0.1} = 0.550$$

The theory has been tested with imipramine and mianserin and the results seem to confirm the predictions (figure 1). The advantages of this method seem to be that less volume of blood samples is used, dilution becomes insignificant, pH is easy to control, and equilibrium is reached within less time. The disadvantages of this method are a somewhat lower precision, and the method has limited application for drugs bound less than 50% in undiluted serum.

PROTEIN BINDING OF IMIPRAMINE IN HEALTHY SUBJECTS

The plasma protein binding studies of most psychotropic drugs have been done with relatively small numbers of subjects and it is not possible to see if age, sex, or other factors influence the degree of drug binding. Therefore, we have studied 145 healthy subjects evenly distributed with respect to age, sex, smoking habits, and use of oral contraceptives.

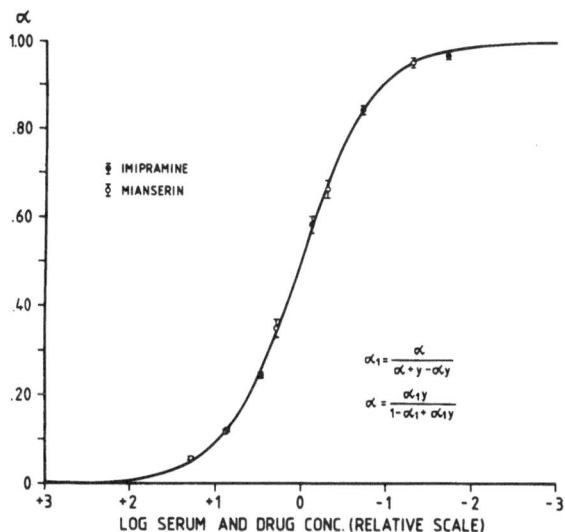

Figure 1. Drug protein binding in diluted serum. The x-axis represents a *relative* log concentration. The curve has been constructed according to equation (1) (see text).

In figure 2, the distribution of free fraction values in men and women is shown. The range of inter-individual variation is less than twofold and the mean value of free fraction is 0.11. In women there was a trend toward higher binding in the elderly (>50 years). No difference between smokers and non-smokers was observed and no definite effects of oral contraceptives could be observed.

To evaluate the impact of inter-individual differences in concentration of 12 plasma proteins these were measured in subjects with relatively high (n = 17) and low (n = 18) binding respectively. Other groups (Bickel, 1975; Piafsky and Borgå, 1977; Brinkschulte and Breyer-Pfaff, 1980) have demonstrated binding of basic drugs to albumin and orosomucoid, but the inter-individual differences in degree of binding have not been explained fully by differences in concentration of these proteins. Other factors thus appear to be involved. These may be binding to other proteins or interference from endogenous compounds such as steroids and electrolytes.

We therefore examined the possible binding to other proteins by measuring the concentration of the following proteins: α_1-antitrypsin, α_2-HS-glycoprotein, ceruloplasmin, prealbumin, β_2-glycoprotein I, complement $C3_c$, haptoglobulin, hemopexin, albumin, α_1-acid-glycoprotein (orosomucoid) and apolipoproteins A and B. The radial immunodiffusion technique (Behring Werke) was used. Significantly higher concentrations of orosomucoid, complement $C3_c$

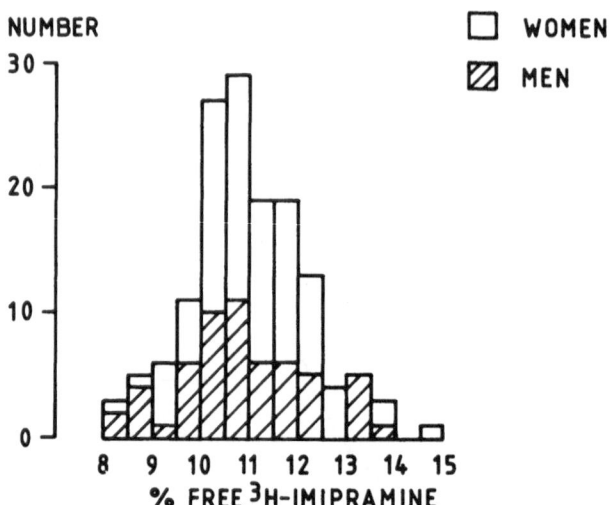

Figure 2. Free fraction of ^{3}H-imipramine in serum from 145 healthy subjects.

and apolipoprotein B were found in the high binding group. No statistically significant difference in concentration of the other proteins was found; in particular, the albumin concentration was the same in the two groups.

In the low binding group, a positive correlation between orosomucoid and apolipoprotein B was found whereas there was a negative correlation in the high binding group. This indicates that in some subjects the high binding may be caused by high concentration of apolipoprotein B and in others by high concentration of α_1-acid-glycoprotein. There was a positive correlation between these two proteins and complement $C3_c$. When the concentration of the three proteins was added (figure 3), the discrimination between the two groups seemed to become better. The results thus indicate significant binding to α_1-acid-glycoprotein and apolipoprotein B. Whether there is a binding to complement $C3_c$ has to be evaluated further because the present results may just as well reflect co-variation with the other two proteins.

MIANSERIN PROTEIN BINDING

Whereas acidic drugs seem to bind almost exclusively to albumin, basic drugs also bind to several other proteins, making the qualitative aspects much more complicated. In order to compare the protein binding of imipramine with the basic, tetracyclic, antidepressive drug mianserin, 43 sera from the imipramine study were tested for mianserin binding (figure 4).

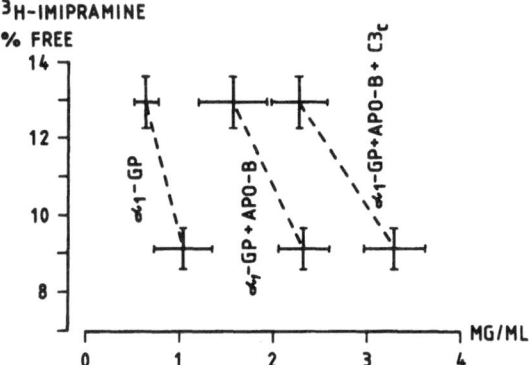

Figure 3. Discrimination between groups of healthy subjects with low and high serum protein binding of ^{3}H-imipramine by addition of concentrations of α_1-acid-glycoprotein (α_1-GP), apolipoprotein B (APO-B) and complement $C3_c$. Mean value ± standard deviation.

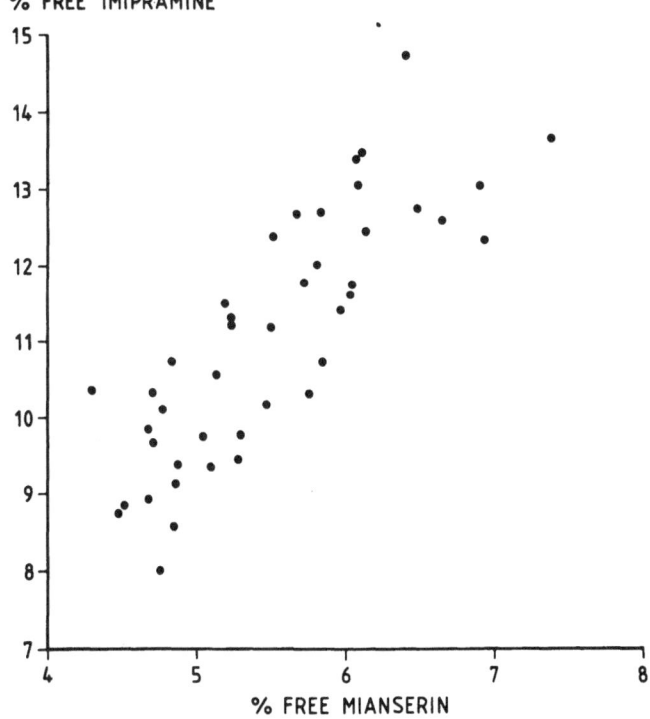

Figure 4. Serum protein binding of imipramine and mianserin in 43 healthy subjects.

A rather high degree of correlation was found between the binding of mianserin and imipramine. There must, however, be some difference in binding of the two compounds because the imipramine-free fraction was, on average, 0.11 and mianserin-free fraction was, on average, 0.055. It is thus indicated that high binding of one basic drug is associated with high binding of another basic drug. This would be expected if the drugs bind to the same proteins, but with different affinity, or to different binding sites on the same protein molecules.

CARBAMAZEPINE AND CARBAMAZEPINE-EPOXIDE

Carbamazepine is used mainly as an anti-epileptic drug, but it is also used for some other purposes, such as treatment of mania (Ballenger and Post, 1978; Okuma *et al.*, 1979). Structurally, it is a tricyclic compound, somewhat related to imipramine. Carbamazepine is weakly acidic and the main metabolite, carbamazepine-epoxide, has an almost neutral reaction. Carbamazepine-epoxide has been shown (Frigerio and Morselli, 1975) to have anticonvulsive activity almost equal to carbamazepine in rats. Attempts (Dam *et al.*, 1977) to evaluate the anticonvulsive effects of the epoxide metabolite by measuring total concentrations of carbamazepine and carbamazepine-epoxide in humans have not been successful. The reason for this might be the variance in plasma level/effect relationship caused by inter-individual variations in protein binding. To study this problem, blood samples were drawn before the morning dose in 17 epileptic patients on long-term carbamazepine monotherapy. The results are shown in figure 5.

A relatively weak linear correlation between total carbamazepine and total epoxide concentrations was found, whereas the free concentration strictly followed a non-linear correlation curve. This curve may be constructed assuming saturable kinetics for the epoxide elimination. This is a rather surprising finding and calls for further investigations, especially larger number of patients. However, the very limited variation in carbamazepine/carbamazepine-epoxide ratio when free fraction was measured indicates little or no genetic variation of this metabolic step. If the hypothesis of saturable kinetics for the epoxide metabolite holds true, it might explain some unexpected effects and side-effects of carbamazepine seen in patients reaching high serum concentrations of carbamazepine (Höppener *et al.*, 1980). A small increase in free carbamazepine concentration may be followed by a large increase in free carbamazepine-epoxide concentration in such patients.

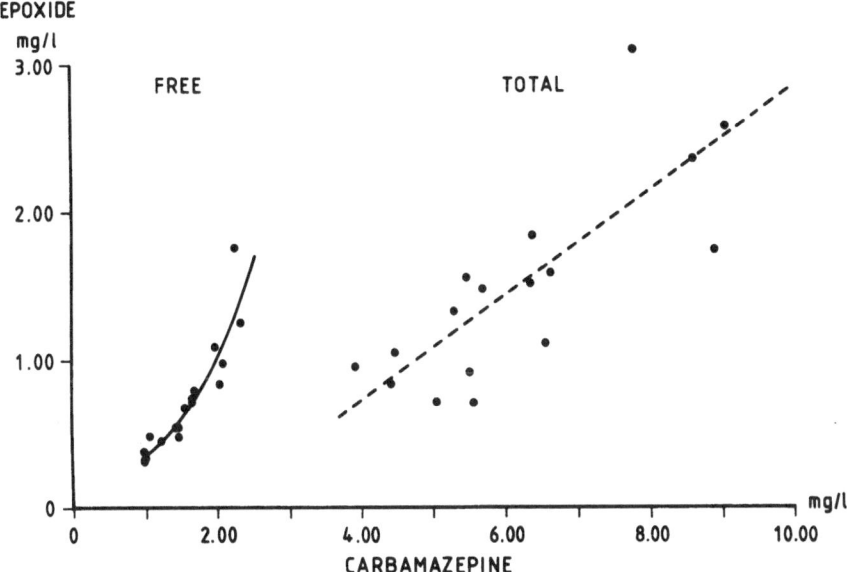

Figure 5. Total and free concentrations of carbamazepine and carbamazepine-epoxide in 17 epileptic patients in chronic treatment with carbamazepine.

CONCLUSION

The inter-individual variation in protein binding of imipramine and related compounds is potentially important from both a pharmacokinetic and a clinical point of view. Both the range of variation in degree of binding and the quality of binding might influence results from studies on plasma level/effect relationships.

One of the difficulties in evaluation of results of protein binding studies is the many different techniques used. Even when the same type of technique is used, different results can be obtained because of the many variables that have to be controlled. This implies that detailed information on the technique used is necessary to evaluate the result.

As described for imipramine and mianserin, the inter-individual variation in binding is less than twofold in healthy subjects. It therefore seems improbable that the degree of protein binding is of importance in clinical practice. The differences in protein concentrations revealed in the imipramine high and low binders indicate, however, that the quality of binding could be of importance. If the binding to a particular protein is strong enough (high affinity) to prevent extraction of the drug by the liver, variation in the concentration of this protein will influence the elimination of the drug. These aspects probably are much more relevant in patients suffering from somatic illnesses leading to abnormal serum protein patter (Piafsky *et al.*, 1977; Kates *et al.*, 1977).

In pharmacokinetic and pharmacogenetic studies it may be an advantage to use concentration of free drug instead of total. As described in the carbamazepine study, the correlation of carbamazepine and the carbamazepine-epoxide free concentrations is much better than the correlation of total concentrations. The 'noise' of inter-individual variance in degree of binding can apparently conceal some inter-relations between parent substance and metabolites.

Acknowledgements

This study was supported in part by grants from the Danish Medical Research Council (Grants Nos. 512-10703 and 12-1626), the Foundation for Advancement of Medical Science (Grants Nos. 31/79 and 58/81) and H. Lundbeck's Foundation for Psychopharmacological Research. Our thanks are due to Mrs Karin Bøjesen Nielsen for excellent technical assistance.

REFERENCES

Ballenger, J.C. and Post, R.M. (1978). Therapeutic effects of carbamazepine in affective illness: a preliminary report. Commun.Psychopharmacol., 2, 159-75

Bickel, M.H. (1975). Binding of chlorpromazine and imipramine to red cells, albumin, lipoproteins and other blood components. J. Pharm. Pharmacol., 27, 733-8

Borgå, O., Azarnoff, D.L., Forshell, G.P. and Sjöqvist, F. (1969). Plasma protein binding of tricyclic antidepressive drugs. Biochem. Pharmacol., 18, 2135-43

Brinkschulte, M. and Breyer-Pfaff, U. (1979). Binding of tricyclic antidepressants and perazine to human plasma. Arch. Pharmacol., 308, 1-7

Brinkschulte, M. and Breyer-Pfaff, U. (1980). The contribution of α_1-acid glycoprotein, lipoproteins, and albumin to the plasma binding of perazine, amitriptyline, and nortriptyline in healthy man. Arch. Pharmacol., 314, 61-6

Dam, M., Sury, J. and Christiansen, J. (1977). Has carbamazepine -10,11-epoxide an independent antiepileptic effect in man? In Epilepsy, The Eighth International Symposium (ed. J.K. Penry), Raven Press, New York, pp. 143-6

Di Salle, E., Pacifici, G.M. and Morselli, P.L. (1974). Studies on the plasma protein binding of carbamazepine. Pharmacol. Res. Commun., 6, 193-202

Frigerio, A. and Morselli, P.L. (1975). Carbamazepine: biotrans-
formation. In Advances in Neurology, vol. 11; (ed. J.K.
Penry and D.D. Daly), Raven Press, New York, pp. 295-308
Glassman, A.H., Hurwic, N.J. and Perel, J.M. (1973). Plasma
binding of imipramine and clinical outcome. Am. J. Psy-
chiatry, 130, 1367-9
Henry, J.A., Dunlop, A.W., Mitchell, S.N., Turner, P. and Adams,
P. (1981). A model for the pH dependence of drug-protein
binding. J. Pharm. Pharmacol., 33, 179-82
Hooper, W.D., Dubetz, D.K., Bochner, F., Cother, L.M., Smith,
G.A., Eadie, M.J. and Tyrer, J.H. (1975). Plasma protein
binding of carbamazepine. Clin. Pharmacol. Ther., 17, 433-40
Höppener, R.J., Kuyer, A., Meijer, J.W.A. and Hulsman, J. (1980).
Correlation between daily fluctuations of carbamazepine serum
levels and intermittant side effects. Epilepsia, 21, 341-50
Johannesen, S.J., Gerna, M., Bakke, J., Strandjord, R.E. and
Morselli, P.L. (1976). CSF concentrations and serum protein
binding of carbamazepine-10,11-epoxide in epileptic patients.
Br. J. Clin. Pharmacol., 3, 575-82
Johannesen, S.J., and Strandjord, R.E. (1972). The concentration
of carbamazepine (Tegretol) in serum and in cerebrospinal
fluid in patients with epilepsy. Acta Neurol. Scand., 48,
Suppl., 445-6
Kates, R.E., Sokoloski, T.D. and Comstock, T.J. (1977). Binding
of quinidine to plasma proteins in normal subjects and in
patients with hyperlipoproteinemias. Clin. Pharmacol. Ther.,
23, 30-5
Kristensen, C.B. and Gram, L.F. (1982). Equilibrium dialysis for
determination of protein binding of imipramine - evaluation
of a method. Acta Pharmacol. Toxicol., 50, 130-6
McAuliffe, J.J., Sherwin, A.L., Leppik, J.E., Fayle, S.A. and
Pippenger, C.E. (1977). Salivary levels of anticonvulsants: a
practical approach to drug monitoring. Neurology, 27, 409-13
Meinardi, H. (1972). Other antiepileptic drugs - carbamazepine.
In Antiepileptic Drugs (ed. Woodbury, Penry and Schmidt),
Raven Press, New York, pp. 487-96
Muscettola, G., Goodwin, F.K., Potter, W.Z., Claeys, M.M. and
Markey, S.P. (1978). Imipramine and desipramine in plasma
and spinal fluid. Arch. Gen. Psychiat., 35, 621-5
Okuma, T., Inanaga, K., Otsuki, S., Sarai, K., Takahashi, R.,
Hazama, H., Mori, A. and Watanabe, M. (1979). Comparison of
the antimanic efficacy of carbamazepine and clorpromazine. A
double-blind controlled study. Psychopharmacology, 66,
211-17
Piafsky, K.M. and Borgå, O. (1977). Plasma protein binding of
basic drugs. II. Importance of α_1-acid glycoprotein for
interindividual variation. Clin. Pharmacol. Ther., 22, 545-9
Piafsky, K.M., Borgå, O., Odar-Cederlöf, I., Johansson, C. and
Sjöqvist, F. (1977). Increased plasma protein binding of

propranolol and chlorpromazine mediated by disease-induced elevation of plasma α_1-acid glycoprotein. <u>New Engl. J. Med.</u>, **299**, 1435-9

Pruitt, A.W. and Dayton, P.G. (1971). A comparison of the binding of drugs to adult and cord plasma. <u>Eur. J. Clin. Pharmacol.</u>, **4**, 59-62

Rawlins, M.D., Collste, P., Bertilsson, L. and Palmer, L. (1975). Distribution and elimination kinetics of carbamazepine in man. <u>Eur. J. Clin. Pharmacol.</u>, **8**, 91-6

Section Five

Receptors and Transmitters Related to the Effects of Antidepressants

Relationships between receptor affinities of different antidepressants and their clinical profiles

Hakan Hall[1]

INTRODUCTION

The mechanism of action of antidepressant drugs is not well understood. The classical tricyclic antidepressant drugs as well as
some newer antidepressants have been developed as inhibitors of
the presynaptical re-uptake of the neurotransmitters norepinephrine (NE) (Glowinski and Axelrod, 1964; Iversen, 1965;
Carlsson et al., 1966) and 5-hydroxytryptamine (5-HT) (Carlsson et
al., 1969; Ross and Renyi, 1969). It has been hypothesized that
the therapeutic action of the antidepressant drugs is due to an
increased availability of NE and 5-HT at postsynaptic receptors in
the brain as the result of the re-uptake blockade (Schildkraut,
1965; Coppen, 1967; van Praag, 1974). However, in recent years
some antidepressants (e.g. mianserin and iprindole) have been
developed which lack effect or have only very slight effect on the
uptake mechanisms.
     Extensive studies of the pharmacological effects of anti-
depressant drugs, tricyclics as well as non-tricyclics, have shown
that several of them exert multiple effects on the pre- and postsynaptic systems in the brain. Thus it has been shown that antidepressants of various structural types inhibit the activation of
histamine-sensitive adenylate cyclase, an effect that was
suggested to be part of the therapeutic effect (Kanof and
Greengard, 1978). Furthermore, a number of antidepressants block
the muscarinic receptors (Snyder and Yamamura, 1977), which has
been suggested to be associated with the well known anticholinergic side-effects rather than with the therapeutic action.
Several of these drugs are, in addition, potent inhibitors of 5-HT
receptors, histaminergic receptors and adrenergic receptors (Hall
and Ogren, 1981). These findings indicate that the increased

[1]Department of Pharmacology, Research and Development Laboratories, Astra
Läkemedel AB, S-151 85 Södertälje, Sweden.

availability of neurotransmitters induced by the inhibition of their re-uptake of neurotransmitters could be counteracted by a simultaneous postsynaptic receptor blockade. The net effect of a drug with these multiple effects is not necessarily an increased neuronal firing in the postsynaptic neuron.

Generally, the depressive syndrome is not alleviated immediately after the administration of antidepressant drugs. There is normally a lag period of one to three weeks before a significant amelioration superior to that of placebo can be seen. This has focused attention on the effect of prolonged treatment on the mechanisms regulating the receptor responses in animals.

It has been observed that several of the antidepressant drugs on repeated administration produce a decreased density of β-adrenoceptors in rat cerebral cortex as studied by NE- or iso-prenaline-stimulated adenylate cyclase (Vetulani *et al.*, 1976) or by radiolabeling of the β-adrenoceptors (Banerjee *et al.*, 1977; Wolfe *et al.*, 1978). Furthermore, $5-HT_1$ and $5-HT_2$ receptors and α_2-adrenoceptors are also affected by long-term treatment with antidepressants (Reisine, 1981). It has been proposed recently that changes in pre- and postsynaptic receptors on long-term treatment are involved in the mechanism of action of the therapeutic effect of the antidepressant drugs (Fuxe *et al.*, 1982). In the present study, I will discuss the effects of antidepressants on receptors, both acutely and subchronically. Emphasis will be put especially on the possibility of predicting the clinical profile, with regard to both wanted effects and unwanted side-effects, based upon the pharmacological profile obtained in animal experiments.

ACUTE EFFECTS ON RECEPTORS

General

It has been shown by several authors that tricyclic antidepressant drugs inhibit the binding of radiolabeled ligands to various receptors in the brain (Hall and Ogren, 1981; Snyder and Yamamura, 1977; U'Prichard *et al.*, 1978). For example, imipramine, desipramine and amitriptyline are potent inhibitors of α_1-adrenoceptors, histamine-H_1 receptors and muscarinic receptors. In addition to these receptors, clomipramine interacts with dopamine-D_2 receptors. Many antidepressants of the non-tricyclic type do not inhibit the neuronal receptors to the same extent as do the tricyclics. Thus, zimelidine, nomifensine and alaproclate do not interact acutely with any receptor studied so far, while other antidepressants of the new generation, such as iprindole and mianserin, do. No antidepressant drug interacts acutely with the β-adrenergic receptor.

We have in an earlier work (Hall and Ogren, 1981) constructed a correlation matrix for comparison of the receptors, based on the above-mentioned results. Correlations were found between several receptor types, indicating similarities in their recognition sites (table 1).

Of special interest for the present study is the close similarity between the muscarinic receptors and the histamine-H_1 receptors, which have both been suggested to be involved in the development of side-effects in the clinical use of antidepressants (Snyder and Yamamura, 1977; Ogren *et al.*, 1981).

Table 1. Correlation coefficients in log-log regression analysis of IC_{50} values of 13 different antidepressants in various receptor binding systems (data from Hall and Ogren, 1981)

Receptor comparison	Correlation coefft.
d-LSD vs 5-HT$_1$	0.94
Muscarinic vs histamine$_1$	0.93
Alpha$_1$ vs dopamine$_2$	0.86
d-LSD vs dopamine$_2$	0.81
d-LSD vs histamine$_1$	0.81
Alpha$_1$ vs muscarinic	0.80

Other comparisons: correlation coefficient < 0.80.

Muscarinic Receptors

One of the main drawbacks in the use of tricyclic antidepressant drugs are the anticholinergic side-effects caused by these drugs. The side-effects related to peripheral anticholinergic action are, for example, dry mouth, constipation, mydriasis and urinary retention. Side-effects related to the central anticholinergic action are, for example, confusion, disturbed concentration, disorientation, delusions and hallucinations. It can be suggested that these side-effects are due to the antagonizing effect of tricyclic antidepressants on the cholinergic receptors in the brain and in the periphery.

The antimuscarinic potencies of drugs can easily be estimated using the ^{3}H-QNB binding assay (Yamamura and Snyder, 1974; Snyder and Yamamura, 1977). The relative potencies of some antidepressants in this assay are shown in table 2 (Hall and Ogren, 1981; see also Snyder and Yamamura, 1977). It is evident that the tricyclic antidepressants and mianserin are potent antimuscarinic drugs while others are more or less devoid of activity on the muscarinic receptor in the CNS.

In the periphery, the anticholinergic effects can be evaluated using the acetylcholine-induced contractions of the guinea-pig ileum. As can be seen from table 2, there is a high corre-

Table 2. Muscarinic receptor binding affinity and anticholinergic effects of some antidepressant drugs

	Inhibition of ^{3}H-QNB binding[a] (IC_{50}, μM)	Blockade of AcCh-induced contractions[b] (ED_{50}, μmol kg^{-1})	Saliva secretion after 150 mg drug[c] (% of placebo)
Alaproclate	79.5	53.8	n.d.
Amitriptyline	0.069	0.48	27.8
Clomipramine	0.184	3.63	35.1
Desipramine	0.848	4.23	n.d.
Imipramine	0.181	3.53	33.2
Iprindole	2.37	18.0	n.d.
Maprotiline	0.650	7.59	44.6
Mianserin	0.566	13.9	53.0*
Nomifensine	48.8	157.0	80.7
Nortriptyline	0.180	2.78	42.2
Norzimelidine	19.8	32.5	n.d.
Zimelidine	33.7	40.9	79.3
	r=0.91, $p < 0.001$	r=0.91, $p < 0.001$	
		r=0.99, $p < 0.001$	

[a] From Hall and Ögren (1981).
[b] From Ögren and Hall (1983).
[c] From Rafaelsen *et al.* (1981).
* dose 60 mg.

Correlation coefficients and p values from regression analysis (logarithms of columns 1 and 2). As mianserin was given in a lower dose in the saliva secretion study, the other values for mianserin were corrected (x 2.5) before the analysis was carried out.

lation between the central muscarinic receptor binding affinity and the peripheral effects (r = 0.91, $p < 0.001$, log-log regression analysis).

Very few studies have been performed to quantify anti-cholinergic side-effects in the clinic. However, Rafaelsen *et al.* (1981) made a quantitative measurement of saliva secretion after the administration of antidepressants to healthy volunteers. I have compared the percent inhibition relative to placebo of whole mouth saliva secretion 10 h after the administration of antidepressants (all 150 mg single dose except mianserin 60 mg single dose). As can be seen from table 2 and figure 1, there was a highly significant correlation between the inhibition of ^{3}H-QNB

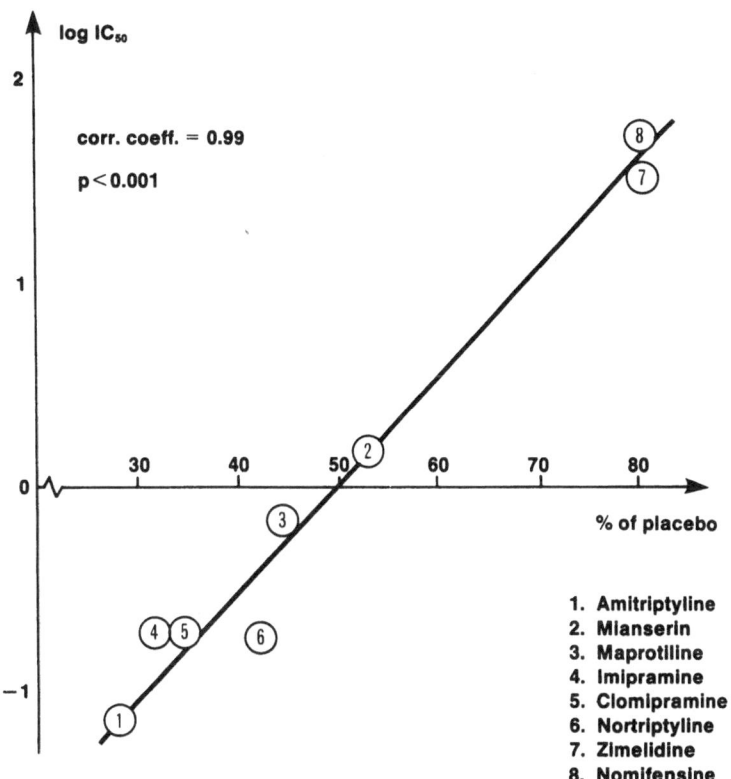

Figure 1.   Inhibition of ^{3}H-QNB binding versus percent inhibition
             of saliva secretion. (Data from Hall and Ogren (1981)
             and from Rafaelsen *et al.* (1981).)

binding in rat brain and the inhibition of whole mouth saliva
secretion in man ($p < 0.001$) and between the inhibition of acetylcholine-induced contractions of the guinea-pig ileum and the
inhibition of the whole mouth saliva secretion in man ($p < 0.001$).
These results imply that ^{3}H-QNB binding experiments can be of
great value for the prediction of antimuscarinic side-effects,
regardless of these being central or peripheral.

Histaminergic Receptors

The effects of drugs on histamine-H_1 receptors in the brain were
assessed by their potency to displace specific ^{3}H-mepyramine
binding from rat cortical homogenates (Hall and Ogren, 1981)
(table 3).   The results show that the tricyclic antidepressants

Table 3. Antihistaminergic effects of some drugs

	Inhibition of ^{3}H-mepyramine binding[a]	Block of histamine-induced contraction of guinea-pig ileum[b]	Inhibition of histamine-sensitive adenylate cyclase[c]
	(IC_{50}, nM)	(IC_{50}, nM)	(IC_{50}, nM)
Alaproclate	23200	42000	>10000
Amitriptyline	6	130	49
Brompheniramine	20	130	1100
Clomipramine	64		53
Desipramine	457	1100	280
Imipramine	29	160	140
Iprindole	250		200
Maprotiline	25	530	
Mianserin	6	330	65
Nomifensine	8870	75000	
Nortriptyline	48		
Norzimelidine	8290	42000	
Zimelidine	2900	24000	>10000

[a] From Hall and Ogren (1981).
[b] From Ogren and Hall (1983).
[c] From Kanof and Greengard (1978) and Dolphin and Greengard (personal communication).

had a high affinity for ^{3}H-mepyramine binding sites, some being approximately as active as brompheniramine.

It is well known that antihistaminergic drugs may be used as sedatives in man. It may reasonably be suggested that anti-depressants cause sedation through inhibition of histamine-H_1 receptors. We have tried to estimate the sedative action of the antidepressant drugs by using a number of different animal tests, such as decrease in locomotor activity, grip strength, passivity, rotarod performance, loss of righting reflex, etc. (Ogren *et al.*, 1981). The drugs were then ranked and the mean rank was used as an estimate of the relative sedative effect of the drug. A correlation ($r = 0.92$, $p < 0.01$) was found between these mean rank orders and the IC_{50} for inhibition of ^{3}H-mepyramine binding (figure 2), which indicates a clear association between the hista-mine-H_1 receptor interaction and sedative effects in animals.

For antidepressant drugs, Ogren *et al.* (1981) have made a rough estimate of the incidence of sedative effects in the clinic

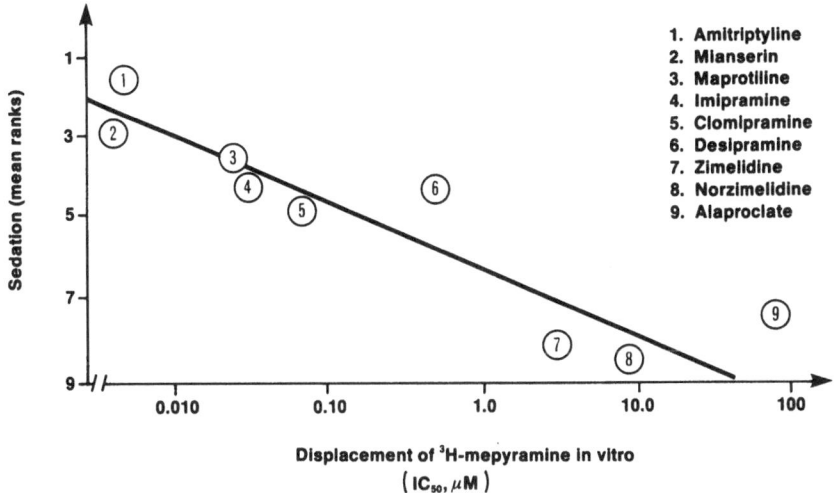

Figure 2. Relationship between sedative effects of antidepressants and central H_1-receptor blocking properties

by interpolation of data from the literature. These data correlate very well ($r = -0.97$) with the inhibition of ^{3}H-mepyramine
binding caused by these drugs. It can thus be suggested that
study of the effects of antidepressants on ^{3}H-mepyramine binding
can predict the incidence of sedative effects in the clinic.

A number of antidepressant drugs have been shown to be potent
inhibitors of histamine-sensitive adenylate cyclase in hippocampal
homogenates of the guinea-pig, an effect that has been suggested
to be mediated by histamine-H_2 receptors (Kanof and Greengard,
1978). Some of the new, non-tricyclic antidepressants, such as
zimelidine and alaproclate, are devoid of activity on histamine-
mediated adenylate cyclase (table 3). This indicates that blockade of histamine-H_2 receptors is not important for antidepressant
activity as was originally suggested (Kanof and Greengard, 1978).

Alpha-Adrenoceptors

The tricyclic antidepressant drugs are generally believed to
enhance NE activity in the brain by increasing the synaptic concentration of NE due to the inhibition of its neuronal uptake.
However, since several antidepressants block α-adrenoceptors at
low concentrations (table 4), it is suggested that several antidepressants in fact may reduce noradrenergic activity in the
brain. However, NE activity could be enhanced by an interaction

Table 4.   Effects of antidepressants on alpha-adrenoceptors and on
NE re-uptake

| | Inhibition of binding of | | Inhibition of |
	[³H]WB4101[a] (IC$_{50}$,µM)	[³H]Clonidine[a] (IC$_{50}$, µM)	NE re-uptake[b] (IC$_{50}$, µM)
Alaproclate	19.1	105	> 34
Amitriptyline	0.022	0.550	0.054
Clomipramine	0.035	4.12	0.060
Desipramine	0.250	10.6	0.003
Imipramine	0.097	5.04	0.028
Iprindole	6.81	6.70	2.6
Maprotiline	0.350	15.5	0.075
Mianserin	0.067	0.126	0.10
Nomifensine	1.27	4.56	0.007
Nortriptyline	0.088	3.87	0.013
Norzimelidine	0.953	9.30	0.76
Zimelidine	1.18	3.35	2.7

[a] From Hall and Ögren (1981).
[b] From Ross and Renyi (1975) and from Ross (personal communication).

of the antidepressants with the presynaptic α_2-adrenoceptor. There is evidence that mianserin, which is a very weak NE uptake inhibitor *in vivo* (Leonard, 1974), might cause an increase of NE release due to this interaction with presynaptic α_2-adrenoceptors (Baumann and Maître, 1977; Harper and Hughes, 1979).

The complexity of the cardiovascular system makes it practically impossible to predict the effect of drugs on, for example, heart rate, ECG and resting blood pressure (table 5) (Burgess, 1981). Nevertheless, it is quite clear that the antidepressants of the new generation, such as nomifensine and zimelidine, elicit fewer side-effects, which could be due to an overall more selective action on uptake with much less effect on the α-receptors.

Blockade of α-adrenoceptors causes a number of effects on the cardiovascular system, such as postural hypotension, tachycardia, increased cardiac output and decreased peripheral resistance (Nickerson and Hollenberg, 1967, cited in Burgess, 1981). However, as pointed out above, the antidepressant drugs may influence the cardiovascular system through other mechanisms, such as anticholinergic effects, blockade of NE or 5-HT re-uptake or local anesthetic effect (table 5). The only cardiovascular effect that might be directly related to α_1-adrenoceptor blockade is postural hypotension (Nickerson and Hollenberg, 1967). No clearcut corre-

Table 5. Potential effects of antidepressants on the CVS.
From Burgess (1981)

(1) Anticholinergic[a]	(1) Sinus bradycardia/tachycardia
	(2) Junctional rhythm
(2) Norepinephrine re-uptake blockade[h]	(1) Sinus bradycardia
	(2) Increase in PR interval
	(3) AV junctional rhythm
	(4) AV dissociation
	(5) Ventricular arrhythmias
	(6) Hypertension
(3) 5-HT re-uptake blockade[c]	(1) Hypertension
	(2) Sinus bradycardia/tachycardia
	(3) Increase in PR interval
	(4) AV junctional tachycardia
(4) Local anesthetic/ quinidine-like activity[d]	(1) Increase in QRS duration
	(2) Increase in Q-Tc duration
	(3) Decreased contractility
(5) α-Adrenoceptor blockade[e]	(1) Postural hypotension
	(2) Tachycardia
	(3) Increased cardiac output
	(4) Decreased peripheral resistance

[a] Gravenstein *et al.*, (1969). [d] Heisenbuttel and Bigger (1970).
[b] Innes and Nickerson (1975). [e] Nickerson and Hollenberg (1967).
[c] James *et al.*, (1975).

lation between the effects of antidepressants on, for example, blood pressure and α_1-adrenoceptor blockade is seen, although most antidepressants with α-adrenoceptor blocking potency cause decreased blood pressure at therapeutic doses. Neither zimelidine nor nomifensine, which are both devoid of activity on the α-adrenoceptors, causes changes in mean arterial blood pressure at doses as low as the tricyclics (Lindbom and Forsberg, 1981). However, mianserin, which is a potent inhibitor of both α_1- and α_2-adrenoceptors (Hall and Ogren, 1981), does not cause any decreased blood pressure, which is probably due to the fact that the inhibition of the presynaptic α_2-adrenoceptors counteracts the effect on the α_1-adrenoceptors.

Peroutka *et al.* (1977) have suggested that there is a significant correlation between the sedative effects of neuroleptic drugs and their ability to block α-adrenoceptors. We can find a significant correlation between the IC_{50} values for α_1-adrenoceptor binding sites (^{3}H-WB4101) and the ED_{50} for suppression of locomotion (Spearman rank correlation coefficient, $r_s = 0.71$,

$p < 0.025$; data on locomotion from Toneby, personal communication). The antidepressants which do not effect locomotion in mice (alaproclate, nomifensine, norzimelidine and zimelidine) were very weak inhibitors of ^{3}H-WB4101 binding in the rat cortex homogenates. However, as is pointed out above, histaminergic blockade is highly correlated to sedation, and the Spearman rank correlation coefficient, r_s, is even higher between ^{3}H-mepyramine binding and suppression of locomotion.

Dopaminergic Receptors

Most antidepressants are weak inhibitors of the dopaminergic receptors. The only antidepressants with some potency are clomipramine (IC_{50} = 268 nM) as seen in ^{3}H-spiroperidol binding tests (Hall and Ogren, 1981) and imipramine (K_i = 180 nM) and mianserin (K_i = 620 nM) in ^{3}H-haloperidol binding tests (Burt *et al.*, 1976). The antidopaminergic effect of these antidepressants cannot be directly related to any clinical effects or side-effects. The inhibition of dopamine uptake caused by nomifensine which increases the activity of dopamine at the receptors may be the cause of the stimulatory effects of nomifensine at higher doses.

Serotonergic Receptors

In acute studies some antidepressant drugs interfere with both central and peripheral $5\text{-}HT_1$ and $5\text{-}HT_2$ receptors. However, for the 5-HT uptake inhibitors, the potencies of postsynaptic blockade are much lower than those of the uptake inhibition (table 6). The newer non-tricyclic 5-HT selective uptake inhibitors are practically devoid of activity on the postsynaptic 5-HT receptors. The acute blockade of serotonergic receptors by some antidepressants has not been related to any effects or side-effects of the antidepressants in the clinic.

Other Receptors

With very few exceptions, the acute administration of antidepressants has been found not to interact with other receptors in the central nervous system (Hall and Ogren, 1981).

UPTAKE BINDING SITES

During recent years, binding of radiolabeled antidepressants has been described. The binding sites involved are probably closely related to the uptake sites of 5-HT (Raisman *et al.*, 1979a, b,

Table 6. Effects of some drugs on 5-HT mechanisms as studied *in vivo* and *in vitro*

	In vitro receptor binding [a] (IC$_{50}$,μM)		*In vivo* block of head twitches[b] (ED$_{50}$,μmol kg^{-1})	Block of serotonin-induced contractions[b] of rat uterus (IC$_{50}$,μM)	Block of 5-HT re-uptake[c] (IC$_{50}$,μM)
	(^{3}H)d-LSD	(^{3}H)5-HT			
Alaproclate	>100	>100	>110	2.96	0.37
Amitriptyline	0.150	1.52	15	0.39	0.18
Clomipramine	0.917	21.2	53	0.15	0.018
Desipramine	3.45	16.1	110	0.30	1.10
Imipramine	1.35	24.6	63	0.29	0.14
Iprindole	5.80	15.2	>110	0.43	10.0
Maprotiline	3.05	15.8	>80	0.23	7.2
Mianserin	0.097	1.21	18	0.0006	11.0
Nomifensine	3.47	9.88	30	0.037	6.6
Nortriptyline	0.302	1.00	30	0.044	0.87
Norzimelidine	14.7	63.1	>110	0.93	0.030
Zimelidine	10.9	33.2	>110	1.12	0.24

[a] From Hall and Ogren (1981).
[b] From Ogren *et al.*, (1979).
[c] From Ross and Renyi (1975) and Ross (personal communication).

1980; Langer and Briley, 1981; Hall *et al.*, 1982b) and of NE (Langer *et al.*, 1981; Lee and Snyder, 1981). The tricyclic anti-depressants and also some new, non-tricyclic, antidepressants have been developed as inhibitors of presynaptic neurotransmitter uptake. A close correlation can therefore also be seen between inhibition of ^{3}H-imipramine binding and the clinical efficacy of the 5-HT uptake inhibitors (Langer and Briley, 1981), as well as between inhibition of ^{3}H-desipramine binding and the clinical efficacy of the NE uptake inhibitors (Lee and Snyder, 1981).

EFFECTS ON RECEPTOR NUMBER

Long-term treatment of rats with antidepressants causes a down-regulation of the central cortical β-adrenoceptor response measured as NE- or isoprenaline-stimulated adenylate cyclase activity (Vetulani *et al.*, 1976; Banerjee *et al.*, 1977; Sulser, 1982). Extensive studies have shown that antidepressants of various types (NE and 5-HT uptake inhibitors, MAO inhibitors, atypical antidepressants) and also other antidepressant treatment (REM sleep deprivation, electroconvulsive treatment) cause subsen-sitivity of the β-adrenergic system in the brain (Sulser, 1982). However, the extent of down-regulation varies greatly between antidepressant drugs and apparently no correlation can be seen between recommended clinical dose and down-regulatory effect of the drugs (table 7).

Recently, other changes in receptor number and affinity have been reported. Thus both $5-HT_1$ and $5-HT_2$ receptors are affected (Peroutka and Snyder, 1980; Fuxe *et al.*, 1979, 1982; Hall *et al.*, 1982a). The $5-HT_2$ receptors are down-regulated similar to the β adrenoceptor, while long-term treatment with both NE and 5-HT

Table 7. Comparison of recommended full daily dose in the clinic and down-regulatory effect on central beta-adrenoceptors upon long-term treatment in rats

	Recommended full daily dose (mg per day)	Effect on beta-adrenoceptors (% of control)†
Amitriptyline	250–300	83.7 (10)
Desipramine	150–200	59.5 (5)
Mianserin	120	85.6 (10)
Zimelidine	200–300	79.0 (10)
Alaproclate*	200–600	96.5 (10)
Amiflamine*	< 5	89.0 (10)

* Drug not yet launched. Possible full daily dose.
† from Hall *et al.*, (1983). Dose (mg/kg per day) given for three weeks to rats within brackets

uptake inhibitors induces one new low-affinity 5-HT$_1$ binding site (Fuxe *et al* , 1979, 1982).

Other receptors that have been reported to be changed upon long-term treatment with antidepressants are α_2-adrenoceptors (up-regulation) (Reisine *et al.*, 1982), α_2-adrenoceptors (down-regulation) (Smith *et al.*, 1981; Vetulani, 1982), dopamine auto-receptors (down-regulation) (Reisine, 1981), and ^{3}H-imipramine binding sites (down-regulation) (Raisman *et al.*, 1980).

The change in various receptor numbers and/or affinities after long-term treatment with antidepressants does not directly correlate to the clinical effect or to any side-effect. However, since most antidepressive treatments so far cause changes in at least one type of receptor (β-adrenoceptors), it has been suggested that this effect may be part of the therapeutic mechanism (Vetulani, 1982).

CONCLUSION

Several antidepressant drugs elicit multiple direct effects on neurotransmitter receptors. Since side-effects often occur directly upon administration in contrast to the therapeutic effect which generally occurs after 2-3 weeks of treatment, it has been suggested that the side-effects are the result of direct receptor blockade. In the present paper, I have tried to correlate the incidence of side-effects with the affinity of the various drugs to neurotransmitter receptors. In a few, obvious cases this has been possible (anticholinergic side-effects vs blockade of muscarinic receptors; sedation vs histamine-H$_1$ blockade; postural hypotension vs α_1-adrenoceptor blockade). Other effects or side-effects seem to be impossible to predict on data from receptor binding studies. This is mainly due to the fact that many drugs are multiple receptor blockers and exert multiple side-effects, while others are very weak overall receptor blockers and elicit very few side-effects. It may, however, be wise to use receptor binding studies in the design of new drugs. The antidepressants of the new generation are a good example of where this technique has led to the development of drugs with more specific action.

REFERENCES

Banerjee, S. P., Kung, L.S., Riggi, S.J., and Chanda, S.K. (1977). Development of β-adrenergic receptor subsensitivity by antidepressants. Nature, 268, 455-6

Baumann, P.A. and Maître, L. (1977). Blockade of presynaptic α-receptors and of amine uptake in the rat brain by the antidepressant mianserine. Naunyn-Schmiedeb. Arch. Pharmacol., 300, 31-7

Burgess, C.D. (1981). Effects of antidepressants on cardiac
    function. Acta Psychiat. Scand., 63, Suppl. 290, 370-9
Burt, D.R., Creese, I. and Snyder, S.H. (1976). Properties of
    [^{3}H]-haloperidol and [^{3}H]dopamine binding associated with
    dopamine receptors in calf brain membranes. Mol. Pharmacol.,
    12, 800-12
Carlsson, A., Corrodi, H., Fuxe, K. and Hökfelt, T. (1969).
    Effect of antidepressant drugs on the depletion of intra-
    neuronal brain 5-hydroxytryptamine stores caused by 4-methyl-
    α-ethyl-*meta*-tyramine. Eur. J. Pharmacol., 5, 357-66
Carlsson, A., Fuxe, K., Hamberger, B. and Lindqvist, M. (1966).
    Biochemical and histochemical studies on the effects of
    imipramine-like drugs and (+)-amphetamine on central and
    peripheral catecholamine neurons. Acta Physiol. Scand., 67,
    481-97
Coppen, A. (1967). The biochemistry of affective disorders.
    Br. J. Psychiatry., 113, 1237-64
Fuxe, K., Ogren, S.O. and Agnati, L.F. (1979). The effects of
    chronic treatment with the 5-hydroxytryptamine uptake blocker
    zimelidine on central 5-hydroxytryptamine mechanisms.
    Evidence for the induction of a low affinity binding site for
    5-hydroxytryptamine. Neurosci. Lett., 13, 307-12
Fuxe, K., Ogren, S.O., Agnati, L.F., Andersson, K. and Eneroth, P.
    (1982). Effects of subchronic antidepressant drug treatment
    on central serotonergic mechanisms in the male rat.   In
    Typical and Atypical Antidepressants. Molecular Mechanisms
    (ed. E.Costa and G. Racagni). (Advances in Biochemical
    Psychopharmacology, Vol. 31) pp. 91-107
Glowinski, J. and Axelrod, J. (1964). Inhibition of uptake of
    tritiated noradrenaline in the intact rat brain by imipramine
    and structurally related compounds. Nature, 204, 1318-19
Gravenstein, J.S., Ariet, M. and Thornby, J.I. (1969). Atropine
    on the electrocardiogram. Clin. Pharmacol. Ther., 10, 660-6
Hall, H. and Ogren, S.O. (1981). Effects of antidepressant drugs
    on different receptors in the brain. Eur. J. Pharmacol., 70,
    393-407
Hall, H., Ross, S.B. and Ogren, S.O. (1982a). Effects of
    zimelidine on various transmitter systems in the brain.   In
    Typical and Atypical Antidepressants. Molecular Mechanisms.
    (ed. E. Costa and G. Racagni). (Advances in Biochemical
    Psychopharmacolocy. Vol. 31) pp 321-5
Hall, H., Ross, S., Ogren, S.O. and Gawell, L. (1982b). Binding
    of a specific 5-HT uptake inhibitor, ^{3}H-norzimelidine, to rat
    brain homogenates. Eur. J. Pharmacol., 80, 281-2
Hall, H., Ross, S.B. and Sällemark, M. (1983). Effect of
    destruction of central noradrenergic and serotonergic nerve
    terminals by systemic neurotoxins on the longterm effects of
    antidepressants on β-adrenoceptors and 5-HT$_2$ in the binding
    sites rat cerebral cortex. To be published

Harper, B. and Hughes, I.E. (1979). Presynaptic α-adrenoceptor blocking properties among tri- and tetra-cyclic antidepressant drugs. Br. J. Pharmacol., 67, 511–17

Heisenbuttel, R. H. and Bigger, J.T. (1970). The effect of quinidine on intraventricular conduction in man. Correlation of plasma quinidine with changes in QRS duration. Am. Heart J., 80, 453–62

Innes, J.R. and Nickerson, M. (1975). Norepinephrine, epinephrine and the sympathomimetic amines. In Pharmacological Basis of Therapeutics (ed. L.S. Goodman and A. Gilman). Macmillan, London, pp.491–2

Iversen, L. (1965). Inhibition of noradrenaline uptake by drugs. J. Pharm. Pharmacol., 17, 62–4

James, T.N., Isobe, J.H. and Urthaler, F. (1975). Analysis of components in a cardiogenic hypertensive reflex. Circulation, 52, 179–92

Kanof, P. D. and Greengard, P. (1978). Brain histamine receptors as targets for antidepressant drugs. Nature, 272, 329–33

Langer, S. Z. and Briley, M. (1981). High affinity imipramine binding: a new biological tool for studies in depression. Trends Neurosci., 2, 28–31

Langer, S.Z., Raisman, R. and Briley, M. (1981). High affinity (^{3}H)-DMI binding is associated with neuronal noradrenaline uptake in the periphery and the central nervous system. Eur. J. Pharmacol., 72, 423–4

Lee, C.-M. and Snyder, S.H. (1981). Norepinephrine neuronal uptake binding sites in rat brain membranes labelled with (^{3}H)-desipramine. Proc. Natl. Acad. Sci., 78, 5250–4

Leonard, B.E. (1974). Some effects of a new tetracyclic antidepressant compound Org GB 94 on the metabolism of monoamines in the rat brain. Psychopharmacologia, 36, 221–36

Lindbom, L.-O. and Forsberg, T. (1981). Cardiovascular effects of zimelidine and other antidepressants in conscious rats. Acta Psychiat. Scand., 63, Suppl. 290, 380–4

Nickerson, M. and Hollenberg, N.K. (1967). Blockade of alpha adrenergic receptors. In Physiological Pharmacology, vol. 4, The Nervous System (ed. W.S. Root and F.G. Hofmann), Academic Press, New York, Part D, autonomic nervous system drugs, pp. 243–305

Ögren, S.O., Cott, J.M. and Hall, H. (1981). Sedative/anxiolytic effects of antidepressants in animals. Acta Psychiat. Scand., 63, Suppl. 290, 277–88

Ögren, S.O., Fuxe, K., Agnati, L.F., Gustafsson, J. A., Jonsson, G. and Holm, A.C. (1979). Reevaluation of the indoleamine hypothesis of depression. Evidence for a reduction of functional activity of central 5-HT systems by antidepressant drugs J. Neural Transm., 46, 85–103

Ögren, S.O. and Hall, H. (1983). Peripheral and central anticholinergic properties of the 5-HT uptake inhibitors zimelidine and alaproclate. To be published

Peroutka, S.J. and Snyder, S.H. (1980). Regulation of serotonin$_2$ (5-HT$_2$) receptors labelled with (^{3}H)-spiroperidol by chronic treatment with the antidepressant amitriptyline. J. Pharmacol. Exp. Ther., 215, 582-7

Peroutka, S.J., U'Prichard, D.C., Greenberg, D.A. and Snyder, S.H. (1977). Neuroleptic drug interactions with norepinephrine α-receptor binding sites in rat brain. Neuropharmacology, 16, 549-56

Rafaelsen, O.J., Clemmesen, L., Lund, H., Mikkelsen, P.L. and Bolwig, T.G. (1981). Comparison of peripheral anticholinergic effects of antidepressants: dry mouth. Acta Psychiat. Scand., 63, Suppl 290, 364-9

Raisman, R., Briley, M. and Langer, S.Z. (1979a). High-affinity [^{3}H]imipramine binding in rat cerebral cortex. Eur. J. Pharmacol., 54, 307-8

Raisman, R., Briley, M. and Langer, S.Z. (1979b). Specific tricyclic antidepressant binding site in rat brain. Nature, 281, 148-50

Raisman, R., Briley, M.S. and Langer, S.Z. (1980). Specific tricyclic antidepressant binding sites in rat brain characterized by high-affinity ^{3}H-imipramine binding. Eur. J. Pharmacol., 61, 373-80

Reisine, T. (1981). Adaptive changes in catecholamine receptors in the central nervous system. Neuroscience, 61, 1471-502

Reisine, T., Johanson, R., Weich, N., Ursillo, R. and Yamamura, H. (1982). Rapid desensitization of central beta-receptors and upregulation of alpha$_2$ receptors following antidepressant treatment. In Typical and Atypical Antidepressants. Molecular Mechanisms. (ed. E. Costa and G. Racagni). (Advances in Biochemical Psychopharmacology, Vol. 31) pp. 63-7

Ross, S. B. and Renyi, A.L. (1969). Inhibition of the uptake of tritiated 5-hydroxytryptamine in brain tissue. Eur. J. Pharmacol., 7, 270-7

Ross, S.B. and Renyi, A.L. (1975). Tricyclic antidepressant agents. I. Comparison of the inhibition of the uptake of [^{3}H]noradrenaline and [^{14}C]5-hydroxytryptamine in slices and crude synaptosome preparations of the midbrain-hypothalamus region of the rat brain. Acta. Pharmacol. Toxicol., 36, 382-94

Schildkraut, J.J. (1965). The catecholamine hypothesis of affective disorders: a review of supporting evidence. Am. J. Psychiatry, 122, 413-18

Smith, C.B., Garcia-Sevilla, J.A. and Hollingsworth, P.J. (1981). Adrenoceptors in rat brain are decreased after long-term tricyclic antidepressant drug treatment. Brain Res., 210, 413-18

Snyder, S.H. and Yamamura, H.I. (1977). Antidepressants and the muscarinic acetylcholine receptor. Arch. Gen. Psychiatry, 34, 236-9

Sulser, F. (1982). Antidepressant drug research, its impact on neurobiology and psychobiology. In Typical and Atypical Antidepressants. Molecular Mechanisms. (ed. E. Costa and G. Racagni). (Advances in Biochemical Psychopharmacology, vol. 31) pp 1-20

U'Prichard, D.C., Greenberg, D.A., Sheehan, P.P. and Snyder, S.H. (1978). Tricyclic antidepressants: therapeutic properties and affinity of α-noradrenergic receptor binding sites in the brain. Science, 199, 197-8

Van Praag, H.M. (1974). Towards a biochemical topology of depression. Pharmacopsychiatry, 7, 281-92

Vetulani, J. (1982). Adaptive changes as the mode of action of antidepressant treatment. In Typical and Atypical Antidepressants. Molecular Mechanisms. (ed. E. Costa and G. Racagni) (Advances in Biochemical Psychopharmacology, vol. 31) pp 27-36

Vetulani, J., Stawarz, R.J., Dingell, J.V. and Sulser, F. (1976). A possible common mechanism of action of antidepressant treatments. Arch. Pharmacol., 293, 109-14

Wolfe, B.B., Harden, T.K., Sporn, J.R. and Molinoff, P.B. (1978). Presynaptic modulation of beta adrenergic receptors in rat cerebral cortex after treatment with antidepressants. J. Pharmacol. Exp. Ther., 207, 446-57

Yamamura, H.I. and Snyder, S.H. (1974). Muscarinic cholinergic binding in rat brain, Proc. Natl. Acad. Sci. USA, 71, 1725-9

Antidepressants and ∝-adrenoceptors

Roger M.Pinder[1]

INTRODUCTION

Although research into the biochemical and pharmacological effects of psychotropic agents has been largely responsible for the development of hypotheses concerning the etiology of depressive illness, the precise mechanism of action of antidepressant drugs is still a matter for conjecture. The widely quoted hypothesis of monoamine deficiency in depression, whereby antidepressants act rapidly to enhance the availability of norepinephrine (NE) and/or serotonin (5-HT) in the brain via decreased catabolism or inhibition of monoamine uptake (Schildkraut, 1965), is now seen to be an oversimplification (Charney *et al.*, 1981b; Sugrue, 1981a; Waldmeier, 1981). Thus, some newer antidepressants neither inhibit monoamine oxidase (MAO) nor significantly affect monoamine uptake, while several highly effective uptake inhibitors appear not to be useful in the treatment of depression. Furthermore, the time course of drug effects on monoamine availability, which are immediate, are inconsistent with the clinical improvement, which may take two to three weeks. In order to accommodate some of these difficulties, the hypothesis has been extended to include dopamine (Randrup and Braestrup, 1977), and research has focused on the effects of chronic administration of antidepressants, particularly the adaptive changes induced in the sensitivity or density of monoamine receptors (Charney *et al.*, 1981b; Waldmeier, 1981).

In addition to their well documented acute effects on monoamine uptake and MAO (Maxwell and White, 1978; Randrup and Braestrup, 1977), antidepressants interact directly with a number of central receptors including muscarinic, histaminergic, serotonergic and adrenergic receptors (Hall and Ogren, 1981; Sugrue, 1981a). Interactions with muscarinic (Snyder and Yamamura, 1977) or histamine H_1-receptors (Richelson, 1979; Diffley *et al.*, 1980)

---

[1]Scientific Development Group, Organon, Oss, The Netherlands.

are probably more associated with the anticholinergic or sedative side-effects respectively of antidepressants than with their therapeutic action. Suggestions that inhibition by antidepressants of H_2-sensitive adenylate cyclase in brain is involved in their therapeutic action (Kanof and Greengard, 1978) are discouraged by the similar potency of neuroleptic phenothiazines in this respect and by the high selectivity of antidepressants for H_1- rather than H_2- receptors (Snyder, 1980). Furthermore, adaptive changes in sensitivity or density have not been observed for muscarinic or histaminergic receptors following chronic treatment with antidepressants (Maggi *et al.*, 1980a; Peroutka and Snyder, 1980). As far as central 5-HT receptors are concerned, many antidepressants behave as classicial 5-HT antagonists in both pharmacological (Maj, 1981) and receptor binding studies (Tang and Seeman, 1980; Hall and Ogren, 1981), while upon chronic administration they appear to reduce the density of 5-HT receptors of the $5-HT_2$ type (Peroutka and Snyder, 1980). It is possible that the therapeutic action of some antidepressants may in part be due to a reduced functional activity of some central serotonergic systems.

Antidepressant drugs exert manifold effects upon central noradrenergic systems (Sugrue, 1981a). Following acute administration or *in vitro*, many antidepressants strongly inhibit neuronal re-uptake of NE, are potent antagonists at postsynaptic α_1-adrenoceptors but in general weak antagonists at presynaptic α_2-adrenoceptors, and do not interact at all with β-adrenoceptors. Chronic administration appears to reduce the density of cortical α_2- and β-receptors leading to a condition of subsensitivity to agonists. The effects of antidepressants on NE uptake (Maxwell and White, 1978) and β-adrenoceptor function (Sulser *et al.*, 1978) have been reviewed elsewhere. It is the purpose of the present paper to review the roles played by α_1- and α_2-adrenoceptors in the mechanisms of action of antidepressants.

CLASSIFICATION AND FUNCTION OF α-ADRENOCEPTORS

There are two basic types of α-adrenoceptor, α_1 and α_2, which differ in their selectivity for the α-antagonists prazosin and yohimbine and for the α-agonists clonidine, α-methylnorepinephrine and phenylephrine (van Zwieten and Timmermans, 1980; Exton, 1982). α_1-Receptors are located postsynaptically, are blocked more potently by prazosin than by yohimbine, and generally have low affinity for clonidine and α-methylnorepinephrine but high affinity for phenylephrine. On the other hand, α_2-adrenoceptors are located both pre- and postsynaptically, are blocked more potently by yohimbine, and have high affinity for clonidine and α-methylnorepinephrine but low affinity for phenylephrine (table 1). The terms pre- and postsynaptic describe the location of α-adrenoceptors, while the α_1/α_2 subdivision is based upon selectivity for

Table 1. Characteristics of α-adrenoceptors

Receptor type	Location	Selective agonists	Selective antagonists
α_1	postsynaptic	phenylephrine	prazosin
α_2	presynaptic	clonidine α-methylnorepinephrine	yohimbine
α_2	postsynaptic	clonidine α-methylnorepinephrine	yohimbine

(1) Receptor binding studies using ^{3}H-clonidine or ^{3}H-yohimbine do not differentiate between pre- and postsynaptic α_2-adrenoceptors. (2) Clonidine acts presynaptically to lower NE turnover, but postsynaptically to lower blood pressure and stimulate growth hormone secretion.

agonists and antagonists. The endogenous catecholamines NE and epinephrine are non-selective agonists, that is they are about equally active at both α_1- and α_2-adrenoceptors.

Postsynaptic α-adrenoceptors are located at the target cell and represent classical receptors in the traditional sense. Their stimulation by an agonist causes a physiological or pharmacological response, involving changes in cell calcium fluxes for α_1-receptors and a decrease in intracellular cyclic AMP for α_2-receptors. Presynaptic α_2-adrenoceptors appear to mediate a negative feedback mechanism which leads to inhibition of transmitter release probably by restricting the calcium available for the excitation-secretion coupling (Langer, 1977; Starke *et al.*, 1977; Westfall, 1977). Thus, stimulation of presynaptic α_2-receptors by agonists, including NE itself, reduces the amount of NE released per nerve impulse from its storage sites in the neuron. Accordingly, NE in the synaptic cleft inhibits its own release, while α-sympatholytic agents increase the amount of NE released per nerve impulse as a result of blockade of presynaptic α_2-receptors. Both α_1- and α_2-adrenoceptors are widely distributed in the brain, particularly in the cortex (Maggi *et al.*, 1980b). However, central postsynaptic α_2-adrenoceptors appear to be mainly involved in mediating hypotensive actions in the brainstem.

ACUTE EFFECTS OF ANTIDEPRESSANTS ON CENTRAL α-ADRENOCEPTORS

α_1-Adrenoceptors

A number of antidepressants have been studied for blockade of central α_1-adrenoceptors, using the antagonistic ligand WB-4101 (tables 2 and 3). The use of different brain areas and species,

Table 2. Inhibition of ³H–WB–4101 binding (α₁-adrenoceptors) by tricyclic antidepressants. All values are given in nM

Drug	Rat brain K_i [a]	Rat cortex		Calf cortex IC_{50} [d]
		K_i [b]	IC_{50} [c]	
Tertiary amines				
Amitriptyline	23	24	22	46
Clomipramine	55	–	35	130
Doxepin	23	23	–	24
Imipramine	58	58	97	160
Trimipramine	–	–	–	67
Secondary amines				
Desipramine	148	150	250	440
Maprotiline	–	–	350	250
Nortriptyline	71	71	88	130
Protriptyline	277	280	–	420
Reference α-antagonists				
Phentolamine (α₁/α₂)	–	3.6	–	–
Prazosin (α₁)	–	0.49	–	–
Yohimbine (α₂)	–	480	–	–

[a] U'Prichard *et al.* (1978).
[b] Maggi *et al.* (1980a).
[c] Hall and Ogren (1981).
[d] Tang and Seeman (1980).

IC_{50} values (nM) for inhibition of NE uptake in rat brain synaptosomes (Randrup and Braestrup, 1977): amitriptyline (20), clomipramine (44), imipramine (20), trimipramine (1000), desipramine (1.5), maprotiline (20), nortriptyline (11), protriptyline (3).

the quoting of results as inhibitory concentrations (IC_{50}) or as inhibition constants (K_i) and the non-standardization of receptor binding techniques suggest that comparisons between antidepressant drugs should be made with confidence only within individual studies. Nevertheless, the different sets of results appear to be consistent.

Most of the drugs studied, particularly tricyclic antidepressants (table 2) had a high affinity for the antagonistic α₁-adrenoceptor. The most potent antidepressants included doxepin, amitriptyline, clomipramine, imipramine and trimipramine, which all have a tertiary amino group in the side chain. These drugs inhibited binding at about the same concentrations as they inhibited NE uptake (table 2), with the exception of trimipramine which was very much more potent as an α₁-antagonist than as an uptake inhibitor. Secondary amino tricyclics, on the other hand, were relatively weak α₁-antagonists and much more effective as inhibitors of NE uptake (table 2).

Table 3. Inhibition of ^{3}H-WB-4101 binding (α_1-adrenoceptors) by
atypical antidepressants. All values are given in nM

Drug	Rat brain K_i [a]	Rat cortex		Calf cortex IC_{50} [d]
		K_i [b]	IC_{50} [c]	
Selective 5-HT uptake inhibitors				
Alaproclate	–	–	19100	–
Fluoxetine	8000	> 1000	–	–
Zimelidine	–	–	1180	1210
Others				
Iprindole	9600	> 1000	6810	6150
Mianserin	–	86	67	56
Nomifensin	–	–	1270	980
Trazodone	–	68	–	–
Reference α-antagonists				
Phentolamine (α_1/α_2)	–	3.6	–	–
Prazosin (α_1)	–	0.49	–	–
Yohimbine (α_2)	–	480	–	–

[a] U'Prichard *et al.* (1978).
[b] Maggi *et al.* (1980a).
[c] Hall and Ogren (1981).
[d] Tang and Seeman (1980).

Of the atypical antidepressants, only mianserin and trazodone
showed inhibition of WB-4101 binding at concentrations below 1 μM
(table 3). Most of the compounds, especially the selective 5-HT
uptake inhibitors alaproclate, fluoxetine and zimelidine, as well
as other atypicals like iprindole and nomifensin, were virtually
inactive. Mianserin and trazodone were intermediate in potency
between the two groups of tricyclic antidepressants.

In assessing the significance of the apparent central α_1-
antagonism displayed by some antidepressants, it is important to
bear in mind that even the most potent compounds like doxepin and
amitriptyline are at least 50-fold less potent than the specific
α_1-antagonist prazosin (table 2). Furthermore, they are about
10-fold less potent in receptor binding studies with WB-4101 than
is the non-selective α-antagonist phentolamine (Maggi *et al.*,
1980a). Nevertheless, it is likely that the α_1-adrenolytic
activity shown by many antidepressants is in part responsible for
their ability to produce hypotensive side-effects. Thus, the
tertiary amines imipramine, amitriptyline and clomipramine, which
are among the most potent antidepressants for central α_1-adreno-
ceptor antagonism, are also more prone to cause orthostatic hypotension than is the secondary amine nortriptyline (Glassman and
Bigger, 1981).

Significant correlations have been noted between the sedative effects of antidepressants and their ability to block α_1-adreno-ceptors, suggesting an involvement of α_1-receptors in the pro-duction of sedation (U'Prichard *et al.*, 1978; Snyder, 1980; Hall and Ogren, 1981). However, a similar rank order of potency exists for the blockade by tricyclic antidepressants of both central (Richelson, 1979; Diffley *et al.*, 1980) and peripheral (Figge *et al.*, 1979) histamine H_1-receptors as holds for blockade of α_1-adrenoceptors, and central H_1-receptors are believed to mediate the production of sedation by antihistamines (Uzan *et al.*, 1979). Suggestions have also been made that an inverse relationship exists between blockade of α_1-adrenoceptors and the ability of antidepressants to produce psychomotor activation (U'Prichard *et al.*, 1978; Snyder, 1980). Some evidence does exist to support this, since those atypical antidepressants which block α_1-adreno-ceptors are also sedative, for example mianserin and trazodone, whereas those which do not block α_1-adrenoceptors tend to be activating, such as nomifensin and zimelidine. Again, however, the so-called activating drugs also happen to have less anti-histamine properties (Hall and Ogren, 1981), which could explain their apparent lack of sedation and tendency toward psychomotor activation.

Table 4. Inhibition of ^3H-clonidine binding (α_2-adrenoceptors) by tricyclic antidepressants. All values are given in nM

Drug	Rat cortex		Calf cortex
	K_1[a]	IC_{50}[b]	IC_{50}[c]
Tertiary amines			
Amitriptyline	630	550	850
Clomipramine	–	5040	7430
Doxepin	890	–	2000
Imipramine	3400	4120	4930
Trimipramine	–	–	1700
Secondary amines			
Desipramine	7600	10600	9400
Maprotiline	–	15500	16770
Nortriptyline	1700	3870	2980
Protriptyline	14000	–	10360
Reference α-antagonists			
Phentolamine (α_1/α_2)	2.5	–	–
Prazosin (α_1)	6400	–	–
Yohimbine (α_2)	73	–	–

[a] Maggi *et al.* (1980a).
[b] Hall and Ogren (1981).
[c] Tang and Seeman (1980).

α_2-Adrenoceptors

Antidepressants are in general weak antagonists at central α_2-adrenoceptors as determined by displacement of binding of the agonistic ligand clonidine (tables 4 and 5). IC_{50} and K_D values tend to be in the 1–10 µM range, comparable to those of prazosin which is pharmacologically inactive at the α_2-receptor (van Zwieten and Timmermans, 1980). All antidepressants are clearly less potent than the non-selective α-antagonist phentolamine and, with the exception of mianserin, they are less potent than the selective α_2-antagonist yohimbine. There appears to be no correlation between the affinities of antidepressants for the α_1-antagonistic and the α_2-agonistic binding sites, except that tertiary amine tricyclics generally tend to be more potent than secondary amine tricyclics at both receptors (table 4). All antidepressants, with the possible exception of mianserin, appear to be selective for the α_1-antagonistic binding site.

In addition to their effects on NE uptake, antidepressants may raise synaptic NE levels by increasing NE release from the presynaptic neuron, that is via presynaptic α_2-adrenoceptor blockade (Collis and Shepherd, 1980). This activity has been confirmed pharmacologically for amitriptyline and mianserin, which are the most potent presynaptic α_2-antagonists in receptor binding experiments (table 5). Thus, mianserin has been shown to raise the

Table 5.   Inhibition of ^{3}H-clonidine binding (α_2-adrenoceptors) by atypical antidepressants. All values are given in nM

Drug	Rat cortex		Calf cortex
	K_i [a]	IC_{50} [b]	IC_{50} [c]
Selective 5-HT uptake inhibitors			
Alaproclate	–	$> 10^5$	–
Fluoxetine	9200	–	–
Zimelidine	–	3350	610
Others			
Iprindole	11400	6700	16000
Mianserin	35	126	12
Nomifensin	–	4560	2480
Trazodone	2100	–	–
Reference α-antagonists			
Phentolamine (α_1/α_2)	2.5	–	–
Prazosin (α_1)	6400	–	–
Yohimbine (α_2)	73	–	–

[a] Maggi *et al.* (1980a).
[b] Hall and Ogren (1981).
[c] Tang and Seeman (1980).

amount of NE released in response to nerve stimulation of tissues previously incubated with ^{3}H-NE, both in central (Baumann and Maître, 1977) and peripheral (Harper and Hughes, 1979; Doggrell, 1980) tissues, and similar effects have been observed for amitriptyline in peripheral tissue (Hughes, 1978; Collis and Shepherd, 1980). Mianserin has also been shown after acute administration to reverse the electrophysiological (Svensson *et al.*, 1981), behavioral (Robson *et al.*, 1978; Clineschmidt *et al.*, 1979; Hunt *et al.*, 1981), cardiovascular (Doxey *et al.*, 1978; Robson *et al.*, 1978; Cavero *et al.*, 1980) and biochemical (Baumann and Maître, 1977; Fludder and Leonard, 1979a; Sugrue, 1980) effects of the α_2-agonist clonidine. However, although mianserin has consistently been shown to be the antidepressant with the most·potent effects at α_2-adrenoceptors, its selectivity for α_2- over α_1-receptors is doubtful. Indeed all of the studies mentioned above have tended to show about equipotency at α_1- and α_2-receptors. Furthermore, while being the most potent of the antidepressants at peripheral α_2-adrenoceptors, mianserin is also somewhat more effective at peripheral α_1-adrenoceptors (table 6). Nevertheless, since mianserin is a very weak inhibitor of NE uptake *in vivo* despite moderately potent effects *in vitro* (Goodlett *et al.*, 1977), presynaptic α_2-blockade could be a way by which the drug raises synaptic NE levels.

CHRONIC EFFECTS OF ANTIDEPRESSANTS ON CENTRAL α-ADRENOCEPTORS

The acute effects of antidepressants on α-adrenoceptors may not be relevant to their therapeutic action, and attention has turned in

Table 6. Antagonistic potencies of antidepressants at peripheral pre- and postsynaptic α-adrenoceptors (Brown *et al.*, 1980)

Compound	Presynaptic activity[a]	Postsynaptic activity[b]	Ratio pre/post
Amitriptyline	8.6×10^{-6}	5.8×10^{-8}	0.007
Nortriptyline	1.1×10^{-5}	8.5×10^{-7}	0.08
Mianserin	6.5×10^{-7}	1.8×10^{-7}	0.28
Trazodone	1.1×10^{-6}	1.8×10^{-7}	0.16
Viloxazine	1.3×10^{-5}	$> 3.5 \times 10^{-5}$	-
Yohimbine	7.9×10^{-9}	8.9×10^{-7}	113
Prazosin	2.9×10^{-6}	1.4×10^{-9}	0.0005

[a] Concentration (M) producing 20% reversal of inhibition by cocaine of electrically induced contractions of rat vas deferens.
[b] Concentration (M) producing 50% inhibition of the effects of NE on rat anoccygeus muscle.

recent years to their influence on receptor systems during chronic administration. The ability of many antidepressants to decrease the binding of postsynaptic β-adrenoceptors and 5-HT receptors in rat brain does not extend to a large extent to α-adrenoceptor binding (Charney *et al.*, 1981b; Sugrue, 1981a).

α_1-Adrenoceptors

Although there are reports of reduced binding of WB-4101 in rat vas deferens following chronic desipramine treatment (Wetzel *et al.*, 1981) and even of increased binding in mouse brain after long-term amitriptyline treatment (Rehavi *et al.*, 1980), the consensus of opinion is that α_1-adrenoceptor binding is largely unaffected by chronic treatment with antidepressants. Thus, chronically administered antidepressants of various classes including desipramine, imipramine, amitriptyline, iprindole, pargyline and fluoxetine fail to alter WB-4101 binding in rat brain (Bergstrom and Kellar, 1979; Rosenblatt *et al.*, 1979; Peroutka and Snyder, 1980; Tang *et al.*, 1981). This conclusion is at variance with both the electrophysiological and behavioral evidence for enhanced responsiveness toward NE at postsynaptic α_1-adrenoceptors. Long-term treatment with imipramine, clomipramine, amitriptyline, desipramine and iprindole has enhanced responses to iontophoretic NE in a number of projection areas of the brain which are mediated through postsynaptic α-adrenoceptors, for example in the dorsal lateral geniculate (Menkes and Aghajanian, 1981) and the facial motor nucleus (Menkes *et al.*, 1980). An enhanced response to iontophoretic NE has also been observed in rat amygdaloid neurons after long-term desipramine, imipramine or iprindole, but the amygdala contains NE neurons which may have both α- and β- characteristics (Wang and Aghajanian, 1980). In behavioral studies (Maj *et al.*, 1979a,b; Charney *et al.*, 1981a,b), chronic antidepressant treatment enhances responsiveness to catecholamine agonists. Despite the lack of changes in binding, it appears that central postsynaptic α_1-adrenoceptors become supersensitive to the effects of NE following long-term treatment with many antidepressants.

α_2-Adrenoceptors

The effects of chronic antidepressant treatment on α_2-adrenoceptors are important *per se*, and because of suggestions that α_2-adrenoceptor sensitivity is mediated by β-receptors in a type of homeostatic control mechanism for central NE function (Maggi *et al.*, 1980b) and that β-receptor desensitization results from a gradually developing subsensitivity of presynaptic α_2-receptors (Crews and Smith, 1978). Central α_2-adrenoceptor subsensitivity, however, is produced by only some and not all antidepressants and is by no means a general mechanism of action. Moreover, supersensitivity has also been reported.

Electrophysiological responses of NE neurons in the locus coeruleus to the α_2-agonist clonidine were reduced by chronic treatment with desipramine, imipramine and zimelidine but not by mianserin, iprindole or clomipramine (Svensson *et al.*, 1981; Svensson and Scuvee-Moreau, 1981). After chronic desipramine treatment, locus coeruleus neurons of rats failed to respond to a single dose of desipramine which in untreated animals markedly decreased neuronal firing (McMillen *et al.*, 1980). However, although chronic desipramine treatment is reported to reduce α_2-adrenoceptor sensitivity in rat heart (Crews and Smith, 1978), the response of brain α_2-receptors is at best equivocal (see Charney *et al.*, 1981a). Certainly, ^{3}H-clonidine binding in rat cortex was unaffected by long-term treatment with desipramine, mianserin or iprindole (Sugrue, 1981b; Tang *et al.*, 1981), although it was reduced by the MAOIs clorgyline, pargyline and tranylcypromine (Cohen *et al.*, 1980; Sugrue, 1981b). There was no evidence that inverse reciprocal modulation of central adrenoceptors occurred, since some of the treatments which failed to alter ^{3}H-clonidine binding were highly effective in reducing β-adrenoceptor density. The effects of amitriptyline on ^{3}H-clonidine binding are equivocal, with reports of unchanged (Tang *et al.*, 1981) or decreased binding (Smith *et al.*, 1981).

Interactions of antidepressants with the behavioral and biochemical effects of clonidine are equivocal because the doses used have sometimes been in excess of those (25–100 μg kg^{-1}, i.p.) required to activate presynaptic α_2-receptors selectively (see Sugrue, 1981a). Long-term treatment with desipramine attenuated suppression of rat locomotor activity induced by a dose of clonidine known to be selective for α_2-adrenoceptors (Spyraki and Fibiger, 1980), and also attenuated the clonidine-induced reduction of rat brain levels of the NE metabolite 3-methoxy-4-hydroxyphenylglycol (MHPG) (McMillen *et al.*, 1980; Sugrue, 1981c). The ability of chronic desipramine to attenuate biochemical responses to clonidine appears to depend upon the frequency (twice daily) and duration (5–9 days) of desipramine administered as well as the dose of clonidine (Sugrue, 1981a,c). The use of low-dose clonidine has also shown that long-term treatment with amitriptyline, trazodone or iprindole does not attenuate the clonidine-induced reduction in MHPG (Sugrue, 1981a).

Mianserin, despite its potent antagonism at presynaptic α_2-adrenoceptors, failed to alter biochemical responses to low-dose clonidine in rats given daily doses of 10 mg kg^{-1} for 9 to 15 days, although it was effective both acutely and after 5 days of treatment (Sugrue, 1980). Reports that chronic mianserin treatment antagonizes both the behavioral and biochemical effects of clonidine involved the use of doses of the α_2-agonist well in excess of 100 μg kg^{-1}, which probably also stimulated α_1-

adrenoceptors (Fludder and Leonard, 1979a,b; Tang *et al.*, 1979). Furthermore, mianserin given chronically failed to reverse the acute hypotensive and biochemical responses to a single dose of 300 μg clonidine in healthy volunteers (Elliott *et al.*, 1981).

There is also evidence that some antidepressants can cause supersensitivity of α_2-adrenoceptors. The density of α_2-receptors has been reported to be increased by long-term desipramine (Johnson *et al.*, 1980). Both desipramine (Schoffelmeer and Mulder, 1982) and mianserin (Cerrito and Raiteri, 1981) appear to increase the release of NE from brain tissue after chronic administration to rats, an action mediated through presynaptic α_2-adrenoceptors.

ANTIDEPRESSANTS AND HUMAN α-ADRENOCEPTORS

Studies of α-adrenoceptors in man have necessarily assessed peripheral rather than brain receptor responses, and have generally had to rely upon indirect and possibly non-specific measures of receptor responses such as blood pressure, growth hormone and cortisol secretion, and NE metabolite levels. The data have been extensively reviewed and lead to opposite conclusions - blood pressure responses appear to support the presence of supersensitive peripheral postsynaptic α-adrenoceptors in depression while the hormone data support a subsensitivity of these same receptors (Cohen *et al.*, 1980; Charney *et al.*, 1981b; Sugrue, 1981a; Waldmeier, 1981). More recent research has concentrated on the role of presynaptic α_2-adrenoceptors in depression, being based upon the hypothesis that such receptors are supersensitive in depression and may be down-regulated or desensitized by antidepressant treatment (Cohen *et al.*, 1980; Smith *et al.*, 1981).

Binding sites for ^{3}H-clonidine or ^{3}H-yohimbine on human platelet membranes seem to satisfy the biochemical and pharmacological requirements of a physiological α_2-adrenoceptor and appear to be similar in nature to central α_2-adrenoceptors in several species including humans (Garcia-Sevilla *et al.*, 1981a,b). Using ^{3}H-clonidine as an agonistic ligand, platelet α_2-adrenoceptor density (B_{max}) in drug-free patients with major depressive disorder was shown to be significantly higher than that in normal subjects, although the affinity of clonidine for the receptor (K_D) was not different between the groups (table 6). There was no relation between values of B_{max} and the severity of depression. Treatment of six patients with imipramine or amitriptyline led to significant decreases in both the density of α_2-receptors and the affinity of clonidine for the receptor (table 6). Since tricyclics competitively inhibit ^{3}H-clonidine binding *in vitro* with an increased K_D and unchanged B_{max} these effects are probably specific for long-term treatment. However, the relevance of these findings to the mechanism of antidepressant action is marred by the observation that similar decreases in B_{max} and K_D were observed in one

Table 7. α₂-Adrenoceptor binding to human platelet membranes[a]

Authors	3H- ligand	Normal subjects		Patients with major depressive disorder[b]			
				Drug-free		After treatment[c]	
		K_D	B_{max}	K_D	B_{max}	K_D	B_{max}
Garcia-Sevilla et al. (1981b)	clonidine	5.0 (n=21)	34.2* (n=21)	5.5 (n=17)	45* (n=17)		
				6.3+ (n=6)	50§ (n=6)	3.3+ (n=6)	34§ (n=6)
Daiguji et al. (1981)	yohimbine	0.92 (n=9)	240 (n=9)	0.97 (n=11)	204 (n=11)	–	–

[a] K_D = dissociation constant (nM), B_{max} = maximal binding capacity (fmol per mg protein), n = number of subjects.

[b] Research Diagnostic Criteria.

[c] Four patients received imipramine 175–250 mg per day for 4 weeks, two patients received amitriptyline, either 125 mg per day for 4 weeks or 150 mg per day for 3 weeks.

* $p < 0.005$; + $p < 0.05$; § $p < 0.005$.

patient who failed to respond to imipramine treatment (Garcia-Sevilla *et al.*, 1981b) and in two other imipramine-treated patients with agoraphobia and panic attacks but no significant depression (Garcia-Sevilla *et al.*, 1981a). Furthermore, using ^{3}H-yohimbine as an antagonistic ligand, Daiguji *et al.* (1981) were unable to demonstrate any differences in K_D or B_{max} values between normal subjects and drug-free depressed patients (table 7). It is also likely that the α_2-adrenoceptors labeled by clonidine and yohimbine are not presynaptic in nature, since the major physiological NE functions of platelets (for example, aggregation) involve postsynaptic α_2-adrenoceptors (Exton, 1982). In a study using the non-selective α-adrenoceptor ligand ^{3}H-dihydroergocryptine, Wood and Coppen (1982) showed that drug-free depressed patients had a reduced number of binding sites (B_{max}) when compared with normal controls.

Some support for the hypothesis of supersensitive α_2-adrenoceptors in depression is provided by a placebo-controlled study in which the effects of clonidine on plasma MHPG levels (a presynaptic effect) and blood pressure (a postsynaptic effect) were evaluated in depressed patients before and after long-term desipramine treatment (Charney *et al.*, 1981a). The effects of a single dose of clonidine (1 to 5 µg kg^{-1}) on both MHPG and blood pressure were attenuated by long-term desipramine treatment, which also significantly reduced plasma MHPG levels. There was no association between therapeutic response, pretreatment MHPG levels and clonidine effects on MHPG levels and blood pressure, during either placebo or drug treatment. However, in a follow-up study by the same group (Charney *et al.*, 1982) the ability of acute clonidine to lower plasma MHPG and reduce blood pressure did not differ between healthy subjects and drug-free depressives but the depressed patients showed a blunted growth hormone response to clonidine, implying normal sensitivity of presynaptic α_2 receptors in depression but decreased sensitivity of postsynaptic α_2-adrenoceptors. Since the same group (Sternberg *et al.*, 1982) has also demonstrated that clonidine fails to lower plasma MHPG levels in schizophrenic patients but does so in healthy subjects, while lowering blood pressure equally in both groups, it is difficult to accept the exclusivity of presynaptic α_2-adrenoceptor subsensitivity for depression. Furthermore, in another placebo-controlled study, but in healthy subjects, biochemical and blood pressure responses to a single 300 µg dose of clonidine were unaffected by chronic treatment with mianserin (Elliott *et al.*, 1981).

COMMENT

Acutely administered antidepressants exert manifold actions on monoaminergic systems. These acute effects may not be relevant to the mechanism of antidepressant activity, because many other drugs

with similar pharmacological actions are not known to be antidepressant and there is no correlation between the doses required
for acute pharmacological effects and those for clinical efficacy.
Thus, as far as α-adrenoceptors are concerned, the moderately
potent α_1-antagonism exhibited by tricyclic antidepressants,
mianserin and trazodone is far exceeded by the classical antagonists prazosin and phentolamine, which are not known to be antidepressant. Furthermore, clinically effective antidepressants
such as nomifensin, iprindole, fluoxetine and zimelidine hardly
interact with α_1-adrenoceptors. It is more likely that such interactions are concerned with the side-effects of some antidepressants. Acute interactions with α_2-adrenoceptors are absent
for most clinically effective antidepressants, which are highly
selective for α_1-adrenoceptors, except for mianserin which, though
non-selective, is more potent at α_2-adrenoceptors than the standard antagonist yohimbine. It is not yet clear whether specific
α_2-antagonists have antidepressant properties.

The delayed onset of therapeutic effects exhibited by all
antidepressants suggests that the pharmacological effects of
long-term treatment may be more important than those following
acute administration. The ability of long-term desipramine treatment to produce α_2-adrenoceptor subsensitivity in rat brain is not
shared by other proven or putative antidepressants, including the
potent α_2-antagonist mianserin, and it is too early to say whether
or not the ability of desipramine to reduce platelet α_2-adrenocep-
tor sensitivity in depressed patients extends to other drugs. The
lack of uniform effects on presynaptic NE function suggests that
such effects cannot explain the clinical activity of all antidepressants.

In contrast to the variable presynaptic actions of chronic
antidepressant treatment, alterations in postsynaptic α_1-adreno-
ceptor sensitivity have been consistently observed with a variety
of drugs, though in the absence of changes in receptor density.
It is possible that the effects of antidepressants on postsynaptic
NE receptors, including α_1- and β-adrenoceptors, represent a final
common pathway for antidepressant activity. These postsynaptic
changes may well be produced by the operation of different mechanisms depending upon the particular antidepressant.

It is tempting to speculate that, leaving aside effects on
serotonergic and possibly other systems, depression is related to
a functional hyperactivity of NE neuronal systems in the brain.
The hypersensitive receptors may serve to amplify incoming stimuli
and thereby result in central excitability. Antidepressant treatment will result in a desensitization of hyper-responsive NE
receptor functioning, leading to a reduction in the amplification
mechanism that translates sensory input into behavioral and
physiological events. Such speculation may necessitate an overhaul
of the original catecholamine hypothesis of depression which
attributed the illness to a deficiency of NE at central synapses.

REFERENCES

Baumann, P. A. and Maitre, L. (1977). Blockade of the presynaptic α-receptors and of amine uptake in the rat brain by the antidepressant mianserin. Naunyn-Schmiedeberg's Arch. Pharmacol., 300, 31-7

Bergstrom, D.A. and Kellar, K.J. (1979). Adrenergic and serotonergic receptor binding in rat brain after chronic desmethylimipramine treatment. J. Pharmacol. Exp. Ther., 209, 256-61

Brown, J., Doxey, J.C. and Handley, S. (1980). Effects of α-adrenoceptor agonists and antagonists and of antidepressant drugs on pre- and postsynaptic α-adrenoceptors. Eur. J. Pharmacol., 67, 33-40

Cavero, I., Gomeni, R., Lefevre-Borg, F. and Roach, A.G. (1980). Comparison of mianserin with desipramine, maprotiline and phentolamine on cardiac presynaptic and vascular postsynaptic α-adrenoceptors and noradrenaline reuptake in pithed normotensive rats. Br. J. Pharmacol., 68, 321-32

Cerrito, F. and Raiteri, M. (1981). Supersensitivity of central noradrenergic presynaptic autoreceptors following chronic treatment with the antidepressant mianserin. Eur. J. Pharmacol., 70, 425-6

Charney, D.S., Heninger, G.R., Sternberg, D.E., Hafstad, K.M., Giddings, S. and Landis, D.H. (1982). Adrenergic receptor sensitivity in depression. Effects of clonidine in depressed patients and healthy subjects. Arch. Gen. Psychiatry, 39, 290-4

Charney, D.S., Heninger, G.R., Sternberg, D.E., Redmond, D.E., Leckman, J.F., Mass, J.W. and Roth, R.H. (1981a). Presynaptic adrenergic receptor sensitivity in depression. Arch. Gen. Psychiatry, 38, 1334-40

Charney, D.S., Menkes, D.B. and Heninger, G.R. (1981b). Receptor sensitivity and the mechanism of action of antidepressant treatment. Arch. Gen. Psychiatry, 38, 1160-80

Clineschmidt, B.V., Flataker, L.M., Faison, E. and Holmes, R. (1979). An *in vivo* model for investigating α_1- and α_2-receptors in the CNS. Studies with mianserin. Arch. Int. Pharmacodyn. Ther., 242, 59-76

Cohen, R.M., Campbell, I.C., Cohen, M.R., Torda, T., Pickar, D., Siever, L.J. and Murphy, D.L. (1980). Presynaptic noradrenergic regulation during depression and antidepressant treatment. Psychiatry Res., 3, 93-105

Collis, M.G. and Shepherd, I.T. (1980). Antidepressant drug action and presynatpic α-receptors. Mayo Clinic Proc., 55, 567-72

Crews, F.T. and Smith, C.B. (1978). Presynaptic alpha-receptor subsensitivity after long-term antidepressant treatment. Science, 202, 322-4

Daiguji, M., Meltzer, H.Y., Tong, C., U'Prichard, D.C., Young, M. and Kravitz, H. (1981). α₂-Adrenergic receptors in platelet membranes of depressed patients: no change in number or ³H-yohimbine affinity. Life Sci., 29, 2059-64

Diffley, D., Tran, V.T. and Snyder, S.H. (1980). Histamine H₁-receptors labelled *in vivo*: Antidepressant and antihistamine interactions. Eur. J. Pharmacol., 64, 177-81

Doggrell, S.A. (1980). Effect of mianserin on noradrenergic transmission in the rat anococcygeus muscle. Br. J. Pharmacol., 68, 241-50

Doxey, J.C., Everitt, J. and Metcalf, G. (1978). Mianserin - an analysis of its peripheral autonomic actions. Eur. J. Pharmacol., 51, 1-10

Elliott, H.L., McLean, K., Summer, D.J. and Reid, J.L. (1981). Pharmacodynamic studies on mianserin and its interaction with clonidine. Eur. J. Clin. Pharmacol., 21, 97-102

Exton, J.H. (1982). Molecular mechanisms involved in α-adrenergic responses. Trends Pharmacol. Sci., 3, 111-15

Figge, J., Leonard, P. and Richelson, E. (1979). Tricyclic antidepressants: potent blockade of histamine H₁-receptors of guinea-pig ileum. Eur. J. Pharmacol., 58, 479-83

Fludder, J.M. and Leonard, B.E. (1979a). The effects of amitriptyline, mianserin, phenoxybenzamine and propranolol on the release of noradrenaline in rat brain *in vivo*. Biochem. Pharmacol., 28, 2333-6

Fludder, J.M. and Leonard, B.E. (1979b). Chronic effects of mianserin on noradrenaline metabolism in rat brain. Evidence for a presynaptic α-adrenolytic action *in vivo*. Psychopharmacology, 64, 329-32

Garcia-Sevilla, J.A., Zis, A.P., Hollingsworth, P.J., Greden, J.F. and Smith, C.B. (1981a). Platelet α₂-adrenergic receptors in major depressive disorder. Arch. Gen. Psychiatry, 38, 1327-33

Garcia-Sevilla, J.A., Zis, A.P., Zelnik, T.C. and Smith, C.B. (1981b). Tricyclic antidepressant drug treatment decreases α₂-adrenoceptors on human platelet membranes. Eur. J. Pharmacol., 69, 121-3

Glassman, A.H. and Bigger, J.T. (1981). Cardiovascular effects of therapeutic doses of tricyclic antidepressants. Arch. Gen. Psychiatry, 38, 815-20

Goodlett, I., Mireylees, S.E. and Sugrue, M.F. (1977). Effects of mianserin, a new antidepressant, on the *in vitro* and *in vivo* uptake of monoamines. Br. J. Pharmacol., 61, 307-13

Hall, H. and Ögren, S.O. (1981). Effects of antidepressant drugs on different receptors in the brain. Eur. J. Pharmacol., 70, 393-407

Harper, B. and Hughes, I.E. (1979). Presynaptic α-adrenoceptor blocking properties among tri- and tetra-cyclic antidepressant drugs. Br. J. Pharmacol., 67, 511-17

Hughes, I.E. (1978). The effect of amitriptyline on presynaptic mechanisms in noradrenergic nerves. Br. J. Pharmacol., 63, 315–21

Hunt, G.E., Atrens, D.M. and Johnson, G.F.S. (1981). The tetracyclic antidepressant mianserin. Evaluation of its blockade of presynaptic α-adrenoceptors in a self-stimulating model. Eur. J. Pharmacol., 70, 59–63

Johnson, R.W., Reisine, T., Spotnitz, S., Wiesch, N., Ursillo, R. and Yamamura, H.I. (1980). Effects of desipramine and yohimbine on α_2- and β-adrenoceptor sensitivity. Eur. J. Pharmacol., 67, 123–7

Kanof, P.D. and Greengard, P. (1978). Brain histamine receptors as targets for antidepressant drugs. Nature, 272, 329–33

Langer, S.Z. (1977). Presynaptic receptors and their role in the regulation of transmitter release. Br. J. Pharmacol., 60, 481–97

McMillen, B.A., Warnack, W., German, D.G. and Shore, P.A. (1980). Effects of chronic desipramine treatment on rat brain noradrenergic responses to α-adrenergic drugs. Eur. J. Pharmacol., 61, 239–46

Maggi, A., U'Prichard, D.C. and Enna, S.J. (1980a). Differential effects of antidepressant treatments on brain monoaminergic receptors. Eur. J. Pharmacol., 61, 91–8

Maggi, A., U'Prichard, D.C. and Enna, S.J. (1980b). β-Adrenergic regulation of α_2-adrenergic receptors in the central nervous system. Science, 207, 645–6

Maj, J. (1981). Serotonergic mechanisms of antidepressant drugs. Pharmacopsychiatry, 14, 35–9

Maj, J., Mogilnicka, E. and Klimek, V. (1979a). The effect of repeated administration of antidepressant drugs on the responsiveness of rats to catecholamine agonists. J. Neural Transm., 44, 221–35

Maj, J., Mogilnicka, E. and Klimek, V. (1979b). Chronic treatment with antidepressant drugs. Potentiation of apomorphine-induced aggressive behavior in rats. Neurosci. Lett., 13, 337–41

Maxwell, R.A. and White, H.L. (1978). Tricyclic and monoamine oxidase inhibitor antidepressants. Structure-activity relationships. In Handbook of Psychopharmacology, vol. 14, Affective Disorders (ed. L.L. Iversen, S.D. Iversen, and S.H. Snyder), Plenum Press, New York, pp. 83–155

Menkes, D.B. and Aghajanian, G.K. (1981). Alpha-1-adrenoceptor mediated responses in the lateral geniculate nucleus are enhanced by chronic antidepressant treatment. Eur. J. Pharmacol., 74, 27–35

Menkes, D.B., Aghajanian, G.K. and McCall, R.B. (1980). Chronic antidepressant treatment enhances α-adrenergic and serotonergic responses in the facial nucleus. Life Sci., 27, 45–55

Peroutka, S.J. and Snyder, S.H. (1980). Long-term antidepressant treatment decreases spiroperidol-labeled serotonin receptor binding. Science, 210, 88-90

Randrup, A. and Braestrup, C. (1977). Uptake inhibition of biogenic amines by newer antidepressant drugs. Relevance to the dopamine hypothesis of depression. Psychopharmacology, 53, 309-14

Rehavi, M., Ramot, D., Yavetz, B. and Sokolovsky, M. (1980). Amitriptyline: long-term treatment elevates α-adrenergic and muscarinic binding in mouse brain. Brain Res., 194, 443-53

Richelson, E. (1979). Tricyclic antidepressants and histamine H_1-receptors. Mayo Clinic Proc., 54, 669-74

Robson, D., Antonaccio, M.J., Saelens, J.K. and Liebman, J. (1978). Antagonism by mianserin and classical α-adrenoceptor blocking drugs of some cardiovascular and behavioural effects of clonidine. Eur. J. Pharmacol., 47, 431-42

Rosenblatt, J.E., Pert, C.B., Tallman, I.E., Pert, A. and Bunney, W.E. (1979). The effect of imipramine and lithium on the α- and β-receptor binding in rat brain. Brain Res., 160, 186-91

Schildkraut, J.J. (1965). The catecholamine hypothesis of affective disorders. A review of the supporting evidence. Am. J. Psychiatry, 122, 509-22

Schoffelmeer, A.N.M. and Mulder, A.H. (1982). ^{3}H-Noradrenaline and ^{3}H-5-hydroxytryptamine release from rat brain slices and its presynaptic α-adrenergic modulation after long-term desipramine treatment. Naunyn-Schmiedeberg's Arch. Pharmacol., 318, 173-80

Smith, C.B., Garcia-Sevilla, J.A. and Hollingsworth, P.J. (1981). Alpha-2-adrenoreceptors in rat brain are decreased after long-term tricyclic antidepressant treatment. Brain Res., 210, 413-18

Snyder, S.H. (1980). Tricyclic antidepressant drug interactions with histamine and α-adrenergic receptors. Pharmacopsychiatry, 13, 62-7

Snyder, S.H. and Yamamura, H.I. (1977). Antidepressants and the muscarinic acetylcholine receptor. Arch. Gen. Psychiatry, 34, 236-9

Spyraki, C. and Fibiger, H.C. (1980). Functional evidence for subsensitivity of noradrenergic $α_2$-receptors after chronic desipramine treatment. Life Sci., 27, 1863-7

Starke, K., Taube, H.D. and Borowski, E. (1977). Presynaptic receptor systems in catecholaminergic transmission. Biochem. Pharmacol., 26, 259-68

Sternberg, D.E., Charney, D.S., Heninger, G.R., Leckman, J.F., Hafstad, K.M. and Landis, D.H. (1982). Impaired presynaptic regulation of norepinephrine in schizophrenia. Effect of clonidine in schizophrenic patients and normal control. Arch. Gen. Psychiatry., 39, 285-9

Sugrue, M.F. (1980). The inability of chronic mianserin to block central α_2-adrenoceptors. Eur. J. Pharmacol., 68, 377–80

Sugrue, M.F. (1981a). Current concepts on the mechanism of action of antidepressant drugs. Pharmacol. Ther., 13, 219–47

Sugrue, M.F. (1981b). Effect of chronic antidepressant administration on rat frontal cortex α_2- and β-adrenoceptor binding. Br. J. Pharmacol., 74, 760P–1P

Sugrue, M.F. (1981c). Effects of acutely and chronically administered antidepressants on the clonidine-induced decrease in rat brain 3-methoxy-4-hydroxyphenylethylene glycol sulphate content. Life Sci., 208, 377–84

Sulser, F., Vetulani, J. and Mobley, P.L. (1978). Mode of action of antidepressant drugs. Biochem. Pharmacol., 27, 257–61

Svensson, T.H., Dahlfof, C., Engberg, G. and Hallberg, H. (1981). Central pre- and post-synaptic monoamine receptors in antidepressant therapy. Acta Psychiatr. Scand., Suppl. 290, 67–78

Svensson, T.H. and Scuvee-Moreau, J. (1981). Sensitivity *in vivo* of central α_2- and opiate receptors after chronic treatment with various antidepressants. Abstracts of Annual Meeting of American College of Neuropsychopharmacology, San Diego, December 1981, p.40

Tang, S.W., Helmeste, D.M. and Stancer, H.C. (1979). Interaction of antidepressants with clonidine on rat brain total 3-methoxy-4-hydroxyphenylglycol. Can. J. Physiol. Pharmacol., 57, 435–7

Tang, S.W. and Seeman, P. (1980). Effect of antidepressant drugs on serotonergic and adrenergic receptors. Naunyn-Schmiedeberg's Arch. Pharmacol., 311, 255–61

Tang, S.W., Seeman, P. and Kwam, S. (1981). Differential effect of chronic desipramine and amitriptyline treatment on rat brain adrenergic and serotonergic receptors. Psychiatry Res., 4, 129–38

U'Prichard, D.C., Greenberg, D.A., Sheehan, P.P. and Snyder, S.H. (1978). Tricyclic antidepressants. Therapeutic properties and affinity for α-noradrenergic binding sites in brain. Science, 199, 197–8

Uzan, A., LeFur, G. and Malgouris, C. (1979). Are antihistamines sedative via a blockade of brain histamine-H_1-receptors? J. Pharm. Pharmacol., 31, 701–2

van Zwieten, P.A. and Timmermans, P.B.M.W.M. (1980). Recent advances in the classification of α-adrenoceptors. Pharmaceut. Weekblad Scient. Edn, 2, 161–71

Waldmeier, P.C. (1981). Noradrenergic transmission in depression. Under- or overfunction? Pharmacopsychiatry, 14, 3–9

Wang, R.Y. and Aghajanian, G.K. (1980). Enhanced sensitivity of amygdaloid neurons to serotonin and norepinephrine after chronic antidepressant treatment. Commun. Psychopharmacol., 4, 83–90

Westfall, T.C. (1977). Local regulation of adrenergic neurotransmission. Physiol. Rev., 30, 133-66

Wetzel, H.W., Briley, M.S. and Langer, S.Z. (1981). ^{3}H-WB 4101
binding in the rat vas deferens. Effects of chronic treatments with desipramine and prazosin. Naunyn-Schmiedeberg's
Arch. Pharmacol., 317, 187-92

Wood, K. and Coppen, A. (1982). α_2-Adrenergic receptors in
depression. Lancet, 1, 1121-2

Antidepressants: effects on histaminic and muscarinic receptors

Elliott Richelson[1]

INTRODUCTION

Antidepressant drugs of many chemical classes are antagonists of several different types of neurotransmitter receptors. Among the first known of these receptor interactions were the antagonisms of histamine H_1 and muscarinic acetylcholine receptors. In fact, the first antidepressant, imipramine hydrochloride, was originally synthesized for use as an antihistamine (Kuhn, 1970). More recently, antidepressants have been shown, in addition, to be antagonists *in vitro* of histamine H_2, α_1-adrenergic, α_2-adrenergic and serotonergic receptors. This paper will present the evidence that antidepressants antagonize histamine H_1, histamine H_2 and muscarinic acetylcholine receptors in brain and elsewhere. In addition the relevance of these data for the treatment of depression and other diseases will be discussed.

It is well established that acetylcholine is a neurotransmitter at nicotinic and muscarinic receptors in the nervous system. An antimuscarinic drug when given to patients may cause a number of effects, most commonly, dry mouth, blurred vision, constipation and sinus tachycardia. Histamine, on the other hand, has a number of different functions in the body and in addition may also serve as a neurotransmitter (Taylor and Richelson, 1981). Histamine causes its effects by activating two different types of receptors (histamine H_1 and histamine H_2). Classically, histamine H_1 receptors are involved with anaphylactic and allergic reactions, while histamine H_2 receptors are involved with the secretion of gastric acid.

When an antihistaminic (H_1) drug is given to patients, sedation and drowsiness often occur. It is presumed that these are effects of histamine H_1 antagonism in the brain and that brain histamine H_1 receptors are involved with mechanisms of arousal.

---

[1] Departments of Psychiatry and Pharmacology, Mayo Foundation, Rochester, MN 55905, USA.

METHODS FOR ASSAY OF HISTAMINIC AND MUSCARINIC RECEPTORS

Histamine H_1 and muscarinic receptors have been successfully assayed by biological techniques as well as by radioligand binding procedures. For histamine H_2 receptors there are a number of different biological assays; however, radioligand binding techniques have not been successful in identifying these receptor sites, despite several attempts to do so.

Ideally, to study a receptor or drug–receptor interaction, both biological and radioligand binding procedures should be used in combination. By using biological assays to corroborate the results from radioligand binding assays, it may be possible to avoid such problems as underestimation of the affinity of a high-affinity ligand for its receptor by having too high a receptor concentration in a binding assay (as discussed below); or the measurement of meaningless binding as, for example, to glass fiber filters or to talcum powder (Hollenberg and Cuatrecasas, 1979).

The classical biological assay for histamine H_1 and muscarinic receptors is the agonist–induced contraction of the guinea-pig ileum *in vitro*. Another, less classical, approach that we have used extensively makes use of cultured murine neuroblastoma cells (clone N1E–115) (Richelson *et al.*, 1978; Richelson, 1978a, b). These cells contain, among other things, histamine H_1 and muscarinic receptors which, when activated, cause a marked and transient increase in intracellular cyclic GMP levels. Because receptor-mediated cyclic GMP synthesis occurs only with intact cells, the availability of a clone that has these properties has greatly aided the study of these receptors and their interactions with psychotropic drugs.

For the histamine H_2 receptor, agonist-induced stimulation of cyclic AMP in tissue slices (Tuong *et al.*, 1980), homogenates (Green and Maayani, 1977; Kanof and Greengard, 1978) or vesicles (Psychoyos, 1981) from brain has been used as a biological assay for this receptor. As discussed later in this paper, the affinities of psychotherapeutic drugs for histamine H_2 receptors in homogenates are different from those for receptors in intact cells (Tuong *et al.*, 1980; Schwartz *et al.*, 1981).

Radiolabeled pyrilamine (also called mepyramine) binds to histamine H_1 receptors in brains of many different species and in smooth muscle with an equilibrium dissociation constant (K_D) of around 1 nM (Hill *et al.*, 1977, 1978; Tran *et al.*, 1978). Recently, [³H]doxepin, a tricyclic antidepressant, and perhaps the most potent histamine H_1 antagonist known (K_D = 20–50 pM), has been shown to identify histamine H_1 receptors in rat brain (Tran *et al*., 1981; Taylor and Richelson, 1982) and in human brain (Kanba and Richelson, unpublished data). Unlike [³H]pyrilamine, this radioligand binds to two classes of sites in rat brain (figure 1) and it is the high-affinity site that has the characteristics of a histamine H_1 receptor.

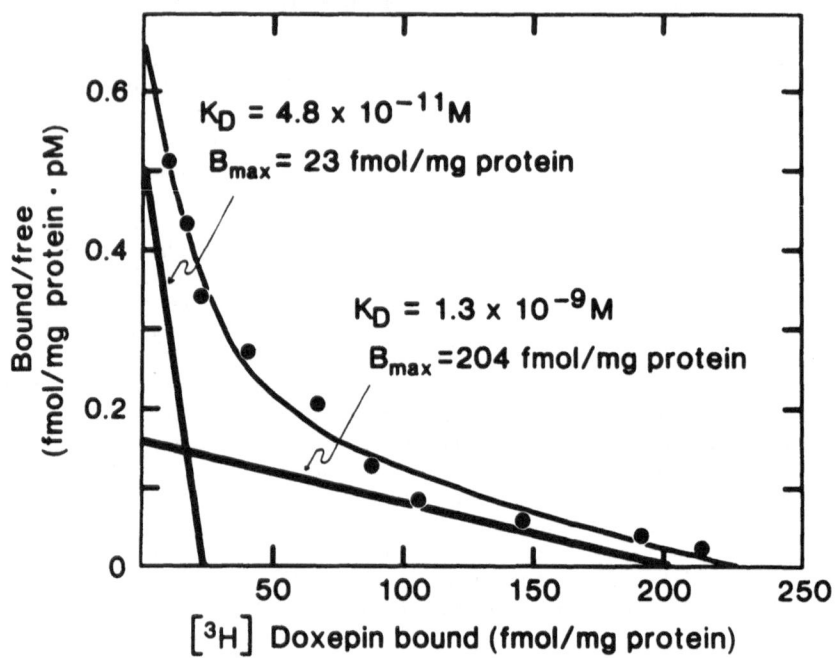

Figure 1. Rosenthal (Scatchard) analysis of [³H]doxepin binding
to rat brain. Reproduced from Taylor and Richelson
(1982) with the permission of Elsevier Biomedical Press.

Radioactively labeled antagonists of histamine H_2 receptors
(mostly [³H]cimetidine) have been used in receptor binding studies
in an attempt to identify these receptors (Rosenfeld *et al.*, 1976;
Burkard, 1978; Devoto *et al.*, 1980; Kendall *et al.*, 1980; Rising
et al., 1980). However, in the reported work, the binding of
[³H]cimetidine lacks the pharmacological characteristics that one
would expect if it were binding to a histamine H_2 receptor; and
this binding is uniformly distributed throughout the brain. Thus,
it is likely that this binding of [³H]cimetidine is not to histamine H_2 receptors.

COMPETITIVE ANTAGONISM BY ANTIDEPRESSANTS OF HISTAMINIC (H_1 AND H_2) AND MUSCARINIC RECEPTORS

Histamine H_1 Receptors

As noted above, it was known from the outset that antidepressants
of the tricyclic type were antihistamines (Kuhn, 1970). Just how

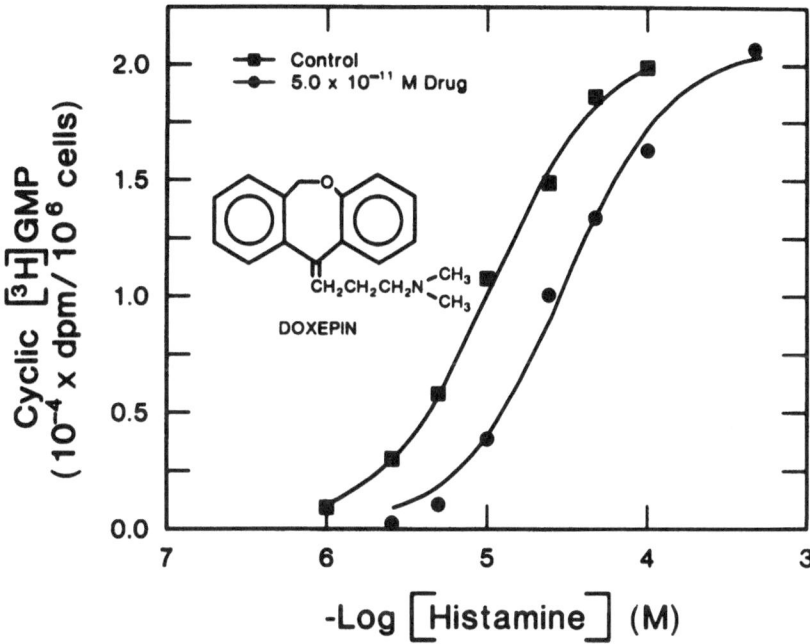

Figure 2. Effect of doxepin on histamine H_1 receptor-mediated cyclic GMP synthesis by murine neuroblastoma cells.

potent these compounds were as histamine H_1 antagonists was learned about 20 years after the first use of these drugs as antidepressants. With our assay using intact cultured nerve cells (Richelson *et al.*, 1978; Richelson, 1978a), we obtained equilibrium dissociation constants for tricyclic antidepressants and histamine H_1 receptors by dose-ratio analyses of dose-response curves (e.g. figure 2) (Richelson, 1978b, 1979). Our results (table 1) showed that all of these antidepressants were competitive antagonists of histamine H_1 receptors and that doxepin (figure 2) was perhaps the most potent histamine H_1 antagonist known (table 1), being, for example, about 800 times more potent than diphenhydramine at histamine H_1 receptors. Since our first reports of these results, we have added to the list of antidepressants studied (table 1) and still find doxepin to be the most potent compound tested.

Because we found that doxepin and amitriptyline were orders of magnitude more potent as antagonists of histamine H_1 receptors than a number of classical antihistaminics, we used another system, the guinea-pig ileum bioassay, to confirm these results (Figge *et al.*, 1979). K_D values for tricyclic antidepressants

Table 1. Antidepressants and related compounds: equilibrium
dissociation constants for histamine H_1 and muscarinic receptors

Compound	Receptor	
	Histamine H_1[a] (pM)	Muscarinic[b] (nM)
Doxepin	32	80
Trimipramine	100	58
Amitriptyline	130	18
Mianserin	310	820
Maprotiline	1000	570
Butriptyline	1800	35
Amoxapine	6800	1000
Nortriptyline	7000	150
Imipramine	10000	90
2-Hydroximipramine	14500	1210
Clomipramine	29600	37
Protriptyline	35000	25
Trazodone	73300	324000
Desipramine	260000	198
Iprindole	320000	2100
Didesmethylimipramine	1090000	590
Diphenhydramine	25000	180
Atropine	> 1000000	2

[a] Data from Richelson (1978b, 1979, and unpublished).
[b] Data from El-Fakahany and Richelson (1983).

determined from their competitive antagonism of histamine-
induced contractions of the guinea-pig ileum were essentially the
same as those found with the use of murine neuroblastoma cells.

After we reported our data for tricyclic antidepressants,
another laboratory (Tran *et al.*, 1978) reported that tricyclic
antidepressants were potent inhibitors of the binding of [³H]-
pyrilamine to histamine H_1 receptors of rat brain. The results
reported by Tran *et al.* (1978) largely confirmed our work. However, there were some interesting discrepancies. For the high-
affinity compounds (doxepin, amitriptyline and nortriptyline),
their calculated equilibrium dissociation constants were at least
one order of magnitude higher (indicating a lower affinity for
these compounds in the binding assays). For the low-affinity
compounds (imipramine, protriptyline and desipramine), our data
from both murine neuroblastoma cells and guinea-pig ileum agreed
very well with their data. In our radioligand binding studies

using [^{3}H]pyrilamine (Taylor and Richelson, 1980), we showed that these discrepant results for the high-affinity compounds resulted from the use in the assay of too high a receptor concentration which results in the overestimation of equilibrium dissociation constants.

In radioligand binding assays this equilibrium dissociation constant is often called an inhibitor constant, K_i, when it is calculated by the Cheng-Prusoff formula (Cheng and Prusoff, 1973) from the concentration of non-radioactively labeled drug giving 50% inhibition of binding (IC$_{50}$) of the radioligand. However, in general, whenever the affinity of the radiolabeled ligand is less than the affinity of the unlabeled ligand (as is the case, for example, of [^{3}H]pyrilamine being displaced by doxepin), incorrect estimates of the relative affinities may be obtained (Munson and Rodbard, 1980). However, even larger discrepancies from the true values occur when the K_D of a non-radioactively labeled compound is in the range of the receptor concentration in the assay, because the IC$_{50}$ then becomes a function of the receptor concentration as well (Taylor and Richelson, 1980). For example, the IC$_{50}$ for the competition between [^{3}H]pyrilamine and doxepin can be increased about 40-fold by increasing the receptor concentration by only threefold!

Using [^{3}H]pyrilamine and relatively low concentrations of histamine H$_1$ receptors from rat brain, we obtained IC$_{50}$ data for six antidepressants (Taylor and Richelson, 1980). The calculated inhibitor constants (K_i) for these compounds showed a significant correlation with their equilibrium dissociation constants derived from the inhibition of either histamine H$_1$ receptor-mediated cyclic GMP formation by murine neuroblastoma cells or histamine H$_1$ receptor-mediated contractions of the guinea-pig ileum. In addition, in [^{3}H]pyrilamine binding studies with homogenates of feline brain (Taylor *et al.*, 1982), K_D values for doxepin, amitriptyline and imipramine were very close to those values obtained with receptors from mouse, rat and guinea-pig. All these data obtained from different species, with the use of vastly different assays, strongly suggest that the true K_D values for the tricyclic antidepressants are as listed in table 1 and that there are no species differences in this characteristic (i.e. binding of tricyclic antidepressants) of histamine H$_1$ receptors.

Since doxepin has such a uniquely high affinity for histamine H$_1$ receptors, we and others have studied the characteristics of its binding to tissue from rat (Tran *et al.*, 1981; Taylor and Richelson, 1982) and human brain (Kanba and Richelson, unpublished data). Rosenthal (Scatchard) analyses of binding data indicated the presence of two distinct binding sites for [^{3}H]doxepin (figure 1) in rat brain. In our studies (Taylor and Richelson, 1982), the K_D of the high-affinity site was 20-50 pM, values similar to those obtained with the several different assays described above. The K_D

for the low-affinity site was about 40 nM and the maximum number of low-affinity binding sites was about 50 times the number of high-affinity sites. The regional distribution of the high-affinity sites correlated with the known distribution of histamine H_1 receptors and, from the results of competition studies between various drugs and [^{3}H]doxepin for the high-affinity site, we demonstrated that [^{3}H]doxepin was binding to histamine H_1 receptors. However, the low affinity site has not been identified.

There were some curious results with our binding studies. The maximum number of high-affinity [^{3}H]doxepin binding sites was about 10% of that found for [^{3}H]pyrilamine binding to histamine H_1 receptors in the same preparations. In addition, various tricyclic antidepressants were very potent competitors at the high-affinity [^{3}H]doxepin site with affinities for this site higher than those for the [^{3}H]pyrilamine site. These data suggested to us that [^{3}H]doxepin is binding to a subclass of histamine H_1 receptors. However, without a biological correlate of these binding studies, we do not know whether this conclusion is valid. It is too soon in our studies of [^{3}H]doxepin binding to human brain to know whether similar results will be obtained with this species.

Histamine H_2 Receptors

Within a short period of time, two different laboratories using essentially similar assays independently reported that tricyclic and other types of antidepressants were more potent than cimetidine as competitive antagonists of histamine H_2 receptors (Green and Maayani, 1977; Kanof and Greengard, 1978). One group (Kanof and Greengard, 1978) even suggested that antagonism of histamine H_2 receptors by antidepressants was responsible for their therapeutic effects, an idea that is unlikely since most neuroleptics are more potent than tricyclic antidepressants in this assay system. In addition, cimetidine causes depression in some patients (Jefferson, 1979).

The assay used for these studies was histamine-stimulated adenylate cyclase activity in homogenates of guinea-pig brain (hippocampus and cortex). Since antidepressants exhibit high affinity for histamine H_2 receptors only in this assay system and not in assays using intact cell preparations from the guinea-pig hippocampus (Tuong *et al.*, 1980) or from porcine skin (Iizuka *et al.*, 1976), there appears to be a major problem with these data. In addition, antidepressants have little or no antagonistic effect in other biological assays of histamine H_2 receptors such as histamine-mediated gastric acid secretion or increase in heart rate (Bohman *et al.*, 1980; Schwartz *et al.*, 1981). The reasons for this discrepancy are unknown. However, it is clear that more research is required to know whether antidepressants are in fact potent histamine H_2 antagonists.

Muscarinic Receptors

Like the antihistaminic (H_1) property of tricyclic antidepressants, the antimuscarinic property of these compounds has been
known since the 1950s. However, the first papers to report equilibrium dissociation constants for some of these compounds were
published only in the last 15 years (Brimblecombe and Green, 1967;
Atkinson and Ladinsky, 1972; Shein and Smith, 1978). These data
were derived in experiments which made use of muscarinic receptor-mediated contractions of the guinea-pig ileum (Brimblecombe
and Green, 1967; Shein and Smith, 1978) or rat fundal strips
(Atkinson and Ladinsky, 1972).

With the advent of radioligand binding technology, many
laboratories have assessed the antagonistic potency of antidepressants at muscarinic receptors of brain from non-human
species. Using a biological assay, we have, in addition, determined the equilibrium dissociation constants for antidepressants
and muscarinic receptors of murine neuroblastoma cells (Richelson
and Divinetz-Romero, 1977; Petersen and Richelson, 1982).

The question frequently arises, however, whether data for
these drugs derived from studies with non-human tissues are applicable to human brain, the true site of action of these psychotherapeutic compounds. Therefore, using human brain tissue, we
determined the equilibrium dissociation constants for a series of

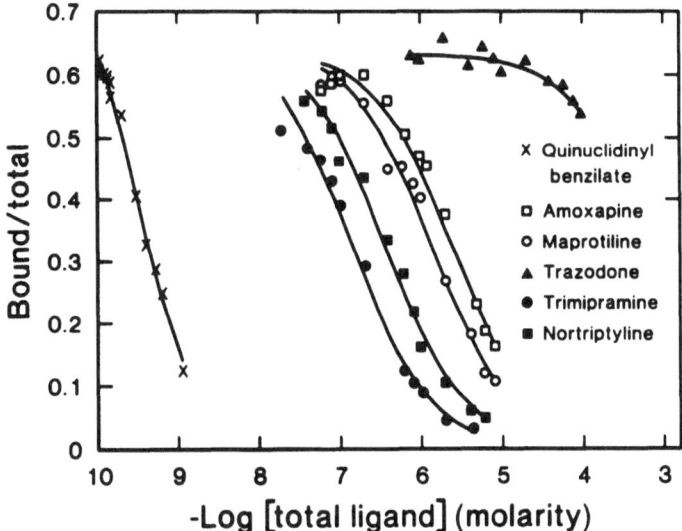

Figure 3. Competition by antidepressants for [^{3}H]quinuclidinyl
benzilate binding to muscarinic receptors of human
caudate nucleus.

antidepressants and related compounds (El-Fakahany and Richelson, 1983). A total of 22 compounds were tested for their ability to antagonize the binding of l-[^{3}H]quinuclidinyl benzilate to muscarinic receptors in homogenates of human caudate nucleus (e.g. figure 3).

Equilibrium dissociation constants for these drugs and muscarinic receptors (table 1 lists 16 of the compounds studied) spanned over four orders of magnitude, with the tertiary amine tricyclic antidepressant amitriptyline (K_D = 324 µM) the least potent.

We compared subsets of the data for antidepressants and related compounds obtained in the human brain studies with data derived by us using the murine neuroblastoma bioassay, with data derived by Shein and Smith (1978) using the guinea-pig ileum bioassay, and with data derived by Golds *et al.*, (1980) using radioligand binding and rat brain. In all three comparisons there was a significant correlation and the slope of the regression lines were all close to 1. We concluded from these analyses that there were no species differences between human, mouse, rat and guinea-pig in the affinities of antidepressants for muscarinic receptors.

CLINICAL IMPLICATIONS OF THE ANTIHISTAMINIC AND ANTIMUSCARINIC PROPERTIES OF ANTIDEPRESSANTS

Treatment of Depression

The histamine H_1 antagonism by antidepressants very likely is responsible for the sedation and drowsiness caused by some of these compounds. This can be a useful property for some patients who are both agitated and depressed and in this sense can be therapeutic. However, for other patients this sedation and drowsiness may become intolerable, necessitating a change to an antidepressant that is low on the list for histamine H_1 antagonism. This property of antidepressants will also potentiate the actions of central depressant drugs such as alcohol and minor tranquilizers.

It has been suggested that the antimuscarinic property of antidepressants is responsible for their mood-elevating effect (Janowsky *et al.*, 1972; Davis *et al.*, 1978). Abuse of antimuscarinic drugs for their euphoriant and other effects also supports this idea (Bluhm and Koller, 1981). Evidence presented here does not support this hypothesis since there is such a broad range of antimuscarinic potencies among the antidepressants with some compounds being practically devoid of activity (table 1).

The antimuscarinic property of antidepressants more likely reflects their propensity to cause adverse effects in patients, such as dry mouth, blurred vision, urinary retention and constipation. When an antimuscarinic side-effect becomes a problem in a patient or when such side-effects are to be avoided, the clinician should choose an antidepressant that has low affinity for muscarinic receptors (table 1).

Treatment of Other Diseases

The remarkable potency of antidepressants at blocking histamine H_1 receptors has led to their use in the treatment of allergic diseases (Sullivan, 1982). In addition, antidepressants are being used to treat peptic ulcer disease (Mangla and Pereira, 1982; Richelson, 1983) and their efficacy for treating ulcers may be related to their antihistaminic (H_2) and antimuscarinic properties.

SUMMARY

In summary, knowledge of the potency of antidepressants at blocking histaminic and muscarinic receptors gives a rational basis for understanding interactions of these drugs with other drugs and for understanding some of their side-effects. In addition, these data from basic research studies are suggesting new uses for these compounds.

Acknowledgement

Supported by Mayo Foundation and U.S.P.H.S. Grant MH27692.

REFERENCES

Atkinson, J. and Ladinsky, H. (1972). A quantitative study of the anticholinergic action of several tricyclic antidepressants on the rat isolated fundal strip. Br. J. Pharmacol., 48, 519-24

Bluhm, R.E. and Koller, W.C. (1981). Anticholinergic abuse – when to suspect it, what to do about it. Drug Ther., 11, 150-5

Bohman, T., Myren, J., Flaten, O. and Schrumpf, E. (1980). The effect of trimipramine, cimetidine, and atropine on gastric secretion. Scand. J. Gastroent., 15, 177-82

Brimblecombe, R.W. and Green, D.M. (1967). Central effects of imipramine-like antidepressants in relation to their peripheral anticholinergic activity. Int. J. Neuropharmacol., 6, 133-42

Burkard, W.P. (1978). Histamine H_2-receptor binding with ^{3}H-cimetidine in brain. Eur. J. Pharmacol., 50, 449-50

Cheng, Y.-C. and Prusoff, W.H. (1973). Relationship between the inhibition constant (K_I) and the concentration of inhibitor which causes 50 per cent inhibition (I_{50}) of an enzymatic reaction. Biochem. Pharmacol., 22, 3099-108

Davis, K.L., Berger, P.A., Hollister, L.E. and Barchas, J.D. (1978). Minireview: cholinergic involvement in mental disorders. Life Sci., 22, 1865-72

Devoto, P., Marchisio, A.M., Carboni, E. and Spano, P.F. (1980). Detection of ^{3}H-cimetidine specific binding in rat anterior pituitary. Eur. J. Pharmacol., 63, 91-3

El-Fakahany, and Richelson, E. (1983). Antagonism by antidepressants of muscarinic acetylcholine receptors of human brain. Br. J. Pharmacol., 78, 97-102

Figge, J., Leonard, P. and Richelson, E (1979). Tricyclic antidepressants: potent blockade of histamine H_1 receptors of guinea pig ileum. Eur. J. Pharmacol., 58, 479-83

Golds, P.R., Przyslo, F.R. and Strange, P.G. (1980). The binding of some antidepressant drugs to brain muscarinic acetylcholine receptors. Br. J. Pharmacol., 68, 541-9

Green, J.P. and Maayani, S. (1977). Tricyclic antidepressant drugs block histamine H_2 receptor in brain. Nature, 269, 163-5

Hill, S.J., Emsons, P.C. and Young, J.M. (1978). The binding of [^{3}H]-mepyramine to histamine H_1 receptors in guinea-pig brain. J. Neurochem., 31, 997-1004

Hill, S.J., Young, J.M. and Marrian, D.H. (1977). Specific binding of ^{3}H-mepyramine to histamine H_1 receptors in intestinal smooth muscle. Nature, 270, 361-3

Hollenberg, M.D. and Cuatrecasas, P. (1979). Distinction of receptor from nonreceptor interactions in binding studies. In The Receptors, vol. 1 (ed. R.D. O'Brien), Plenum, New York, pp. 193-214

Iizuka, H., Adachi, K., Halprin, K.M. and Levine, V. (1976). Histamine (H_2) receptor-adenylate cyclase system in pig skin (epidermis). Biochim. Biophys. Acta, 150-7

Janowsky, D.S., El-Yousef, M.K., Davis, J.M. and Sekerke, H.J. (1972). A cholinergic-adrenergic hypothesis of mania and depression. Lancet, ii, (Sept. 23), 632-35

Jefferson, J.W. (1979). Central nervous system toxicity of cimetidine: a case of depression. Am. J. Psychiatry, 136, 346

Kanof, P.D. and Greengard, P. (1978). Brain histamine receptors as targets for antidepressant drugs. Nature, 272, 329-33

Kendall, D.A, Ferkany, J.W. and Enna, S.J. (1980). Properties of ^{3}H-cimetidine binding in rat brain membrane fractions. Life Sci., 26, 1293-302

Kuhn, R. (1970). The imipramine story. In Discoveries in Biological Psychiatry, (ed. F.J. Ayd Jr and B. Blackwell), J.B. Lippincott Co., Philadelphia, pp. 205-17

Mangla, J.C. and Pereira, M. (1982). Tricyclic antidepressants in the treatment of peptic ulcer disease. Arch. Intern. Med., 142, 273-5

Munson, P.J. and Rodbard, D. (1980). LIGAND: a versatile computerized approach for characterization of ligand-binding systems. Anal. Biochem., 107, 220-39

Petersen, R.C. and Richelson, E. (1982). Anticholinergic activity of imipramine and some analogs at muscarinic receptors of cultured mouse neuroblastoma cells. Psychopharmacology, 76, 26-8

Psychoyos, S. (1981). Antidepressant inhibition of H_1- and H_2-histamine-receptor-mediated adenylate cyclase in [2-^{3}H]-adenine-prelabeled vesicular preparations from guinea pig brain. Biochem. Pharmacol., 30, 2182-5

Richelson, E. (1978a). Histamine H_1 receptor-mediated guanosine 3',5'-monophosphate formation by cultured mouse neuroblastoma cells. Science, 201, 69-71

Richelson, E. (1978b). Tricyclic antidepressants block histamine H_1 receptors of mouse neuroblastoma cells. Nature, 274, 176-7

Richelson, E. (1979). Tricyclic antidepressants and histamine H_1 receptors. Mayo Clinic Proc., 54, 669-74

Richelson, E. (1983). Antimuscarinic and other receptor blocking properties of antidepressants. Mayo Clinic Proc., 58, 40-6

Richelson, E. and Divinetz-Romero, S. (1977). Blockade by psychotropic drugs of the muscarinic acetylcholine receptor in cultured nerve cells. Biol. Psychiatr., 12, 771-85

Richelson, E., Prendergast, F.G. and Divinetz-Romero, S. (1978). Muscarinic receptor-mediated cyclic GMP formation by cultured nerve cells: ionic dependence and effects of local anesthetics. Biochem. Pharmacol., 27, 2039-48

Rising, T.J., Norris, D.B., Warrander, S.E. and Wood, T.P. (1980). High affinity ^{3}H-cimetidine binding in guinea-pig tissues. Life Sci., 27, 199-206

Rosenfeld, G.C., Jacobson, E.D. and Thompson, W.J. (1976). Re-evaluation of the role of cyclic AMP in histamine-induced gastric acid secretion. Gastroenterology, 70, 832-5

Schwartz, J.-C., Garbarg, M. and Quach, T.T. (1981). Histamine receptors in brain as targets for tricyclic antidepressants. Trends Pharmacol. Sci., May, 122-5

Shein, K. and Smith, S.E. (1978). Structure-activity relationships for the anticholinoceptor action of tricyclic antidepressants. Br. J. Pharmacol., 62, 567-71

Sullivan, T.J. (1982). Pharmacologic modulation of the whealing response to histamine in human skin: identification of doxepin as a potent *in vivo* inhibitor. J. Allergy Clin. Immunol., 69, 260-7

Taylor, J.E. and Richelson, E. (1980). High-affinity binding of tricyclic antidepressants to histamine H_1 receptors: fact and artifact. Eur. J. Pharmacol., 67, 41-6

Taylor, J.E. and Richelson, E. (1981).   Histamine receptors in
    neural tissue.   In Neurotransmitter Receptors, pt 2, ser. B,
    vol. 10, of Receptors and Recognition, (ed. H.I. Yamamura and
    S. Enna), Chapman and Hall, London, pp. 71-100
Taylor, J.E. and Richelson, E. (1982).   High affinity binding of
    [^{3}H]doxepin to histamine H_1 receptors in brain.   Eur. J.
    Pharmacol., 78, 279-85
Taylor, J.E., Yaksh, T.L. and Richelson, E. (1982).   Histamine H_1
    receptors in the brain and spinal cord of the cat.   Brain
    Res., 243, 391-4
Tran, V.T., Chang, R.S.L. and Snyder, S.H. (1978).   Histamine H_1
    receptors identified in mammalian brain membranes with [^{3}H]-
    mepyramine.   Proc. Natl. Acad. Sci. USA, 75, 6290-4
Tran, V.T., Lebovitz, R., Roll, L. and Snyder, S.H. (1981).
    [^{3}H]Doxepin interactions with histamine H_1-receptors and
    other sites in guinea pig and rat brain homogenates.   Eur. J.
    Pharmacol., 70, 501-9
Tuong, M.D.T., Garbarg, M. and Schwartz, J.C. (1980).
    Pharmacological specificity of brain histamine H_2-receptors
    differs in intact cells and cell-free preparations.   Nature,
    287, 548-51

Antidepressants and components of the beta adrenoceptor system: studies on zimelidine

R.Klysner[1], A.Geisler[1] and P.Andersen[1]

INTRODUCTION

Treatment of rats with a number of antidepressants for one to several weeks leads to a decrease in the density of beta adrenoceptors in the cerebral cortex and other brain regions (Bergstrom and Kellar, 1979; Maggi *et al.*, 1980). This reduction is accompanied by a concomitant decrease in the beta adrenoceptor-mediated cyclic AMP accumulation (Vetulani *et al.*, 1976; Wolfe *et al.*, 1978). Similar beta adrenoceptor alterations are also evoked by other antidepressant treatments. Thus, treatment with electro-convulsive therapy and monoamine oxidase inhibitors also induce beta adrenoceptor down-regulation (Gillespie *et al.*, 1979; Sellinger-Barnette *et al.*, 1980). The antidepressant treatments, however, have to be administered for a clinically relevant period of time before the changes are observable, whereas a single treatment does not change the number of beta adrenoceptors nor the associated cyclic AMP accumulation (Sarai *et al.*, 1978; Vetulani *et al.*, 1976; Wolfe *et al.*, 1978). We have found that deprivation of REM sleep, which is as effective as imipramine in the allevi-ation of depression (Vogel *et al.*, 1975), causes a reduction of beta adrenoceptor-mediated cyclic AMP accumulation in rat 'limbic' forebrain, without changing the density of beta adrenoceptors in this brain region (Klysner and Geisler, 1983). In these animals that were submitted to deprivation of REM sleep for one week, no change in either beta adrenoceptor number or cyclic AMP synthesis was observed in the cerebral cortex or in the cerebellum. In contrast, Mogilnicka *et al.* (1980) found that 72 h of REM sleep deprivation leads to a reduced density of beta adrenoceptors in the rat cerebral cortex.

[1] Department of Pharmacology, University of Copenhagen, Juliane Maries vej 20, DK-2100 Copenhagen, Denmark.

Treatment with reserpine, which in some persons may provoke a serious depression, causes an opposite change, i.e. the number of cerebral beta adrenoceptors is increased after reserpine administration. Concomitant treatment of rats with reserpine and lithium, giving a plasma lithium concentration of approximately 1 mmol 1^{-1}, prevents the increase in beta adrenoceptor density due to reserpine treatment (Treiser and Kellar, 1979), an effect which has been proposed to be related to the ability of lithium to prevent the occurrence of depressive episodes. Concomitant treatment with lithium and imipramine does not prevent the beta adrenoceptor down-regulation brought about by imipramine (Rosenblatt *et al.*, 1979). We have observed that chronic treatment of rats with lithium, giving a plasma lithium concentration of 0.5-0.6 mmol 1^{-1}, has no effect on the alteration in the number of ^{3}H-dihydro-alprenolol (^{3}H-DHA) binding sites in the cerebral cortex after reserpine and imipramine treatment, although this lithium treatment does counteract the rise in isoprenaline-stimulated cyclic AMP accumulation after reserpine treatment (A. Geisler and R. Klysner, unpublished).

Such studies suggest a relationship between down-regulation of beta adrenoceptors and alleviation of depression, and suggest that the function of these receptors may be increased in the brain of patients suffering from depressive illness. A few studies have focused on determination of beta adrenoceptor number and function in blood cells from depressed patients. Thus, Pandey *et al.* (1979) found that isoprenaline-stimulated cyclic AMP formation in a mixed leukocyte preparation was significantly reduced in patients with major depressive disorders in comparison to the isoprenaline-induced response in leukocytes from normal subjects. In a study performed by Extein *et al.* (1979) the number of beta adrenoceptors in isolated lymphocytes was lower in both depressed and manic patients compared to euthymic patients and control persons, and the same pattern of changes was observed when isoprenaline-stimulated cyclic AMP production was studied. The treatments given, i.e. desipramine and lithium, did not significantly alter ^{3}H-DHA binding to the beta adrenoceptors, nor did they alter isoprenaline-stimulated cyclic AMP formation in the blood cells. However, in a study by Lerer *et al.* (1981), it was found that salbutamol given as an antidepressant did reduce beta adrenoceptor-mediated rise in the blood level of cyclic AMP. This cyclic AMP is thought to originate from beta adrenoceptors in blood vessels. It should be remembered, however, that alterations in the number and function of beta adrenoceptors in blood cells and blood vessels may depend on such local factors as the level of beta adrenoceptor agonists in the blood (epinephrine and salbutamol), and may therefore not give a true reflection of beta adrenoceptor function in the brain of these patients. An indication that beta adrenoceptor alterations after antidepressant treatments may in fact be confined to the brain comes from the study of Frazer *et al.* (1978) in which no changes in isoprenaline-stimulated cyclic AMP formation was evident in the heart and diaphragm of animals treated with desipramine, although the same response was clearly reduced in the cerebral cortex.

The molecular events leading to a down-regulation of beta adrenoceptors in rat brain after antidepressant treatments are unknown. It is possible that increased availability of norepinephrine (NE) at the beta adrenoceptor due to inhibition by antidepressants of presynaptic NE uptake mechanisms, or due to a decreased number of alpha$_2$ adrenoceptors during antidepressant treatment, leading to increased NE release, may eventually result in a down-regulation of the beta adrenoceptors. In line with the latter assumption is the observation that a combined treatment with an antidepressant and an alpha adrenoceptor blocking drug results in a faster down-regulation of cerebral beta adrenoceptors than treatment with the antidepressant drug alone (Crews *et al.*, 1981; Wiech and Ursillo, 1980). However, Sugrue (1981) found that, although beta adrenoceptors in the cerebral cortex were down-regulated by various antidepressant treatments, only some of these treatments led to a reduction in alpha$_2$ adrenoceptor binding in this tissue. With regard to the notion that inhibition of presynaptic NE uptake by antidepressants results in beta adrenoceptor down-regulation, it is difficult to explain why treatment with cocaine does not decrease the number of beta adrenoceptors (Sellinger-Barnette *et al.*, 1980), even when given as chronic infusion (Sethy and Harris, 1981).

In addition, it seems complicating that some antidepressant treatments down-regulate both the number of beta adrenoceptors and associated cyclic AMP formation, while other treatments reduce the beta adrenoceptor-mediated cyclic AMP accumulation without altering the number of receptors. As mentioned above, we have found that deprivation of REM sleep decreased isoprenaline-mediated cyclic AMP accumulation in rat 'limbic' forebrain without affecting the number of beta adrenoceptors and, also, that low plasma lithium levels antagonized the effect of reserpine on beta adrenoceptor-mediated cyclic AMP formation without counteracting the reserpine-induced increase in beta adrenoceptor density. Furthermore, Mishra *et al.* (1979) observed a decreased NE-stimulated cyclic AMP accumulation in rat cerebral cortex after nisoxetine treatment without alteration of beta adrenoceptor binding, and Mishra *et al.* (1980) found that treatment with the new antidepressant zimelidine (Coppen *et al.*, 1979; Aberg-Wistedt *et al.*, 1981) had no effect on the density of beta adrenoceptors in rat cerebral cortex, yet inhibiting NE-stimulated cyclic AMP accumulation. In contrast, Ross *et al.* (1981) found that zimelidine dose-dependently reduced the number of beta adrenoceptors in rat cerebral cortex, and also Sethy and Harris (1981) found a down-regulation of beta adrenoceptor density after zimelidine treatment.

Since such discrepancies may arise from the use of beta adrenoceptor antagonists to determine the number of beta adrenoceptors and the use of beta adrenoceptor agonists to assess cyclic AMP accumulation, we have in the present study investigated the effect of zimelidine treatment on components of the beta adrenoceptor system, i.e. the binding of agonist and antagonist to the receptor and the associated cyclic AMP accumulation. Further, we have evaluated the fluoride-stimulated adenylate cyclase activity in order to assess possible changes in the GTP-binding protein (Citri and Schramm, 1980), which participates in the receptor-mediated cyclic AMP formation.

MATERIALS AND METHODS

Male Wistar rats weighing 180–200 g were treated twice a day with 10 mg kg^{-1} zimelidine dihydrochloride monohydrate, intraperitoneally. Controls received a corresponding volume of saline. After 14 days the treatment was discontinued and 24 h after the last zimelidine administration the rats were decapitated and dissected in a cold room (4°C). Most of the cerebral cortex on the dorsal and lateral aspect of the brain was used. Tissue for binding studies and fluoride-stimulated adenylate cyclase activity was frozen and stored at -80°C, while tissue for isoprenaline-stimulated cyclic AMP formation was processed immediately.

^{3}H-DHA Binding

Binding of ^{3}H-DHA was essentially as described by Bylund and Snyder (1976). The tissue was diluted to approximately 5 mg ml^{-1}. However, the incubation at 23°C was extended to 25 min, and non-specific binding was defined as the binding of ^{3}H-DHA that could be displaced by 0.3 μmol l^{-1} L-propranolol. When studying agonist binding, GTP was added to a final concentration of 0.3 mmol l^{-1}. The number of beta adrenoceptor sites (B_{max}) and their affinity for ^{3}H-DHA was assessed by Scatchard analysis (Scatchard, 1949). The Scatchard analysis was made by linear regression.

Fluoride-Stimulated Adenylate Cyclase

Tissue for fluoride-stimulated cyclic AMP formation was thawed at 4°C and processed as previously described (Laursen *et al.*, 1977) with the following exceptions: the tissue was diluted in 50 volumes of buffer and incubated for 40 min at 0°C followed by addition of NaF or water. The incubation continued for 20 min at 30°C and then cyclic AMP formation was started by addition of ATP (final concentration, 0.5 mmol l^{-1}). After 2.5 min, incubation

was stopped by boiling for 3 min. The boiled tissue was centrifuged at 4°C and the supernatant was stored at -20°C until determination of cyclic AMP.

Isoprenaline-Stimulated Cyclic AMP Accumulation

Cerebral tissue for determination of cyclic AMP accumulation was
chopped with a microtome to a thickness of 300 μm. After a 45°
rotation of the table the tissue was chopped again. Thereafter
the tissue was suspended in 20 ml of a Krebs-Ringer buffer with
the following composition: NaCl, 122 mM; KCl, 3 mM; $CaCl_2$, 1.3 mM;
$MgSO_4$, 1.2 mM; KH_2PO_4, 0.4 mM; D-glucose, 10 mM; $NaHCO_3$, 25 mM;
Na_2EDTA, 10 mM. This buffer had previously been gassed with 95%
O_2 - 5% CO_2 to a pH value of 7.3-7.4. The tissue preparation was
then pre-incubated for 60 min at 37°C in an atmosphere of 95% O_2 -
5% CO_2 with changes of buffer every 20 min. After 60 min the
tissue suspension was diluted and 500 μl aliquots were transferred
to beakers continuously gassed with 95% O_2 - 5% CO_2. Buffer or
isoprenaline and buffer or Rolipram were added and the incubation
was continued for 15 min. The incubation was stopped by boiling
the tissue for 10 min. The samples were then spun in the cold and
the clear supernatant was stored at -20°C until determination of
cyclic AMP. Cyclic AMP was determined by a competitive protein
binding method (Geisler *et al.*, 1977). The protein content in the
preparations was determined by the method of Lowry *et al.* (1951).
Statistical analysis was performed by the Mann-Whitney rank sum
test for unpaired samples. ^{3}H-Dihydroalprenolol was obtained from
New England Nuclear, Boston, Mass., DL-isoproterenol sulfate from
Sigma Chemical Corp., St Louis, Mo., and guanosine 5'-triphosphate
(GTP) was obtained from Boehringer, Mannheim, FRG. L-Propranolol
was a generous gift from Imperial Chemical Industries, UK, and
zimelidine dihydrochloride monohydrate was generously supplied by
Astra Läkemedel AB, Södertälje, Sweden. All other agents used
were of reagent grade. Rolipram (ZK 62.711) was generously supplied by Schering AG, Berlin/Bergkamen, FRG.

Table 1. Effect of 14 days of zimelidine treatment on ^{3}H-DHA
binding to rat cerebral cortex

	B_{max} (fmol/mg protein)	K_d (nmol/mg protein)
Control	256 ± 19	0.76 ± 0.07
Zimelidine	220 ± 13 (N.S.)	0.84 ± 0.10 (N.S.)

Means ± S.E.M. There were six animals in each group. Treated animals received
zimelidine (10 mg kg[-1] b.i.d.) and controls received 0.9% NaCl.
N.S. = not significant compared to corresponding controls.

RESULTS

Treatment with zimelidine for 14 days was not found to change the affinity of beta adrenoceptors in the cerebral cortex for ^{3}H-DHA, and although there was a trend toward a decrease in receptor density after the treatment, this did not, however, reach statistical significance (table 1). For both animals treated with zimelidine and control animals, displacement of specifically bound

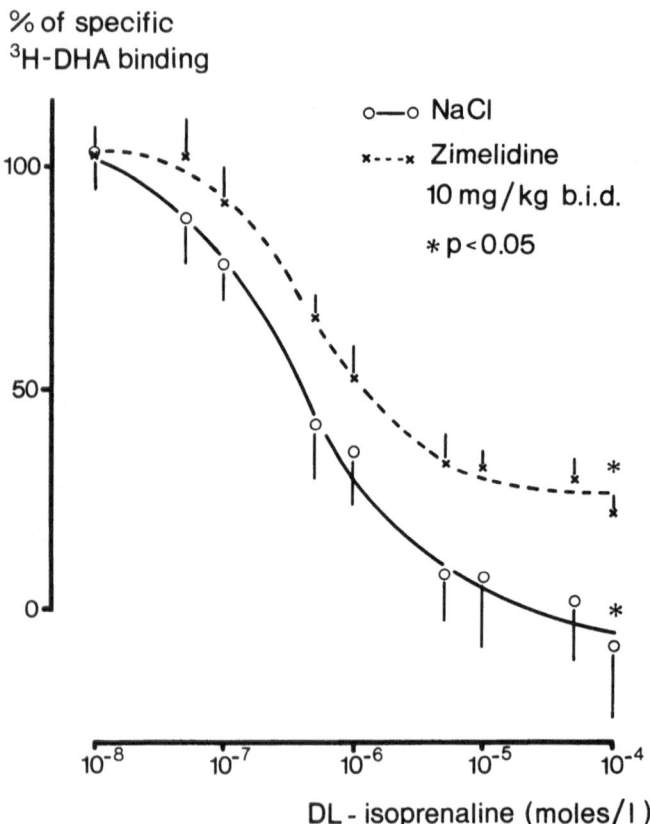

Figure 1. Displacement of specifically bound ^{3}H-DHA (4 nmol 1^{-1}) by increasing concentrations of DL-isoprenaline. Means ± S.E.M. There were six animals in each group. Rats were treated with zimelidine 10 mg kg^{-1} b.i.d. or saline. The specific binding of ^{3}H-DHA was defined for each animal as the binding that could be displaced by 0.3 μmol 1^{-1} of L-propranolol.

^{3}H-DHA (4 nmol l^{-1}) was performed with increasing concentrations of DL-isoprenaline. The specifically bound ^{3}H-DHA was defined for each animal as the binding that could be displaced by 0.3 μmol l^{-1} of L-propranolol. By this approach it was found that high concentrations of isoprenaline (0.1 mmol l^{-1}) displaced less specifically bound ^{3}H-DHA in the zimelidine-treated group than in the control group, indicating a reduction of agonist binding sites after zimelidine treatment (figure 1). The affinity for isoprenaline, however, did not seem to be altered by the treatment, since IC$_{50}$ values were the same in the zimelidine-treated and in the control group. Zimelidine treatment was found to reduce isoprenaline-stimulated cyclic AMP accumulation in slices of cerebral cortex when measured as percent stimulation over basal values (table 2). This effect was only evident when the potent phosphodiesterase inhibitor Rolipram (Schwabe *et al.*, 1976) was present in the assay medium. The effect of zimelidine treatment on cyclic AMP formation was not due to a direct effect of zimelidine, since zimelidine added *in vitro* (0.1 mmol l^{-1}) had no effect on isoprenaline-stimulated cyclic AMP accumulation with Rolipram added to the assay medium. The same changes in cyclic AMP accumulation after zimelidine treatment as described above were seen when the absolute values were considered, although the changes did not reach statistical significance (table 3). Stimulation of cyclic AMP formation in homogenized cerebral cortex by NaF (10 mmol l^{-1}) was not changed by zimelidine treatment. Thus, in control animals the basal adenylate cyclase activity was 101 ± 7 pmol cyclic AMP/mg protein (mean ± S.E.M.), while the corresponding value for zimelidine-treated animals was 102 ± 7. The fluoride-stimulated activity was 317 ± 26 and 299 ± 27 pmol cyclic AMP/mg protein for control and zimelidine-treated animals, respectively. Each group comprised 16 animals.

Table 2. Effect of 14 days of zimelidine treatment on cyclic AMP accumulation in slices of rat cerebral cortex

	Isoprenaline 1x10^{-4} M	Isoprenaline 1x10^{-4} M + Rolipram 1x10^{-5} M
Control	236 ± 40	203 ± 35
Zimelidine	176 ± 27 (N.S.)	102 ± 10*

* $p<0.02$ compared to NaCl.
Results are expressed as percent stimulation above the basal level.
Means ± S.E.M. There were 13-14 animals in each group. Rats received zimelidine 10 mg kg^{-1} b.i.d. or 0.9% NaCl.

Clinical Pharmacology in Psychiatry

Table 3. Effect of 14 days of zimelidine treatment on cyclic AMP accumulation in slices of rat cerebral cortex

	Basal	Isoprenaline 1×10^{-4} M	Rolipram 1×10^{-5} M	Isoprenaline 1×10^{-4} M + Rolipram 1×10^{-5} M
Control	7.7 ± 1.2	15.0 ± 2.2	19.6 ± 2.5	32.9 ± 3.6
Zimelidine	10.0 ± 1.0	15.9 ± 2.1	24.3 ± 1.4	25.3 ± 1.9
	(N.S.)	(N.S.)	(N.S.)	(N.S.)

Results are expressed as pmol cAMP/mg protein.
Means ± S.E.M. Rats received zimelidine 10 mg kg^{-1} b.i.d. or 0.9% NaCl. There were 13–14 animals in each group.
The figures for isoprenaline and isoprenaline + Rolipram give increase above basal values.
N.S. = not significant compared to corresponding controls.

DISCUSSION

In this study it was found that chronic treatment with zimelidine leads to a decreased beta adrenoceptor-mediated cyclic AMP accumulation in rat cerebral cortex. This supports the notion that all antidepressant treatments decrease beta adrenoceptor-mediated cyclic AMP formation in the rat cerebrum. The diminished cyclic AMP synthesis after zimelidine treatment is accompanied by a reduced binding of agonist to the beta adrenoceptor, and although the agonist binding was assessed indirectly by displacement of an antagonist, the data indicate a reduction of the number of agonist binding sites, but unaltered affinity for the agonist. In contrast, the antagonist binding was not found to be significantly changed by the zimelidine treatment. Determination of agonist binding sites may be more physiologically relevant, but it should be emphasized that in other studies antidepressants have been able to bring about a decreased beta adrenoceptor antagonist binding, although in many cases not of the same magnitude as the decrease in cyclic AMP formation. Consequently, the lack of correlation between the reduced antagonist binding and the reduction of cyclic AMP accumulation may be due to different changes in agonist and antagonist binding.

This study dose not give any indication of alterations in GTP binding proteins associated with cyclic AMP formation after zimelidine treatment, since the fluoride stimulation of cyclic AMP production did not differ between the control group and the zimelidine-treated group. It cannot, however, be excluded that a change did take place in the GTP binding proteins associated with beta adrenoceptor function, since these probably only constitute a minor part of the GTP binding proteins present in the cerebral cortex.

In most studies on the influence of antidepressant treatments on beta adrenoceptor-mediated cyclic AMP accumulation, inhibitors of cyclic AMP degradation have not been included in the assay medium. It is therefore not clear if changes in phosphodiesterase occur after antidepressant treatments, either as an adaptation to the altered beta adrenoceptor function or as a direct effect of antidepressants on phosphodiesterases. This possibility should be borne in mind since it has been shown that antidepressants can bind to calmodulin, a phosphodiesterase regulator (Reynolds and Claxton, 1982).

In the present study it has been necessary to include the potent phosphodiesterase inhibitor Rolipram in order to demonstrate the changes in isoprenaline-stimulated cyclic AMP accumulation after zimelidine treatment. Therefore, further studies on the effects of zimelidine and other antidepressants on the various components of the beta adrenoceptor system may serve to elucidate the changes occurring in beta adrenoceptor function after antidepressant treatment.

SUMMARY

The antidepressant drug zimelidine given for 2 weeks decreased agonist binding to beta adrenoceptors without significantly affecting antagonist binding in rat cerebral cortex. Further, zimelidine lowered the isoprenaline-stimulated cyclic AMP accumulation in slices of cerebral cortex, but only when a phosphodiesterase inhibitor was included in the assay medium. This study supports the assumption that antidepressant drugs reduce beta adrenoceptor function in the brain, but differences in the effect of various antidepressants on the functional components of the beta adrenoceptor system may occur.

REFERENCES

Aberg-Wistedt, A., Jostell, K.-G., Ross, S. and Westerlund, D. (1981). Effects of zimelidine and desipramine on serotonin and noradrenaline uptake mechanisms in relation to plasma concentrations and to therapeutic effects during treatment of depression. Psychopharmacology, 74, 297-305

Bergstrom, D.A. and Kellar, K.J. (1979). Adrenergic and serotonergic receptor binding in rat brain after chronic desmethylimipramine treatment. J. Pharmacol. Exp. Ther., 209, 256-61

Bylund, D.B. and Snyder, S.H. (1976). Beta adrenergic receptor binding in membrane preparations from mammalian brain. Mol. Pharmacol., 12, 568-80

Citri, Y. and Schramm, M. (1980). Resolution, reconstitution and kinetics of the primary action of a hormone receptor. Nature, 287, 297-300

Coppen, A., Rama Rao, V.A., Swade, C. and Wood, K. (1979). Zimelidine: a therapeutic and pharmacokinetic study in depression. Psychopharmacology, 63, 199-202

Crews, F.T., Paul, S.M. and Goodwin, F.K. (1981). Acceleration of beta-receptor desensitization in combined administration of antidepressants and phenoxybenzamine. Nature, 290, 787-9

Extein, I., Tallman, J., Smith, C.C and Goodwin, F.K. (1979). Changes in lymphocyte beta-adrenergic receptors in depression and in mania. Psychiatry Res., 1, 191-7

Frazer, A., Hess, M.E., Mendels, J., Gable, B., Kunkel, E. and Bender, A. (1978). Influence of acute and chronic treatment with desmethylimipramine on catecholamine effects in the rat. J. Pharmacol. Exp. Ther., 206, 311-19

Geisler, A., Klysner, R,. Thams, P. and Christensen, S. (1977). A simple and inexpensive protein binding assay for cyclic AMP in biological materials. Acta Pharmacol. Toxicol., 40, 356-68.

Gillespie, D.D., Manier, D.H. and Sulser, F. (1979). Electroconvulsive treatment: rapid subsensitivity of the norepinephrine receptor coupled adenylate cyclase system in brain linked to down-regulation of beta-adrenergic receptors. Commun. Psychopharmacol., 3, 191-5

Klysner, R. amd Geisler, A. (1983). Effect of REM sleep deprivation on beta-adrenergic receptors in rat brain. Submitted for publication

Laursen, H., Klysner, R. and Geisler, A. (1977). Adenylate cyclase activity in corpus striatum of rats with porto-caval anastomosis. Acta Physiol. Scand., 100, 282-7

Lerer, B., Ebstein, R,P, and Belmaker, R.H. (1981). Subsensitivity of human beta-adrenergic adenylate cyclase after salbutamol treatment of depression. Psychopharmacology, 75, 169-72

Lowry, O.H., Rosebrough, N.J., Farr, A.L. and Randall, R.J. (1951). Protein measurement with the folin phenol reagent. J. Biol. Chem., 193, 265-75

Maggi, A., U'Prichard, D.C. and Enna, S.J. (1980). Differential effects of antidepressant treatment on brain monoaminergic receptors. Eur. J. Pharmacol., 61, 91-8

Mishra, R., Janowsky, A. and Sulser, F. (1979). Subsensitivity of the norepinephrine receptor-controlled adenylate cyclase system in brain: effects of nisoxetine versus fluoxetine. Eur. J. Pharmacol., 60, 379-82

Mishra, R., Janowsky, A. and Sulser, F. (1980). Action of mianserin and zimelidine on the norepinephrine receptor coupled adenylate cyclase system in brain: subsensitivity without reduction in beta-adrenergic receptor binding. Neuropharmacology, 19, 983-7

Mogilnicka, E., Arbilla, S., Depoortere, H. and Langer, S.Z. (1980). Rapid-eye-movement sleep deprivation decreases the density of ^{3}H-dihydroalprenolol and ^{3}H-imipramine binding sites in the rat cerebral cortex. Eur. J. Pharmacol., 65, 289-92

Pandey, G.N., Dysken, M.W., Garver, D.L. and Davis, J.M. (1979). Beta-adrenergic receptor function in affective illness. Am. J. Psychiatry, 136, 675-8

Reynolds, C.H. and Claxton, P.T.J. (1982). Inhibition of calmodulin-activated cyclic nucleotide phosphodiesterase: Multiple binding-sites for tricyclic drugs on calmodulin. Biochem. Pharmacol., 31, 419-21

Rosenblatt, J.E., Pert, C.B., Tall, J.F., Pert, A. and Bunney, W.E. (1979). The effect of imipramine and lithium on alpha- and beta-receptor binding in rat brain. Brain Res., 160, 186-91

Ross, S.B., Hall, H., Renyi, A.L. and Westerlund, D. (1981). Effects of zimelidine on serotonergic and noradrenergic

neurons after repeated administration in the rat. <u>Psycho-
pharmacology</u>, 72, 219-25

Sarai, K., Frazer, A., Brunswick, D. and Mendels, J. (1978).
Desmethylimipramine-induced decrease in beta-adrenergic
receptor binding in rat cerebral cortex. <u>Biochem. Pharmacol.</u>, 27, 2179-81

Scatchard, G. (1949). The attraction of proteins for small
molecules and ions. <u>Ann. NY Acad. Sci.</u>, 51, 660-72

Schwabe, U., Miyake, M., Ohga, Y. and Daly, J.W. (1976). 4-(3-
Cyclopentyloxy-4-methoxyphenyl)-2-pyrrolidone (ZK 62711): a
potent inhibitor of adenosine cyclic 3',5'-monophosphate
phosphodiesterases in homogenates and tissue slices from rat
brain. <u>Mol. Pharmacol.</u>, 12, 900-10

Sellinger-Barnette, M.M., Mendels, J. and Frazer, A. (1980). The
effect of psychoactive drugs on beta-adrenergic receptor
binding sites in rat brain. <u>Neuropharmacology</u>, 19, 447-54

Sethy, V.H. and Harris, D.W. (1981). Effect of norepinephrine
uptake blocker on beta-adrenergic receptors of the rat cerebral cortex. <u>Eur. J. Pharmacol.</u>, 75, 53-6

Sugrue, M.F. (1981). Effect of chronic antidepressant administration on rat frontal cortex alpha$_2$- and beta-adrenoceptor
binding. <u>Br. J. Pharmacol.</u>, 74, 760P-1P

Treiser, S. and Kellar, K. (1979). Lithium effects on adrenergic
receptor supersensitivity in rat brain. <u>Eur. J. Pharmacol.</u>,
58, 85-6

Vetulani, J., Stawarz, R.J., Dingell, J.V. and Sulser, F. (1976).
A possible common mechanism of action of antidepressant
treatments. <u>Naunyn-Schmiedeberg's Arch. Pharmacol.</u>, 293,
109-14

Vogel, G.W., Thurmond, A., Gibbons, P., Sloan, K., Boyd, M. and
Walker, M. (1975). REM sleep reduction effects on depression
syndromes. <u>Arch. Gen. Psychiatry.</u>, 32, 765-77

Wiech, N.L. and Ursillo, R.C. (1980). Acceleration of desipra-
mine-induced decrease of rat corticocerebral beta-adrenergic
receptors by yohimbine. <u>Commun. Psychopharmacol.</u>, 4, 95-100

Wolfe, B.B., Harden, T.K., Sporn, J.R. and Molinoff, P.B. (1978).
Presynaptic modulation of beta-adrenergic receptors in rat
cerebral cortex after treatment with antidepressants. <u>J.
Pharmacol. Exp. Ther.</u>, 207, 446-57

ß-Adrenoceptor agonists enhance the functional activity of brain 5-hydroxytryptamine: relationship to antidepressant activity

D.G.Grahame-Smith[1], P.J.Cowen[1], A.R.Green[1], D.J.Heal[1] and
V.Nimgaonkar[1]

INTRODUCTION

Salbutamol, a β_2-adrenoceptor agonist, has been reported to be a
clinically effective antidepressant (Jouvent *et al.*, 1977;
Lecrubier *et al.*, 1980; Lerer *et al.*, 1981). It has been suggested
that salbutamol may be producing its therapeutic effect by an
action on brain β-adrenoceptors (Lerer *et al.*, 1981; Kostowski,
1981). The question arises as to how such an action might be
translated into an antidepressant effect and whether other β-
adrenoceptor agonists might have a neuropharmacological spectrum
of activity similar to that of salbutamol.

Repeated electroconvulsive shock given as electroconvulsive
therapy is an effective antidepressant treatment in man (see
Kendell, 1981). Repeated electroconvulsive shock in animals
produces enhanced 5-hydroxytryptamine-mediated (5-HT) behavioral
responses in experimental animals (see Costain *et al.*, 1979).
There is also some evidence (Stolz and Marsden, 1982) that chronic
tricyclic antidepressant administration, given the right experimental conditions, can produce enhancement of some 5-HT-mediated
behaviors.

Salbutamol has been shown to increase 5-HT-mediated behavior
in rats (Ortmann *et al.*, 1981; Cowen *et al.*, 1982). Here we wish
to describe some of the effects of salbutamol and other β-adreno-
ceptor agonists on 5-HT-mediated behaviors and to describe in
greater detail the effects of clenbuterol [4-amino-L-(*tert*-butyl-
amine)methyl-3,5-dichlorobenzylalcohol-hydrochloride] which is
also a β_2-adrenoceptor agonist (Engelhardt, 1976). It is very
liposoluble and therefore enters the brain with ease (von Kopitar
and Zimmer, 1976).

---

[1]MRC Unit and University Department of Clinical Pharmacology, University of
Oxford, Radcliffe Infirmary, Oxford, UK.

METHODS

Animals

Adult male Sprague-Dawley derived rats and male C_{57} Bl Ola mice
were used. Animals were housed in groups of six in a 0800-2000 h
light-dark cycle at constant temperature (20 ± 1°C) and fed on an
ad libitum diet of modified 41B pellets and tap water. Behavioral
studies were performed between 0930 and 1730 h.

Behavioral Studies

5-HT-mediated behaviors in rats were examined in the following
ways. Groups of three rats were pre-treated with the β-adrenoceptor agonist simultaneously with tranylcypromine (10 mg kg^{-1})
and 30 min later given L-tryptophan (50 mg kg^{-1}). In other experiments, pairs of rats were pre-treated with the appropriate β-
adrenoceptor agonist and 15 min later given either quipazine (25
mg kg^{-1}) or 5-MeODMT (2 mg kg^{-1}). Hyperactivity responses produced
by these treatments were measured on Automex meters. Results were
analyzed using Student's unpaired t test.

Individual behavioral changes which occur following quipazine
administration were rated separately. Forepaw treading, headweaving, hindlimb abduction and Straub tail were scored by the method
described by Deakin and Green (1978) and Green *et al.* (1981); i.e
0 = absent, 1 = equivocal, 2 = present, 3 = severe. Results were
analyzed using Wilcoxon non-parametric statistics.

Dopamine-mediated behavioral responses were tested using the
unilateral nigrostriatal-lesioned rat model of Ungerstedt (1971a,
b). 6-Hydroxydopamine (8 µg) was infused unilaterally into the
substantia nigra as previously described by Heal *et al.* (1980).
Circling activity to both apomorphine and metamphetamine was
measured in glass rotameter bowls. Circling during 1 min was
recorded at 10 min intervals following injection. Only rats which
circled more than 5 turns per min to both apomorphine (2 mg kg^{-1})
and metamphetamine (2 mg kg^{-1}) were used. Results were analyzed
using Student's paired t test and analysis of variance.

The 5-hydroxytryptophan-induced (5-HTP) head twitch responses
were determined as follows: Mice received carbidopa (25 mg kg^{-1}
i.p.) followed 15 min later by clenbuterol (0.5 mg kg^{-1}) and 5-HTP
(10 mg kg^{-1} i.p.) after a further 15 min. Control animals received
saline instead of clenbuterol. Head twitches were counted for 2
min every 15 min during the 60 min period following 5-HTP.

Brain 5-HT and 5-hydroxyindoleacetic acid (5-HIAA) were
measured by the method of Curzon and Green (1970). The concentration of brain 5-HT was measured 60 min after administration of

the monoamine oxidase inhibitor tranylcypromine (5 mg kg^{-1}i.p.) in rats given either saline or clenbuterol (0.5 mg kg^{-1} or 5 mg kg^{-1} i.p.) 60 min earlier and the rate of 5-HT synthesis calculated by the method of Neff and Tozer (1968). Plasma total and ultra-filterable tryptophan was determined as previously described (Curzon *et al.*, 1972).

DRUGS

All drugs were administered i.p. dissolved in 0.9% saline or suspended in 1% carboxymethylcellulose in saline. Carbidopa (5 mg ml^{-1}) and 5-HTP (20 mg ml^{-1}) were dissolved in a small volume of 0.1 N HCl before being diluted with normal saline to give a final concentration of 30 mM HCl.

RESULTS

Effect of β-Adrenoceptor Agonists on 5-HT-Mediated Behaviors

None of the β-adrenoceptor agonists administered alone, at doses employed in these experiments, stimulated locomotor activity or produced stereotyped behaviors. Therefore, the β-agonists themselves are not capable of producing the various behavioral syndromes produced by increased functional activity of 5-HT.

Clenbuterol at a dose of 5 mg kg^{-1} administered 15 min before quipazine (25 mg kg^{-1}) produced marked enhancement of the behav-

Table 1. The effect of β-adrenoceptor agonists on the 5-HT-mediated hyperactivity produced by quipazine

Pre-treatment	Activity counts (mean ± S.D.)		(*n*)
Saline	2344	± 265	(7)
Clenbuterol (0.25 mg kg^{-1})	3093	± 191	(4)†
Clenbuterol (5 mg kg^{-1})	3516	± 238	(3)†
Saline (pH 3)	2183	± 372	(7)
Salbutamol (5 mg kg^{-1})	2396	± 623	
Terbutaline (5 mg kg^{-1})	2203	± 359	(3)
Salbutamol (20 mg kg^{-1})	3030	± 178	(3)*
Terbutaline (20 mg kg^{-1})	3541	± 785	(3)*

The β-adrenoceptor agonist was injected intraperitoneally (i.p.) 15 min before quipazine, 25 mg kg^{-1} i.p. Activity counts are the number of counts for the 50 min following quipazine administration recorded by pairs of rats placed on Automex meters. Bracketed figure is number of pairs of animals tested.

Different from appropriate saline control: *$p < 0.01$, †$p < 0.001$.

ioral response. This enhancement was detected by an increase in automated counts recorded on the Automex meters and also by scoring the behavioral responses of headweaving, forepaw treading and hindlimb abduction.

Clenbuterol was effective in increasing 5-HT-mediated behavioral responses at a dose of 0.25 mg kg^{-1}. In contrast, neither salbutamol nor terbutaline enhanced the 5-HT hyperactivity syndrome produced by quipazine at a dose of 5 mg kg^{-1}. At a dose of 20 mg kg^{-1} they did, however, produce an enhanced response (see table 1).

Clenbuterol (5 mg kg^{-1}) given 15 min *after* quipazine produced significant enhancement of the hyperactivity syndrome. At a lower dose (0.5 mg kg^{-1}), it failed to do so. The timing of the clenbuterol administration in relation to its potency in enhancing 5-HT-mediated behaviors may, therefore, be crucial.

Clenbuterol (5 mg kg^{-1}) also enhanced the hyperactivity produced by the 5-HT agonist, 5-MeODMT (0.2 mg kg^{-1}) and also that produced by tranylcypromine (10 mg kg^{-1}) with L-tryptophan (50 mg kg^{-1}), a combination known to increase brain 5-HT and its spillover into functional activity (see table 2).

Table 2. The effect of clenbuterol on the hyperactivity syndromes produced by 5-methoxy-N,N-dimethyltryptamine (5-MeODMT), and tranylcypromine (TCP) and L-tryptophan

Treatment			Activity counts (mean ± S.D.)			(n)
Saline	+	5-MeODMT	807	±	65	(4)
Clenbuterol	+	5-MeODMT	1152	±	92	(4)†
Saline	+	TCP/L-tryptophan	2306	±	420	(4)
Clenbuterol	+	TCP/L-tryptophan	3492	±	393	(4)*

Clenbuterol (5 mg kg^{-1}) was injected 15 min before 5-MeODMT (2 mg kg^{-1}) or together with TCP (10 mg kg^{-1}) 30 min before L-tryptophan (40 mg kg^{-1}). Results show the mean ± S.D. of activity counts in the 20 min following 5-MeODMT, or the 90 min following tryptophan. Animals were tested either in pairs (5-MeODMT) or in groups of three (TCP/L-tryptophan). The bracketed figure refers to the number of groups of animals tested.

Different from appropriate saline control: *p <0.01, †p < 0.001.

Effect of Clenbuterol on 5-HTP-Induced Head Twitches in Mice

Clenbuterol (0.5 mg kg^{-1}) injected 15 min before 5-HTP (100 mg kg^{-1}) produced a significant enhancement of the mouse head twitch.

Effect of β-Adrenoceptor Antagonists on Clenbuterol-Induced
Enhancement of Quipazine Hyperactivity

The β-adrenoceptor antagonists were administered 15 min before the
s.c. injection of clenbuterol (2 mg kg^{-1}). Quipazine (25 mg kg^{-1})
was administered 15 min later.
    Metoprolol (5 mg kg^{-1}) blocked the clenbuterol-induced en-
hancement of quipazine hyperactivity. Atenolol (5 mg kg^{-1}) and
butoxamine (5 mg kg^{-1}) were without effect (table 3). None of the
β-adrenoceptor antagonists significantly reduced the baseline
responses to quipazine (table 3).

Table 3. Effect of β-adrenoceptor antagonists on
clenbuterol-induced enhancement of quipazine hyperactivity

Pre-treatment			Activity counts (mean ± S.D.)			(n)
Saline	+	saline	2108	±	448	(3)
Saline	+	clenbuterol	2908	±	189	(4)*
Metoprolol	+	saline	2005	±	333	(5)
Metoprolol	+	clenbuterol	2298	±	310	(5)
Butoxamine	+	saline	1723	±	372	(3)
Butoxamine	+	clenbuterol	3355	±	570	(3)†
Atenolol	+	saline	2090	±	74	(3)
Atenolol	+	clenbuterol	2671	±	230	(3)†

The β-adrenoceptor antagonists were injected i.p. in a dose of 5 mg kg^{-1} 15 min
before either saline or clenbuterol 2 mg kg^{-1} subcutaneously. Quipazine 25 mg
kg^{-1} i.p. was administered 15 min later. Activity counts were recorded as
described in table 1. The bracketed figure is the number of pairs of animals
tested.

Different from appropriate saline control: *$p < 0.05$, †$p < 0.02$.

Effect of Clenbuterol Pre-Treatment on Dopamine-Mediated
Behavioral Responses

Rats with unilateral lesions of the substantia nigra were first
pre-treated with clenbuterol (5 mg kg^{-1}). After 15 min the circling responses were tested with either metamphetamine (0.5 mg kg^{-1})
or apomorphine (0.5 mg kg^{-1}). Clenbuterol administration did not
alter the ipsilateral circling response to metamphetamine. The
contralateral circling response to the dopamine agonist apomorphine did not differ from controls at any timepoint or in total
rotations during the 60 min period of the experiment. However,
the rate of decline of response to apomorphine appeared to be
slower in the clenbuterol-treated rats.

Table 4. Effect of clenbuterol on brain tryptophan and indoleamine concentration and metabolism

Brain concentration (g/g brain)	Saline	Clenbuterol (0.5 mg kg^{-1})	Clenbuterol (5.0 mg kg^{-1})
Tryptophan	2.03 ± 0.20 (10)	3.86 ± 0.23 (10)†	9.14 ± 0.97 (4)†
5-Hydroxyindoleacetic acid	0.50 ± 0.02 (9)	0.59 ± 0.03 (5)*	0.61 ± 0.01 (8)§
5-Hydroxytryptamine	0.32 ± 0.01 (7)	0.32 ± 0.02 (5)	0.36 ± 0.01 (5)*
5-HT after tranylcypromine	0.48 ± 0.01 (10)	0.56 ± 0.02 (6)†	0.58 ± 0.01 (6)§
Synthesis rate (μg g^{-1}h^{-1})	0.16	0.24	0.22

Results expressed as mean ± S.E.M. with the number of observations in brackets. Tryptophan, 5-HT and 5-HIAA concentrations were measured 60 min after clenbuterol. Brain 5-HT concentration was also measured 60 min after tranylcypromine.

Different from saline-treated controls: *$p < 0.025$, †$p < 0.01$, §$p < 0.001$.

Effect of *p*-Chlorophenylalanine (PCPA) Pre-Treatment on Clenbuterol-Induced Enhancement of Quipazine-Mediated Hyperactivity

Rats were injected with PCPA (200 mg kg^{-1} i.p.) at 1530 h on day 1 and day 2. On day 3 the animals were injected with clenbuterol (0.5 mg kg^{-1} i.p.) or saline followed 15 min later by quipazine (25 mg kg^{-1} i.p.).

Pre-treatment with PCPA did not affect the enhancement by clenbuterol of quipazine-induced hyperactivity. Biochemical investigations showed that pre-treatment with PCPA produced a 65% reduction in whole brain 5-HT concentrations.

Effect of Prazosin Pre-Treatment on the Clenbuterol-Induced Enhancement of Quipazine-Mediated Hyperactivity

Prazosin (3 mg kg^{-1} i.p.) was administered 15 min before clenbuterol (0.5 mg kg^{-1} i.p.) or saline and quipazine (25 mg kg^{-1}) after a further 15 min. Although prazosin pre-treatment reduced the quipazine-induced hyperactivity response in its own right, an enhancement of this quipazine response was still seen in rats pre-treated with clenbuterol. Thus, α_1-adrenoceptor inhibition had no effect on the enhancement of 5-HT function by clenbuterol.

Brain and Plasma Indole Concentrations Following Clenbuterol

Clenbuterol (0.5 mg kg^{-1}) did not alter whole brain 5-HT concentrations 50 min later but a dose of 5 mg kg^{-1} produced a modest increase (table 4). Both doses increased brain 5-HIAA concentration. There was an increase in whole brain 5-HT content following tranylcypromine which was greater in rats pre-treated with clenbuterol, suggesting that there was an increase in brain 5-HT turnover.

Both doses of clenbuterol increased the concentration of tryptophan in the brain.

Clenbuterol produced about a doubling of plasma free fatty acid concentration, a marked decrease in plasma total tryptophan concentration, a small but not statistically significant increase in plasma free tryptophan concentration and a 170% increase in the plasma free tryptophan as a percentage of plasma total tryptophan (table 5).

Since clenbuterol increased brain tryptophan and brain 5-HIAA concentrations, the effect of the peripheral β_1-adrenoceptor antagonist atenolol (5 mg kg^{-1}) given 15 min before clenbuterol (5 mg kg^{-1}) on the increase in brain 5-HIAA concentration was examined. Atenolol alone did not alter brain 5-HIAA concentration but it completely blocked the rise produced by clenbuterol (table 6).

Table 5. Plasma free fatty acid and tryptophan concentration 30 min after clenbuterol (5 mg kg^{-1})

Plasma concentration	Saline ($n = 6$)			Clenbuterol (5 mg kg^{-1}) ($n = 6$)		
Free fatty acid (mEq l^{-1})	0.57	±	0.07	1.17	±	0.08*
Total tryptophan (µg ml^{-1})	17.41	±	1.1	8.75	±	0.7*
Free tryptophan (µg ml^{-1})	3.26	±	0.30	4.32	±	0.60
Free tryptophan (%)	18.72	±	1.5	48.47	±	4.4*

Different from saline-treated controls: *$p < 0.001$.

Table 6. Effect of atenolol on the clenbuterol-induced rise of brain 5-HIAA

	Brain 5-HIAA concentration (µg/g brain)			
Saline	0.50	±	0.02	(9)
Clenbuterol (5 mg kg^{-1})	0.61	±	0.01	(8)*
Atenolol (5 mg kg^{-1})	0.53	±	0.02	(4)
Atenolol (5 mg kg^{-1}) + clenbuterol	0.49	±	0.03	(4)

Brain 5-HIAA concentration was measured 60 min after clenbuterol. Different from saline, atenolol or atenolol plus clenbuterol: *$p < 0.001$.

DISCUSSION

Although salbutamol and terbutaline both enhanced 5-HT-mediated behaviors, they were less potent in doing so than clenbuterol. This is probably because they are less lipid-soluble and therefore do not enter the brain as readily as clenbuterol. Delini-Stula *et al.* (1979) showed that salbutamol potentiated 5-HTP-induced head twitch. Fenoterol and terbutaline were also shown to enhance this behavior (Ortmann *et al.*, 1981). We have now shown that clenbuterol is active in enhancing head twitch behavior.

Metoprolol, which enters the brain, blocked the clenbuterol-induced enhancement of quipazine hyperactivity while atenolol, which has limited brain penetration (Day *et al.*, 1977), did not. The precise nature of the receptor upon which clenbuterol may be acting to enhance 5-HT-mediated behaviors is difficult to interpret. While clenbuterol, salbutamol and related agonists are classified as β$_2$-adrenoceptor agonists, the effect of clenbuterol was blocked by metoprolol, which is a relatively selective β_1-adrenoceptor antagonist, but not by the β_2-adrenoceptor antagonist butoxamine. Although the selectivity of β-adrenoceptor agonists is not absolute and may be dose-related, it is odd that butoxamine was inactive. From these limited experiments, it seems that clenbuterol may produce enhancement of 5-HT-mediated responses by activation of central β_1-adrenoceptors, but more experiments need to be done on this point.

It is important to note that none of the β-adrenoceptor agonists administered alone induced behaviors like those produced by increasing brain 5-HT function. It seems unlikely, therefore, that the β-adrenoceptor agonists produce their enhancement of 5-HT-mediated responses by acting directly upon 5-HT receptors. This possibility has to be considered because non-selective β-adrenoceptor antagonists reduce 5-HT-mediated responses (Costain and Green, 1978), perhaps by direct blockade of 5-HT receptors (Middlemiss *et al.*, 1977).

The effect upon dopamine-mediated behaviors of clenbuterol was insignificant compared with its effect upon 5-HT-mediated behaviors. There was a slight slowing of the rate of decline of apomorphine-induced circling; in other experiments, clenbuterol has been known to increase slightly apomorphine-induced hyper-activity, but the effects are minor as compared with the effects on 5-HT-mediated behaviors.

Careful observation showed that clenbuterol enhanced those quipazine-induced behaviors thought to be specifically mediated by 5-HT, i.e. headweaving, forepaw treading and hindlimb abduction, as well as more generalized hyperactivity. In addition, clen-buterol has now been shown to enhance the 5-HTP-induced head twitch, as does salbutamol (Ortmann *et al.*, 1981), so that clen-buterol is active in various behavioral models of central 5-HT function.

Waldmeier (1981) found increased levels of 5-HIAA in rat brain, striatum and cortex after clenbuterol (0.3 mg kg^{-1} i.v.) and also found increased 5-HT levels in the striatum. Erdö *et al.* (1982) found no change in rat whole brain 5-HT and 5-HIAA levels after salbutamol administration. In the present study, clenbuterol has been shown to elevate whole brain 5-HT concen-trations (at the high dose of 5 mg kg^{-1}) and to increase brain 5-HT synthesis rate. Our investigations imply that increased plasma level of non-esterified (or free) fatty acids probably displace tryptophan from plasma albumin binding sites, increase plasma free tryptophan concentrations, and result in an increase in brain tryptophan concentrations, producing a resulting increase in brain 5-HT synthesis and metabolism (Curzon and Fernando, 1976). An alternative explanation might be that, if clenbuterol causes increased secretion of insulin by stimulation of pancreatic cell β-adrenoceptors, the increased plasma levels of insulin may produce a fall in the plasma concentration of branched-chain amino acids competing with tryptophan for transport in the brain, which may then facilitate tryptophan transport into the brain (Munro *et al.*, 1975), with subsequent increase in 5-HT synthesis and turnover.

We believe, though, that there is little causative relationship between clenbuterol-induced changes in brain 5-HT metabolism and the clenbuterol-induced enhancement of 5-HT-mediated behaviors. Behavioral enhancement still occurs in rats treated with PCPA to lower brain 5-HT concentrations. Additionally, the action of direct 5-HT agonists, such as quipazine and 5-methoxy-*N*,*N*-dimethyltryptamine, which are also enhanced by clenbuterol, speak against the involvement of a presynaptic increase in 5-HT synthesis and release from nerve terminals in the phenomenon of enhancement of 5-HT-mediated behavioral responses by clenbuterol. Atenolol blocked the clenbuterol-induced rise in brain 5-HIAA concentration but not the enhancement of quipazine-mediated behaviors and it seems likely that atenolol blocks the metabolic effects of clenbuterol on plasma free fatty acid concentrations and the changes in plasma and brain tryptophan.

It is not yet clear how β-adrenoceptor agonists such as salbutamol and clenbuterol enhance 5-HT-mediated behavioral responses. The experiments reported here seem to suggest that clenbuterol is not acting on presynaptic mechanisms involved in 5-HT synthesis and release. This is not to say that β-agonists by acting on norepinephrine (NE) receptors in 5-HT cell bodies might not influence the activity of 5-HT neurons and increase the turnover of 5-HT (Baraban and Aghajanian, 1981), but this does not seem to be the mechanism by which clenbuterol enhances 5-HT behavioral responses.

One must, therefore, ask whether clenbuterol could increase the sensitivity of 5-HT receptors. As far as the brain is concerned, we have no information on that point.

It seems more likely, however, that clenbuterol acts upon that sequence of neural mechanisms by which activation of 5-HT receptors is translated into a behavioral response. We have seen no impressive enhancement of dopamine-mediated behaviors by clenbuterol. Therefore, the enhancement of 5-HT-mediated behaviors does not seem to involve a dopaminergic mechanism despite the known interactions of dopaminergic and serotonergic mechanisms in the production of the 5-HT hyperactivity syndrome (Green and Grahame-Smith, 1974).

It will be necessary, however, to define those receptors upon which clenbuterol is acting before we can understand the mechanisms by which it enhances 5-HT-mediated behaviors. It is distinctly odd that a β-agonist with predominantly β_2 activity should be blocked by an antagonist with mainly β_1-antagonist activity. Simplistically this might mean that either the brain receptors responsible for interacting with the so-called β_2-agonists are unlike those receptors classified as β_1 or β_2 in the periphery, or that clenbuterol, a so-called β_2-agonist, is not actually acting on β-adrenoceptors, i.e. NE or epinephrine receptors, but on some other related type of amine receptor which, fortuitously, is blocked by metoprolol.

Apart from these neuropharmacological speculations, how do the findings described in this paper have relevance to the antidepressant action of β_2-agonists? The most information on clinical efficacy is on salbutamol and no adequate trials of the antidepressant activity of clenbuterol have yet been reported. If, however, the antidepressant activity of salbutamol is related to enhancement of brain 5-HT function, then clenbuterol should be a more potent antidepressant than salbutamol. Many lines of investigation suggest that there may be abnormalities of 5-HT function in the brains of endogenously depressed patients and that in certain patients treatments which enhance 5-HT function, such as L-tryptophan, tryptophan plus a monoamine oxidase inhibitor, 5-HTP, 5-HTP plus a specific 5-HT uptake inhibitor (such as chlorimipramine), are effective antidepressant therapies. Because of these lines of evidence, it is of great interest to observe that the so-called β_2-agonists have a degree of selectivity in enhancing 5-HT function. Assuming that the β_2-agonists are acting on some type of NE receptor in an area of the brain, it would be of great interest in terms of the various monoamine theories of depression to sort out neuropharmacologically the way in which noradrenergic mechanisms are modulating 5-HT functional activity.

There are further interesting analogies and paradoxes. The functional activity of rat brain 5-HT is increased by repeated electroconvulsive shock, yet in these circumstances cortical β-adrenoceptor number and their function (i.e. NE-sensitive adenylate cyclase activity) are decreased. This would not be expected if the 'degree' of 5-HT-mediated behavior was directly dependent on β-adrenoceptor sensitivity and activity. In addition, the functional activity of brain 5-HT is inhibited by non-selective lipophilic β-adrenoceptor antagonists, such as propranolol (Costain and Green, 1978). This does fit the hypothesis that in some way β-adrenoceptor function is positively correlated to 5-HT function. Against this, however, is the observation that, although lesions of the locus coeruleus and ventral and dorsal noradrenergic bundles prevent the enhancement of 5-HT-mediated behaviors by repeated ECS, such lesions do not in themselves inhibit or alter the 5-HT-mediated behaviors described (Green and Deakin, 1980). Thus these 5-HT-mediated behaviors are not dependent upon the functioning of the noradrenergic projections to the cortex.

At the moment we cannot construct an overall hypothesis which fits together the following points:

(1) β_2-Agonists enhance behavioral responses to 5-HT agonists.
(2) This enhancement is blocked by a β_1-antagonist but not by a β_2-antagonist.

(3) Repeated electroconvulsive shock (given like ECT) down-regulates cortical β-adrenoceptor function but enhances 5-HT function. Antidepressant drug administration down-regulates cortical β-adrenoceptor function but enhances certain aspects of 5-HT function.

(4) Non-selective lipophilic β-adrenoceptor antagonists (e.g. propranolol) inhibit 5-HT-mediated behavioral responses.

Within these analogies and paradoxes, a great deal remains to be revealed about the inter-relationships of brain 5-HT and nor-adrenergic function.

REFERENCES

Baraban, J.M. and Aghajanian, G.K. (1981). Noradrenergic innervation of serotonergic neurons in the dorsal raphe: demonstration by electron microscopic autoradiography. Brain Res. 204, 1-11

Costain, D.W. and Green, A.R. (1978). β-Adrenoceptor antagonists inhibit the behavioural responses of rats to increased brain 5-hydroxytryptamine. Br. J. Pharmacol., 64, 193-200

Costain, D.W., Green, A.R. and Grahame-Smith, D.G. (1979). Enhanced 5-hydroxytryptamine-mediated behavioural responses in rats following repeated electroconvulsive shock: relevance to the mechanism of the antidepressant effect of electroconvulsive therapy. Psychopharmacology, 61, 167-70

Cowen, P.J., Grahame-Smith, D.G., Green, A.R. and Heal, D.J. (1982). β-Adrenoceptor agonists enhance 5-hydroxytryptamine-mediated behavioural responses. Br. J. Pharmacol., 76, 265-70

Curzon, G. and Fernando, J.C.R. (1976). Effect of aminophylline on tryptophan and other aromatic amino acids in plasma, brain and other tissues and on brain 5-hydroxytryptamine metabolism. Br. J. Pharmacol., 58, 533-45

Curzon, G. and Green, A.R. (1970). Rapid method for the determination of 5-hydroxytryptamine and 5-hydroxyindoleacetic acid in small regions of rat brain. Br. J. Pharmacol., 39, 653-5

Curzon, G., Joseph, M.H. and Knott, P.J. (1972). Effects of immobilization and food deprivation on rat brain tryptophan metabolism. J. Neurochem., 19, 1967-74

Day, M.D., Hemsworth, B.A. and Street, J.A. (1977). The central uptake of β-adrenoceptor antagonists. J. Pharm. Pharmacol., 29, 52P

Deakin, J.F.W. and Green, A.R. (1978). The effects of putative 5-hydroxytryptamine antagonists on the behaviour produced by administration of tranylcypromine and L-tryptophan or tranylcypromine and L-dopa to rats. Br. J. Pharmacol., 64, 201-9

Delini-Stula, A., Vassout, A., Radeke, E. and Ortmann, R. (1979). Psychopharmacological profile of β2-receptor stimulants. Naunyn-Schmiedeberg's Arch. Pharmacol., 307, R65

Engelhardt, G. (1976). Pharmakologisches wirkungsprofil von NAB 365 (clenbuterol), einem neuen broncholytikum mit einer selektiven wirkung auf die adrenergen β₂-rezeptoren. Arzneim-Forsch., 26, 1404-20

Erdö, S.L., Kiss, B. and Rosdy, B. (1982). Effect of salbutamol on the cerebral levels, uptake and turnover of serotonin. Eur. J. Pharmacol., 78, 357-61

Green, A.R. and Deakin, J.F.W. (1980). Brain noradrenaline depletion prevents ECS-induced enhancement of serotonin and dopamine-mediated behaviour. Nature, 285, 232-3

Green, A.R. and Grahame-Smith, D.G. (1974). The role of brain dopamine in the hyperactivity syndrome produced in rats after the administration of L-tryptophan and a monoamine oxidase inhibitor. Br. J. Pharmacol., 50, 442-3

Green, A.R., Hall, J.E. and Rees, A.R. (1981). A behavioural and biochemical study in rats of 5-hydroxytryptamine receptor agonists and antagonists, with observations on structure activity requirements for the agonists. Br. J. Pharmacol., 73, 703-19

Heal, D.J., Green, A.R. and Buylaert, W.A. (1980). Inhibition of apomorphine-, bromocriptine-, and lergotrile-induced circling behaviour in rats by subsequent haloperidol administration. Neuropharmacology, 19, 133-7

Jouvent, R., Lecrubier, Y., Pusch, A-J., Frances, H., Simon, P. and Widlöcher, D. (1977). De l'étude expérimentale d'un stimulant bêta-adrénergique á la mise en évidence de son activité antidépressive chez l'homme. Encéphale, 3, 285-93

Kendell, R. (1981). The present status of electroconvulsive therapy. Br. J. Psychiatry, 139, 265-83

Kostowski, W. (1981). Brain noradrenaline, depression and antidepressant drugs: facts and hypothesis. Trends Pharmacol. Sci., 2, 314-17

Lecrubier, Y., Pusch, A-J., Jouvent, R., Simon, P. and Widlöcher, D. (1980). A beta adrenergic stimulant (salbutamol) versus clomipramine in depression: a controlled study. Br. J. Psychiatry, 136, 354-8

Lerer, B., Ebstein, R.P. and Belmaker, R.H. (1981). Subsensitivity of human β-adrenergic adenylate cyclase after salbutamol treatment of depression. Psychopharmacology, 75, 169-72

Middlemiss, D.N., Blakeborough, L. and Leather, S.R. (1977). Direct evidence for an interaction of β-adrenergic blockers with the 5-HT receptor. Nature, 267, 289-90

Munro, H.N., Fernstrom, J.D. and Wurtman, R.J. (1975). Insulin, plasma amino acid inbalance, and hepatic coma. Lancet, i, 722-4

Neff, N.H. and Tozer, T.N. (1968). In vivo measurement of brain serotonin turnover. Adv. Pharmacol., A, 6, 97-109

Ortmann, R., Martin, S., Radeke, E. and Delini-Stula, A. (1981). Interation of β-adrenoceptor agonists with the serotonergic system in rat brain. Naunyn-Schmiedeberg's Arch. Pharmacol., 316, 225-30

Stolz, J.F. and Marsden, C.A. (1982). Withdrawal from chronic treatment with metergoline, di-propranolol and amitriptyline enhances serotonin receptor mediated behavior in the rat. Eur. J. Pharmacol., 79, 17-22

Ungerstedt, J. (1971a). Striatal dopamine release after amphetamine on nerve degeneration revealed by rotational behaviour. Acta Physiol. Scand., 367, Suppl., 49-68

Ungerstedt, J. (1971b). Postsynaptic supersensitivity after 6-hydroxydopamine induced degeneration of the nigro-striatal dopamine system. Acta Physiol. Scand., 367, Suppl., 69-93

Von Kopitar, Z. and Zimmer, A. (1976). Pharmakokinetic und metaboliten muster von clenbuterol bei der ratte. Arzneim-Forsch., 26, 1435-41

Waldmeier, P.C. (1981). Stimulation of central serotonin turnover by β-adrenoceptor agonists. Naunyn-Schmeideberg's Arch. Pharmacol., 317, 115-19

Effects of antidepressant treatments on 'whole body' norepinephrine turnover

Markku Linnoila[1], Farouk Karoum[2] and William Z. Potter[1]

INTRODUCTION

Monoamine theories of depression postulate that a relative lack of either norepinephrine (Schildkraut, 1965; Bunney and Davis, 1965) or serotonin (Ashcroft et al., 1966; Coppen, 1967) at certain critical synapses in the central nervous system (CNS) are associated with symptoms of 'endogenous' depression. Based on these theories, Prange et al. (1974) have developed a 'permissive monoamine' hypothesis of bipolar affective disorders. They suggest that a continuously low serotonergic tone permits wide fluctuations in CNS norepinephrinergic activity, low activity being associated with depressive and high with manic symptoms. Janowsky et al. (1972) have emphasized that a cholinergic-norepinephrinergic imbalance may be important in generating affective symptoms. In their view, an increased cholinergic tone and a reduced norepinephrinergic activity is characteristic of depression, whereas a relatively low cholinergic tone and a high norepinephrinergic activity is associated with mania.

The possible role of monoamines in affective disorders was originally suggested by side-effects of antihypertensive treatments such as reserpine, which deplete CNS monoamines (Brodie and Costa, 1962) and produce depressions in susceptible individuals (Achor et al., 1955). Moreover, the classic antidepressant drugs, tricyclics and monoamine oxidase inhibitors (MAOIs), block, respectively, the re-uptake (Carlsson et al., 1969a, b) or enzymatic degradation of norepinephrine, serotonin and several other monoamines.

[1]Clinical Psychobiology Branch, National Institute of Mental Health, Bethesda, Maryland 20205, USA.
[2]Adult Psychiatry Branch, National Institute of Mental Health, Bethesda, Maryland 20205, USA.

Maas (1975) summarized the literature concerning the biochemistry and pharmacology of affective disorders and concluded that there could be two biochemical subtypes of depressions: one associated with a relative lack of norepinephrine and another with a relative lack of serotonin. Two clinical studies, which involved treatment with desipramine or zimelidine, relatively specific uptake inhibitors of norepinephrine or serotonin respectively, in an intended crossover design failed to support this postulate (Stewart *et al.*, 1980; Aberg, 1981). In both studies, a large majority of patients responded well to the first active treatment regardless of its transmitter specificity.

Animal experiments investigating receptor changes in the CNS produced by different chronic antidepressant treatments have demonstrated desensitization of norepinephrinergic postsynaptic β and presumed presynaptic α_2 adrenoceptors, serotonin receptors and, in some instances, presynaptic dopamine autoreceptors (for review, see Charney *et al.*, 1981). The most recent studies have found that direct manipulations of the norepinephrine or serotonin neuronal systems at the specific receptor level can cause secondary functional changes in the other system (Przegalinsky *et al.*, 1981; Hallberg *et al.*, 1982; Grahame-Smith *et al.*, 1982).

Thus, contrary to earlier suggestions, the transmitter specificity of certain antidepressants may not be helpful in parceling out the significance of a given neurotransmitter to the pathology of depression in a given patient. Consequently, attempts to define 'norepinephrine and serotonin depressions' may be futile. Indeed, our recent data in schizophrenics and murderers which follow upon previous findings in other groups of subjects support that low 5-hydroxyindoleacetic acid, already reported to be associated with suicidal depressions and impulsive psychopathy (Asberg *et al.*, 1976; Brown *et al.*, 1979), is not characteristic of depression, but rather is primarily associated with violent behavior toward oneself or others (Ninan *et al.*, unpublished; Virkkunen *et al.*, unpublished).

In light of the above uncertainties concerning the role of serotonin and the preponderance of norepinephrine theories in the field, we focused our efforts to quantitate effects of antidepressant treatments on norepinephrine metabolism in depressed patients. We are measuring indices of dopamine and serotonin metabolism as well, because of the above-mentioned animal and clinical data suggestive of important interactions between the monoaminergic neuronal systems. This communication, however, deals mainly with the results involving norepinephrine. Our strategy has been to use the most specific monoamine re-uptake inhibiting antidepressants clinically available (Carlsson *et al.*, 1969a,b; Ogren *et al.*, 1981), and to compare them with clorgyline, a specific MAO type A inhibitor (Johnston, 1968) and the 'non-specific' treatments, lithium and electroconvulsive therapy. All patients were followed longitudinally during a lengthy pre-drug placebo period and during steady-state kinetics on each drug. We measured the monoamines and their main metabolites in the urine, because this is currently the best way to investigate the turnover of these transmitters in man.

PATIENTS AND METHODS

Twenty-one severely depressed patients, 17 women and four men, participated in our studies (Linnoila *et al.*, 1982a, b, 1983, and unpublished). All of them underwent a minimum 5-week initial placebo period and were subsequently treated with either clorgyline, desipramine, ECT, lithium or zimelidine. Clorgyline was administered in doses of 5 or 10 mg per 24 h to four women with a primary, major bipolar affective disorder (Spitzer *et al.*, 1978). Three men and nine women, six unipolar and six bipolar, participated in the desipramine-zimelidine trial. Based on single dose kinetics, the dose of desipramine was titrated to produce plasma levels between 300 and 450 μmol l^{-1} (Potter *et al.*, 1981). Zimelidine was administered as a 200-300 mg/24 h dose. Seven women and one man, four bipolar and four unipolar, took part in the ECT-lithium study. In all studies, where a crossover design was partially used (four patients in the desipramine-zimelidine trial and three patients in the ECT-lithium study), an adequate washout period was allowed between the treatments. Three patients participated in more than one study on separate admissions. Throughout the studies, all patients were maintained on a strictly controlled low monoamine diet (Muscettola *et al.*, 1977).

The severities of depression, mania and psychosis were rated every morning and night by trained psychiatric nurses with the Bunney and Hamburg (1963) scale.

Urinary norepinephrine, normetanephrine, 3-methoxy-4-hydroxy-phenylglycol (MHPG) and vanilmandelic acid (VMA) were quantified with mass fragmentography (Karoum and Neff, 1982). Twenty-four hour urine samples (7 a.m. - 7 a.m.), with volumes in excess of 900 ml, obtained during the last two weeks of placebo treatment and during steady-state kinetics on the antidepressants as well as between days 7 to 14 after the ECTs, were stored at -20°C and preserved with 3% sodium metabisulfite until analyzed. The means of three to four urine collections were used in the statistical analyses. Urinary norepinephrine, normetanephrine, MHPG and VMA outputs were added to produce an indicator of 'whole body' norepinephrine turnover (Linnoila *et al.*, 1982a).

The urinary norepinephrine and metabolite outputs and 'whole body' norepinephrine turnovers during placebo and active treatments were compared by parametric analysis of variance for repeated measurements, when appropriate, and with Student's *t*-test for related samples. The mood ratings were compared using the Mann-Whitney *U*-test. Two-tailed probabilities were used in all comparisons.

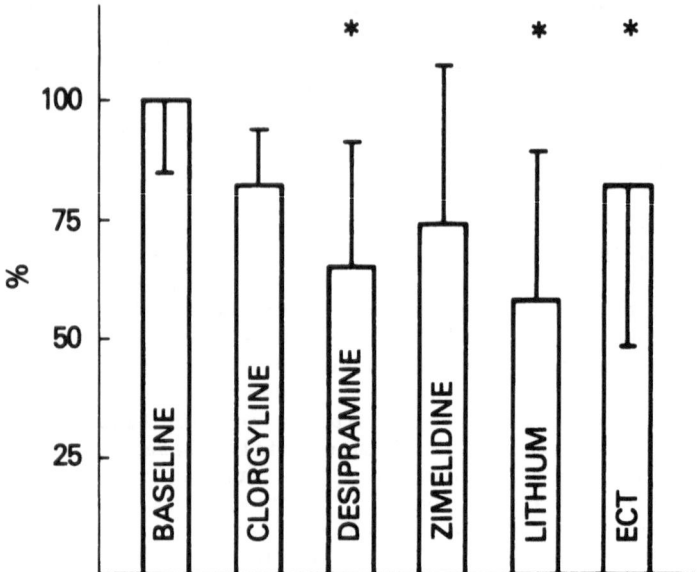

Figure 1.   Effect of antidepressants on 24-hour mean ± S.D.
urinary norepinephrine (NE) output. *$p < 0.05$,
Student's t-test for related samples, two-tailed
probability.

RESULTS

Clorgyline significantly reduced urinary MHPG and VMA output and
'whole body' norepinephrine turnover, but it increased normetanephrine output (Figures 1–5). Desipramine significantly
reduced urinary norepinephrine, MHPG and VMA output and whole body
norepinephrine turnover, but zimelidine reduced urinary MHPG
output only (Figures 1–5). Lithium reduced all indices of norepinephrine metabolism to a significant degree, and ECT reduced
norepinephrine and normetanephrine output and tended to reduce
'whole body' norepinephrine turnover as well.
    Clorgyline, ECT and lithium reduced mean depression ratings
significantly ($p < 0.01$) but only two depressed patients responded
to treatment with desipramine or zimelidine, respectively.
Furthermore, clorgyline tended to stabilize mood in rapidly cycling bipolar patients (Potter *et al.*, 1982). No differences could
be found in the antidepressant-induced changes of urinary norepinephrine and metabolite outputs between the responders and non-
responders. However, the patients showing a favorable therapeutic
outcome during desipramine and zimelidine treatments had relatively low pre-treatment MHPG outputs.

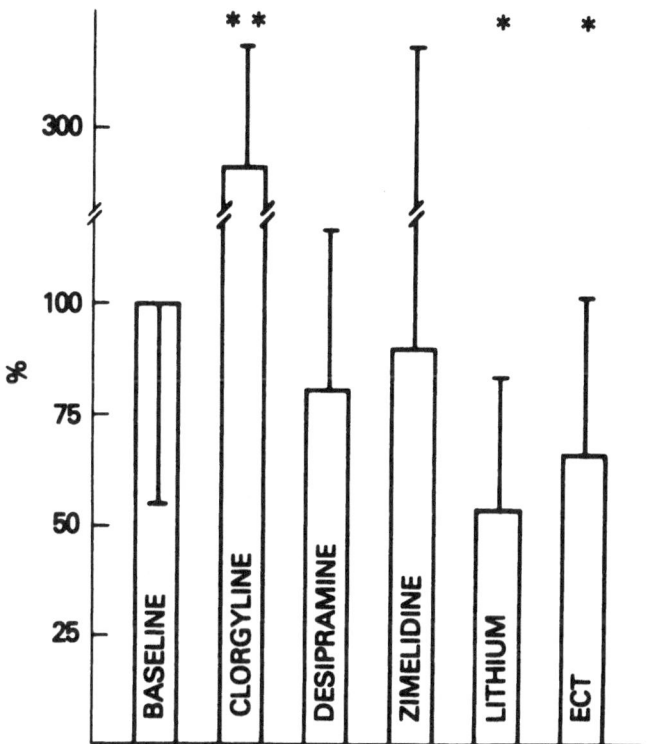

Figure 2. Effect of antidepressants on 24-hour mean ± S.D.
urinary normetanephrine (NM) output. *$p < 0.05$;
**$p < 0.01$; Student's t-test for related samples,
two-tailed probability.

DISCUSSION

The main finding of this series of studies was that five different
antidepressant treatments all affected norepinephrine metabolism
in man. Moreover, the different effects of some of these treatments on the relative amounts of norepinephrine and its main
metabolites excreted in the urine allowed us to 'fingerprint'
their mechanism of action in depressed patients.

Seemingly our results are hard to reconcile with the norepinephrine theory of depression and the animal studies demonstrating
desensitization of β and $α_2$ adrenoceptors during administration of
antidepressants (Charney *et al.*, 1981). After all, neither the
theory nor the animal experiments necessarily predict that antidepressants would reduce total norepinephrine metabolism as a
result of reduced presynaptic release of the transmitter (Linnoila

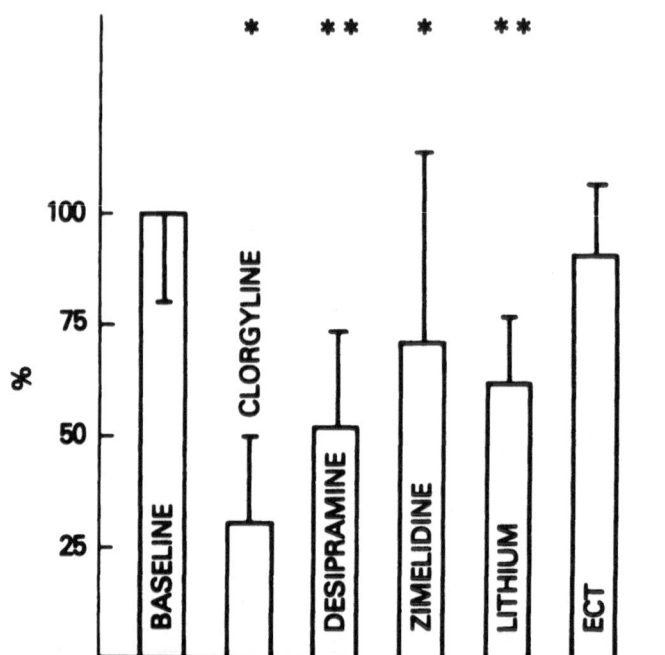

Figure 3.   Effect of antidepressants on 24-hour mean ± S.D.
urinary 3-methoxy-4-hydroxyphenylglycol (MHPG) output.
*$p < 0.05$; **$p < 0.01$; Student's *t*-test for related
samples, two-tailed probability.

et al., 1982b). However, in spite of reducing 'whole body' norepinephrine turnover, desipramine may actually increase the amount of
intrasynaptic norepinephrine and potentiate its effects in man, as
indicated by an increased plasma norepinephrine concentration,
heart rate and blood pressure in healthy volunteers receiving the
drug (Ross *et al.*, unpublished). Thus, the reduced 'whole body'
norepinephrine turnover, in depressed patients on desipramine, is
consistent with an adaptation of the noradrenergic neuron system
to increased intrasynaptic transmitter. The mechanism of this
adaptation could involve both a reduced firing rate of presynaptic
norepinephrine neurons and subsensitization of presynaptic α_2
adrenoceptors as observed in experimental animals treated with
desipramine (Svensson and Usdin, 1978), depending on the balance
of intrasynaptic norepinephrine increase and α_2 adrenoceptor
subsensitivity.

Over and beyond the absolute reduction in 'whole body' norepinephrine turnover produced by desipramine, the drug modestly
increased the relative amount of norepinephrine excreted as normetanephrine.   This finding is compatible with a blockade of nor-

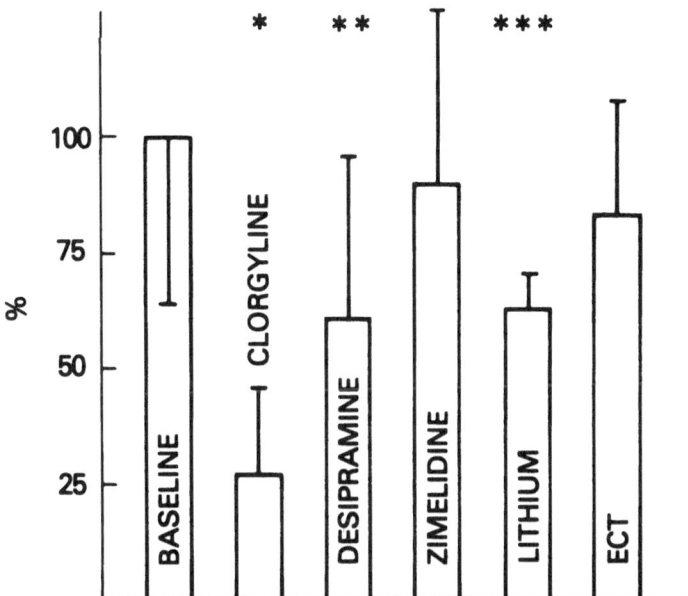

Figure 4. Effect of antidepressants on 24-hour mean ± S.D.
urinary vanilmandelic acid (VMA) output. *p < 0.05;
**p < 0.01; ***p < 0.001, Student's t-test for related
samples, two-tailed probability.

epinephrine re-uptake, which is maintained even during chronic
administration (Linnoila *et al.*, 1983; Ross *et al.*, unpublished).

Clorgyline reduced 'whole body' norepinephrine turnover more
than any other antidepressant that we have studied (Linnoila *et
al.*, 1982a). This drug has been demonstrated to increase the
cerebrospinal fluid ratio of norepinephrine to dopamine-β-hydroxylase in man. The relative decrease of dopamine-β-hydroxylase
has been suggested to indicate a reduced firing of norepinephrinergic neurons (Lerner *et al.*, 1979). Our findings are in
agreement with this interpretation. Furthermore, like desipramine, clorgyline presumably increases intrasynaptic norepinephrine
concentration as indicated by the greatly enhanced normetanephrine
output during clorgyline treatment. Thus, the mechanism by which
clorgyline could reduce presynaptic norepinephrine neuronal firing
would be similar to that of desipramine.

Clorgyline most markedly reduced the absolute and relative
outputs of the deaminated metabolites of norepinephrine. These
effects on norepinephrine and metabolite output pattern are consistent with MAO inhibition. Moreover, the drug did not change
the urinary output of phenylethylamine, which is a preferred
substrate of MAO type B. Therefore, our data with multiple para-

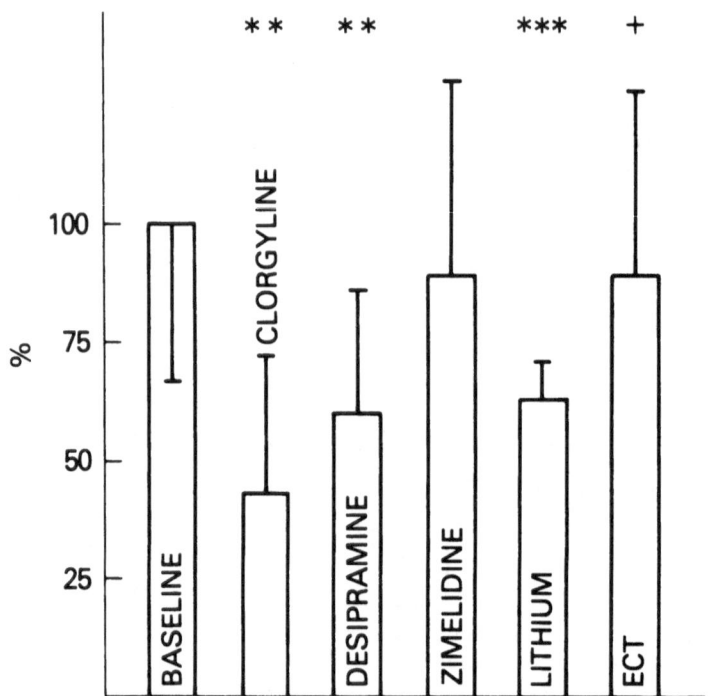

Figure 5.   Effect of antidepressants on mean ± S.D. 'whole body'
norepinephrine (N) turnover. ^+p < 0.07; $**p$ < 0.01;
$***p$ < 0.001, Student's t-test for related samples,
two-tailed probability.

meters (Linnoila *et al.*, 1982a) provide direct support for the
previous conclusion that clorgyline is a specific MAO type A
inhibitor *in vivo* which was based on measures of MHPG and platelet
MAO type B (Murphy *et al.*, 1979).

Lithium reduced the urinary outputs of norepinephrine and all
of the measured metabolites. The reduction of 'whole body'
norepinephrine turnover produced by lithium was only slightly less
than that produced by clorgyline. Interestingly, the two drugs
that have mood stabilizing effects in bipolar patients (lithium
and clorgyline (Potter *et al.*, 1982)), produced no more reduction
in 'whole body' norepinephrine turnover than desipramine, which
may even precipitate mood cycles (Extein *et al.*, 1979). Because
lithium reduced proportionately both the extracellular and intracellular metabolites of norepinephrine, our data do not provide
evidence for lithium-induced increases of norepinephrine re-uptake
in depressed patients as has been suggested in animal experiments
(Schildkraut, 1974). Rather, lithium may inhibit tyrosine hyd-

roxylase, since it reduces 'whole body' dopamine turnover as well as that of norepinephrine (Linnoila, Karoum and Potter, unpublished). If this finding holds, then our attempts to elucidate the relative importance of dopamine and norepinephrine in bipolar affective disorders by measuring urinary catecholamines during lithium treatment will be futile.

ECT reduced urinary norepinephrine and normetanephrine outputs and tended to reduce 'whole body' norepinephrine turnover. The mechanism by which ECT produces these changes remains obscure. Interestingly, depressed patients have been reported to 'spillover' more norepinephrine from sympathetic nervous system synapses than volunteers (Esler *et al.*, 1982). Our data suggest that such 'spillover' may be specifically reduced by ECT.

It is also unclear how zimelidine might reduce urinary MHPG output without altering ratios between norepinephrine and its metabolites. We currently speculate that this could be secondary to a zimelidine-mediated increase of inhibitory serotonergic input to the locus coeruleus - a speculation for which we are attempting to provide experimental evidence.

Although our results can be interpreted to indicate that the five antidepressant treatments reduce presynaptic norepinephrine release, we cannot conclude that this effect is a necessary component of their antidepressant mechanism of action. This is because the clinical antidepressant effect of these treatments usually does not appear until at least two weeks of administration whereas our animal and healthy volunteer data (Garrick *et al.*, unpublished; Ross *et al.*, unpublished) suggest that the effects of clorgyline and desipramine on norepinephrine metabolism are immediate. Thus, an adaptation of the CNS to a reduced presynaptic norepinephrine release could be involved in producing an antidepressant effect. In phobic patients, who often respond to antidepressants within days, the reduction of presynaptic norepinephrine release can be postulated to be therapeutic *per se*. In hyperactive children who respond rapidly to treatment with tricyclic antidepressants but lose the favorable therapeutic effect within weeks, an adaptation to the reduced release of presynaptic norepinephrine can be postulated to be counter-therapeutic (Linnoila *et al.*, 1980). Further parallel biochemical studies in depressed and phobic patients as well as hyperactive children should help us to understand better the ultimate mechanisms of action of current antidepressant treatments.

REFERENCES

Aberg, A. (1981). Controlled cross-over study of a 5HT uptake inhibiting and a NA uptake inhibiting antidepressant. Acta Psychiatr. Scand, **63**, Suppl.290, 244-55

Achor, R. W. P., Hanson, N. O. and Gifford, R. W. (1955).
    Hypertension treated with rauwolfia serpentina (whole root)
    and with reserpine. J. Am. Med. Assoc., 159, 841-7
Asberg, M., Thoren, P., Träskman, L., Bertilsson, L. and
    Ringberger, V. (1976). Serotonin depression - a biochemical
    subgroup within the affective disorders. Science, 191,
    478-80
Ashcroft, G. W., Crawford, T. B. B., Eccleston, D., Sharman,
    D. F., MacDougall, E. J., Stanton, B. and Bims, J. K. (1966).
    5-Hydroxy indole compounds in the cerebrospinal fluid of
    patients with psychiatric or neurological disease. Lancet,
    ii, 1049-51
Brodie, B. B. and Costa, E. (1962). Some current views on brain
    monoamines. Psychopharmacol. Bull., 2, 1-22
Brown, G. L., Goodwin, F. K., Ballenger, J. C., Goyer, P. F. and
    Major L. F. (1979). Aggression in humans correlates with
    cerebrospinal fluid amine metabolites. Psychiatry Res., 1,
    131-9
Bunney, W. E. Jr. and Davis, J. M. (1965). Norepinephrine in
    depressive reactions. Arch. Gen. Psychiatry, 13, 483-94
Bunney, W. E. Jr. and Hamburg, D. A. (1963). Methods for reliable
    longitudinal observation of behavior. Arch. Gen. Psychiatry,
    9, 280-94
Carlsson, A., Corrodi, H., Fuxe, K. and Hökfelt, T. (1969a).
    Effect of antidepressant drugs on the depletion of intra-
    neuronal brain 5-hydroxy-tryptamine stores caused by 4-
    methyl-α-ethyl-meta-tyramine. Eur. J. Pharmacol., 5, 357-66
Carlsson, A., Corrodi, H., Fuxe, K. and Hökfelt, T. (1969b).
    Effects of some antidepressant drugs on the depletion of
    intraneuronal brain catecholamine stores caused by 4-α-di-
    methyl-meta-tyramine. Eur. J. Pharmacol., 5, 367-73
Charney, D. S., Menkes, D. B. and Heninger, G. R. (1981). Receptor
    sensitivity and the mechanism of action of antidepressant
    treatments. Arch. Gen. Psychiatry, 38, 1160-72
Coppen, A. (1967). The biochemistry of affective disorders. Br.
    J. Psychiatry, 113, 1237
Esler, M., Turbott, J., Schwarz, R., Leonard, P., Bobik, A., Skews
    H. and Jackman G. (1982). The peripheral kinetics of norepi-
    nephrine in depressive illness. Arch. Gen. Psychiatry, 39,
    295-300
Extein, I., Potter, W. Z., Wehr, T. A. and Goodwin, F. K. (1979).
    Rapid mood cycles after noradrenergic but not serotonergic
    antidepressant. Am. J. Psychiatry, 136, 1602-4
Grahame-Smith, D.G., Cowen, P.J., Green, A.R., Heal, D.J. and
    Nimgaonkar, V (1982). β-Adrenoceptor agonists enhance the
    functional activity of brain 5-hydroxytryptamine: relation-
    ship to antidepressant activity. This volume, pp. 313-26
Hallberg, H., Almgren, O. and Svensson, T. H. (1982). Reduced

brain serotonergic activity after repeated treatment with β-adrenoceptor antagonists. Psychopharmacology, 76, 114-19

Janowsky, D., El-Yousef, K., Davis, M. and Sekerke, H. J. (1972). A cholinergic-adrenergic hypothesis of mania and depression. Lancet, ii, 632-4

Johnston, J. P. (1968). Some observations upon a new inhibitor of monoamine oxidase in brain tissue. Biochem. Pharmacol., 17, 1285-93

Karoum, F. and Neff, N. H. (1982). Quantitative gas chromatography-mass spectrometry (GC-MS) of biogenic amines: theory and practice. In Handbook of Analytical Methods in Pharmacology, (ed. S. Spector), Raven Press, New York, in press

Lerner, P., Major, F. P., Murphy, D. L., Lipper, S., Lake, C. R. and Lovenberg, W. (1979). Dopamine-β-hydroxylase and norepinephrine in human cerebrospinal fluid: effects of monoamine oxidase inhibitors. Neuropharmacology, 18, 423-8

Linnoila, M., Karoum, F., Calil, H. M., Kopin, I. J. and Potter, W. Z. (1983). Alteration of norepinephrine metabolism with desimipramine and zimelidine in depressed patients. Arch. Gen. Psychiatry, in press

Linnoila, M., Karoum, F. and Potter, W. Z. (1982a). Effect of low-dose clorgyline on 24-hour urinary monoamine excretion in patients with rapidly cycling bipolar affective disorder. Arch. Gen. Psychiatry, 39, 513-16

Linnoila, M., Karoum, F. and Potter, W. Z. (1982b). High correlation of norepinephrine and its major metabolite excretion rates. Arch. Gen. Psychiatry, 39, 521-3

Linnoila, M., Seppala, T., Mattila, M. J., Vihko, R., Pakarinen, A. and Skinner T. (1980). Clorimipramine and doxepin in depressive neurosis. Arch. Gen. Psychiatry, 37, 1295-9

Maas, J. W. (1975). Monoamines in affective disorders. Arch. Gen. Psychiatry, 32, 1159-63

Murphy, D. L., Lipper, S., Slater, S., and Shiling, D. (1979). Selectivity of clorgyline and pargyline as inhibitors of monoamine oxidases A and B *in vivo* in man. Psychopharmacology, 62, (2), 129-32

Muscettola, G., Wehr, T. and Goodwin, F. K. (1977). Effect of diet on urinary MHPG excretion in depressed patients and in normal controls. Am. J. Psychiatry, 134, 914-17

Ogren, S. O., Ross, S. B., Hall, H., Holm, A. C. and Renyi, A. L. (1981). The pharmacology of zimelidine: a 5-HT-selective reuptake inhibitor. Acta Psychiatr. Scand., 63, Suppl. 290, 127-51

Potter, W. Z., Calil, H. M., Extein, I., Gold, P. W., Wehr, T. A. and Goodwin, F. K. (1981). Specific norepinephrine and serotonin uptake inhibitors in man: a crossover study with pharmacokinetic, biochemical, neuroendocrine and behavioral parameters. Acta Psychiatr. Scand., 63, Suppl. 290, 152

Potter, W. Z., Murphy, D. L., Wehr, T. A., Linnoila, M. and Goodwin, F. K. (1982). Clorgyline: a new treatment for patients with refractory rapid-cycling disorder. Arch. Gen. Psychiatry, 39, 505-15

Prange, A., Wilson, I., Lynn, C. W., Alltop, L. B. and Stikeleather, R. A. (1974). L-tryptophan in mania: contribution to a permissive hypothesis of affective disorders. Arch. Gen. Psychiatry, 30, 56-63

Przegalinsky, E., Kordecka-Magrera, A., Mogihuka, E. and Maj, S. (1981). Chronic treatment with some atypical antidepressants increases the brain level of 3-methoxy-4-hydroxyphenylglycol (MHPG) in rats. Psychopharmacology, 74, 187-91

Schildkraut, J. J. (1965). The catecholamine hypothesis of affective disorders: a review of supporting evidence. Am. J. Psychiatry, 122, 509-22

Schildkraut, J. J. (1974). The effects of lithium on norepinephrine turnover and metabolism: basic and clinical studies. J. Nerv. Ment. Dis., 158, 348-60

Spitzer, R. L., Endicott, T. and Robbins, E. (1978). Research diagnostic criteria: rationale and validity. Arch. Gen. Psychiatry, 35, 773-82

Stewart, J. W., Quitkin, F. and Fyer, A. (1980). Efficacy of desmethylimipramine in endogenomorphically depressed patients. Psychopharmacol. Bull., 16, 52-3

Svensson, T. H. and Usdin, T. (1978). Feedback inhibition of brain noradrenaline neurons by tricyclic antidepressants: α-receptor mediation. Science, 202, 1089-92

Association of ³H-imipramine binding with serotonin uptake and of ³H-desipramine binding with norepinephrine uptake: potential research tools in depression

S.Z.Langer[1], M.Sette[1] and R.Raisman[1]

INTRODUCTION

The study of the classical pharmacological receptors with receptor binding techniques is by now a well established methodology. Receptor binding techniques have also been successfully employed to study and characterize sites of drug action which possess the properties of pharmacological receptors. One such example concerns the discovery and characterization of the high-affinity binding sites for ³H-diazepam which are related to the site of action of benzodiazepines in the central nervous system (Squires and Braestrup, 1977; Möhler and Okada, 1977). Using the same approach, we have recently studied the high-affinity binding of two radio-actively labeled tricyclic antidepressants, ³H-imipramine and ³H-desipramine, with the aim of investigating the mechanism of action of tricyclic antidepressant drugs and to attempt to identify their sites of action and their possible relationship to the biochemistry of affective disorders.

CHARACTERIZATION OF THE ³H-IMIPRAMINE BINDING SITE

The high-affinity binding site for ³H-imipramine is present in membranes prepared from various regions of the brain of several species, including man (Raisman *et al.*, 1979a,b, 1980; Langer *et al.*, 1981a, 1982). ³H-Imipramine also binds saturably and with high affinity to human platelets (Briley *et al.*, 1979; Langer *et al.*, 1980a).

As shown in table 1, the high-affinity binding of ³H-imipramine to membranes of the rat cerebral cortex is inhibited by tricyclic antidepressants and by non-tricyclic inhibitors of neuronal uptake of 5-HT in the nanomolar range. Serotonin is the

[1] Department of Biology, Laboratoires d'Etudes et de Recherches - Synthélabo, 58 rue de la Glacière, 75013 Paris, France.

Table 1.   Inhibition of ^{3}H-imipramine binding in membranes of
the rat cerebral cortex

	IC_{50} (nM)	Hill coefficient
Imipramine	7	0.91
Desipramine	177	1.11
Chlorimipramine	25	1.19
Nortriptyline	200	0.92
Amitriptyline	25	0.96
Citalopram	30	0.64
Fluoxetine	50	0.58
Norzimelidine (Z)	200	0.55
Serotonin	2000	0.49

[3]H-Imipramine binding was measured in rat cortical membranes at 2.5 nM ^{3}H-imipramine in the presence of various concentrations of the drugs. IC50's were calculated from semilog plots, and Hill coefficients according to Braestrup and Nielsen (1980). Each value was calculated from 8 to 10 points, which were repeated at least three times.

Table 2.   Stereospecific inhibition of ^{3}H-imipramine binding by
the optical isomers of femoxetine and paroxetine

	IC_{50} (nM)	n
Paroxetine α (−)	6.2 ± 0.25	7
Paroxetine α (+)	63.5 ± 6.8	4
Paroxetine β (−)	288.0 ± 17.0	4
Paroxetine β (+)	66.4 ± 18.9	4
Femoxetine α (−)	135.0 ± 35.0	4
Femoxetine α (+)	68.7 ± 7.6	4

[3]H-Imipramine binding was measured in rat cortical membranes at 2.5 nM ^{3}H-imipramine in the presence of various concentrations of the drugs. IC50's were calculated from semilog plots and are given as means ± S.E.M. n = number of determinations.

only neurotransmitter that inhibits the high-affinity binding of
[3]H-imipramine (table 1).   While the tricyclic antidepressants
inhibit the binding of ^{3}H-imipramine competitively, 5-HT and the
non-tricyclic inhibitors of 5-HT uptake inhibit the binding of
[3]H-imipramine in a complex manner (Sette *et al.*, 1983), with Hill
coefficients significantly below unity (table 1).   Studies using
the optical isomers of paroxetine and femoxetine (table 2) have
confirmed that ^{3}H-imipramine binding is stereoselective for the

isomers which are active at inhibiting the uptake of serotonin. Similar results were previously reported for the (Z) and (E) isomers of zimelidine and norzimelidine (Langer *et al.*, 1980c).

A significant correlation was reported between the potency of 17 antidepressant and non-antidepressant drugs to inhibit neuronal uptake of 5-HT and ³H-imipramine binding in the rat hypothalamus (Langer *et al.*, 1980b). No such correlation was obtained between the inhibition of norepinephrine (NE) uptake and ³H-imipramine binding (Langer *et al.*, 1980b). Compatible with these results is the fact that the distribution of ³H-imipramine binding sites in the brain is closely correlated with the density of serotonergic innervation, in the rat brain (Palkovits *et al.*, 1981) and in the human brain (Langer *et al.*, 1981a).

Following electrolytic lesions of the dorsal raphe in the rat and subsequent to degeneration of serotonergic nerve terminals in the hypothalamus, striatum and cerebral cortex the endogenous levels of 5-HT are reduced by approximately 50% (Sette *et al.*, 1981) while the levels of dopamine (DA) and NE remain essentially unchanged. In these three areas of the brain and following the electrolytic lesions of the dorsal raphe the B_{max} of ³H-imipramine binding was reduced in parallel with the decrease in 5-HT levels, indicating that these binding sites are located on serotonergic nerve terminals (Sette *et al.*, 1981). Similar results were obtained when the neurotoxin 5,7-dihydroxytryptamine was used to produce selective degeneration of serotonergic nerve terminals (Gross *et al.*, 1981; Brunello *et al.*, 1982).

Our results suggest that ³H-imipramine binds to sites associated with the 5-HT uptake system but different from the substrate recognition site for 5-HT as shown schematically in figure 1. It is possible that a site modulating the neuronal uptake of 5-HT is present on serotonergic nerve endings, and that this site (labeled by ³H-imipramine) is different from the substrate recognition site for the transmitter, 5-HT (figure 1). One can envisage the existence of a presynaptic site that modulates neuronal uptake in analogy with the presynaptic autoreceptors which modulate the release of their neurotransmitter (Langer, 1980). While the release-modulating presynaptic autoreceptors are acted upon by the neurotransmitter itself, the sites modulating 5-HT uptake may be acted upon by a co-transmitter or by an, as yet, unknown endogenous substance probably acting like imipramine (figure 1) and present at the synapse or in the circulation. The possible significance of this substance which inhibits the uptake of ³H-5-HT and the binding of ³H-imipramine remains to be established. It would certainly be of interest to isolate and determine the chemical properties of this endogenous factor (IDF = imipramine displacing factor) which inhibits ³H-imipramine binding and ³H-5-HT uptake. At present, it remains to be clarified whether the IDF is a known or a novel substance.

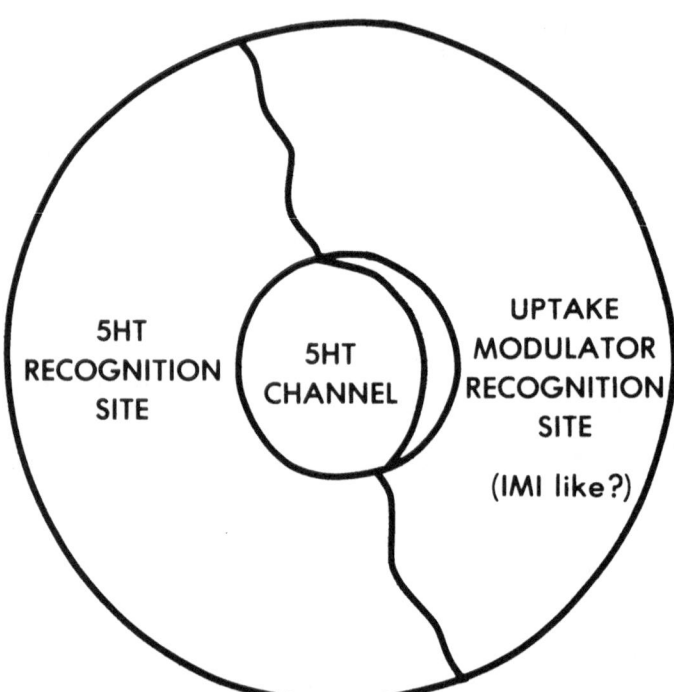

Figure 1. Schematic representation of the recognition sites at the
level of the transporter for serotonin. Two different
recognition sites appear to be present for the transporter of serotonin at the level of the nerve terminals.
One is the substrate recognition site for serotonin and
the second, where ^{3}H-imipramine binds with high affinity, may be a site which modulates the uptake of serotonin. The ^{3}H-imipramine binding site may be activated
by an endogenous ligand which could be different from
serotonin.

CHARACTERIZATION OF THE ^{3}H-DESIPRAMINE BINDING SITE

Following the discovery that ^{3}H-imipramine binds with high affinity to sites located on 5-HT nerve terminals and associated with
the uptake mechanism for 5-HT (for review, see Langer *et al.*,
1981c) the question arose as to whether antidepressants which are
selective for the inhibition of neuronal uptake of NE, like desipramine, could bind with high affinity to specific sites on
noradrenergic nerve endings, possibly associated with the neuronal
uptake of NE.

As shown in table 3, the high-affinity binding site for [3]H-
desipramine is present in the peripheral and the central nervous

Table 3. Localization and density of ^{3}H-imipramine and
^{3}H-desipramine binding sites in the rat

	^{3}H-Imipramine binding		^{3}H-Desipramine binding	
	K_d (nM)	B_{max} (fmol/mg prot.)	K_d (nM)	B_{max} (fmol/mg prot.)
Hypothalamus	5.2	279	2.6	156
Cerebral cortex	4.0	249	2.4	101
Striatum	2.8	164	3.4	29
Cerebellum	8.0	60	1.5	80
Heart	N.D.		1.5	63
Submaxillary gland	N.D.		2.3	308
Vas deferens	N.D.		2.6	1015
Platelets	2.3	1750	N.D.	

K_d and B_{max} values for ^{3}H-imipramine and ^{3}H-desipramine binding
were determined with the method described by Raisman et $al.$
(1980) and Langer et $al.$ (1981b). N.D. = non-detectable.

system (CNS) with a tissue distribution which follows the density
of noradrenergic innervation. Table 3 also shows the differences
between the distribution of ^{3}H-imipramine and ^{3}H-desipramine
binding sites: in peripheral tissues with a dense noradrenergic
innervation like the vas deferens, the heart and salivary glands
^{3}H-desipramine binding is present while ^{3}H-imipramine binding is
non-detectable. On the other hand, in platelets, which have an
active transport mechanism for 5-HT, but not for NE, there are
^{3}H-imipramine binding sites but no ^{3}H-desipramine binding sites
(table 3). In the CNS the lowest density of ^{3}H-desipramine binding
sites is in the striatum, which lacks noradrenergic innervation,
while for ^{3}H-imipramine binding the cerebellum is the region with
the lowest density of binding sites (table 3). The density of both
^{3}H-imipramine and ^{3}H-desipramine binding sites are high in the
hypothalamus and cerebral cortex. While chemical sympathectomy
with 6-hydroxydopamine leads to a reduction of ^{3}H-desipramine
binding sites in the CNS (Hrdina et $al.$, 1981) it does not affect
the density of ^{3}H-imipramine binding sites in the brain (Gross et
$al.$, 1981). In the periphery, surgical sympathetic denervation of
the rat heart or salivary glands leads to a pronounced decrease
in the B_{max} of ^{3}H-desipramine binding (Langer et $al.$, 1981b;
Raisman et $al.$, 1982b). These results support the view that the
^{3}H-desipramine binding sites are localized on noradrenergic nerve
endings.
    The profile of inhibition of ^{3}H-desipramine binding by drugs
is also different from that of ^{3}H-imipramine (compare tables 1 and
4). Compounds known to act at classical neurotransmitter receptors
are generally inactive at inhibiting ^{3}H-desipramine binding
(Raisman et $al.$, 1982b). Drugs which inhibit neuronal uptake of

Table 4. Inhibition of ^{3}H-desipramine binding in membranes of the rat vas deferens

	IC_{50} (nM)
Desipramine	5
Nisoxetine	8
Imipramine	117
D-Imafen	80
L-Imafen	400
Fluoxetine	4600
(-)-Norepinephrine	112000
Metaraminol	34500

[3]H-Desipramine binding was measured in membranes of the rat vas deferens at 2.5 nM ^{3}H-desipramine in the presence of various concentrations of the drugs. IC50's were calculated from semilog plots. Each value was obtained from 8 to 10 points which were repeated at least three times.

NE all inhibit ^{3}H-desipramine binding with high affinity (table 4). As shown for ^{3}H-imipramine binding, the inhibition of ^{3}H-desipramine binding is stereoselective when the two optical isomers of oxaprotiline are compared (Raisman *et al.*, 1982b). Similar results were obtained with the two optical isomers of imafen (table 4). It should be noted that D-imafen is the isomer active at inhibiting ^{3}H-NE uptake (Laduron *et al.*, 1982) and it was 5 times more potent than the inactive isomer, L-imafen, at inhibiting ^{3}H-desipramine binding (table 4).

These results are at variance with those of Laduron *et al.* (1982), who failed to find a stereospecific inhibition of ^{3}H-desipramine binding with the L- and D-enantiomers of imafen in the rat cerebral cortex. The discrepancy between our results (table 4) and those of Laduron *et al.* (1982) may reflect either tissue or methodological differences.

Comparison of the potency of a number of drugs on the inhibition of ^{3}H-desipramine binding and the inhibition of the uptake of NE gives a highly significant correlation (Raisman *et al.*, 1982b). While 5-HT is weakly active at the ^{3}H-imipramine binding site (table 1), the natural substrate for the NE uptake mechanism is inactive at inhibiting ^{3}H-desipramine binding (table 4). Similar results were obtained for other substrates of the NE uptake mechanism such as metaraminol (table 4), dopamine and tyramine (Raisman *et al.*, 1982b).

While denervation experiments clearly indicate that the ^{3}H-desipramine binding sites are localized on noradrenergic nerve terminals, the failure of pre-treatment with reserpine to change either the K_d or the B_{max} of ^{3}H-desipramine binding indicates that the binding site is not associated with the granular storage sites for norepinephrine (Raisman *et al.*, 1982b). Consequently, it appears that ³H-desipramine binds to a presynaptic site, different from the uptake-substrate recognition site for NE but associated with the neuronal uptake of NE. Since neuronal uptake is the main inactivating mechanism for released NE, the modulation of neuro-transmitter uptake may play an important role in the regulation of neurotransmission.

CONCLUSIONS

The high-affinity binding sites for ³H-imipramine and ³H-desipra-mine label different sites with pharmacological profiles and tissue distribution corresponding to an association with the neuronal uptake mechanisms for 5-HT and NE respectively. Both binding sites have most of the characteristics of the recognition site of a pharmacological receptor or a site of drug action (Langer and Briley, 1981).

It appears that the ³H-imipramine binding site may represent a new biological marker in depression. Studies carried out in platelets from severely depressed untreated patients have revealed a significant decrease in B_{max} of ³H-imipramine, without changes in K_d (Langer et al., 1980d, 1981c, 1982; Briley et al., 1980; Raisman et al., 1981). These observations have recently been confirmed by other groups (Asarch et al., 1981; Paul et al., 1981). It is of interest that a recent study carried out in *post-mortem* brains of suicide victims revealed a significant decrease in B_{max} of ³H-imipramine binding in the frontal cortex, when compared with matched control brains (Stanley et al., 1982). These results would suggest that the changes in ³H-imipramine binding observed in the platelets of depressed patients may indeed reflect similar changes in the brain, as previously suggested (Langer et al., 1981c, 1982). In support of this view, it was recently reported that chronic treatment of cats with imipramine produces a down-regulation of ³H-imipramine binding in the brain as well as in platelets (Briley et al., 1982).

It is of interest to note that the decrease in B_{max} of ³H-imipramine binding observed in the platelets of severely depressed untreated patients co-exists with a decrease in V_{max} of uptake of ³H-5-HT (Tuomisto et al., 1979; Raisman et al., 1982a). The exist-ence in plasma of a substance which inhibits both ³H-5-HT uptake and ³H-imipramine binding, IDF, might be associated with the above-mentioned findings in depressed patients. Although this suggestion is highly speculative, it is possible that IDF may turn out to be an endogenous substance which plays a significant role in the biochemical changes linked to affective disorders.

The ³H-desipramine binding site is likely to become a useful tool for studies related to the neuronal uptake of NE. This binding site is, however, not present in platelets, red blood cells or lymphocytes, making its determination in human tissues less easily available.

Both for human and animal experimental studies in affective disorders, the ^{3}H-imipramine and ^{3}H-desipramine binding sites represent new biochemical tools in relation to the role of the neuronal uptake of 5-HT and NE. Finally, we cannot exclude the possibility that endogenous ligands may exist which act on these high-affinity binding sites to modulate the neuronal uptake of both monoamines.

Acknowledgements

We are grateful to Catherine Barrier for careful typing of the manuscript.

REFERENCES

Asarch, K.B., Shih, J.C. and Kulesar, A. (1981). Decreased ^{3}H-imipramine binding in depressed males and females. Commun. Psychopharmacol., 4, 425-32

Braestrup, C. and Nielsen, M. (1980). Multiple benzodiazepine receptors. Trends Neurosci., 3, 301-3

Briley, M.S., Langer, S.Z., Raisman, R., Sechter, D. and Zarifian, E. (1980). Tritiated imipramine binding sites are decreased in platelets of untreated depressed patients. Science, 209, 303-5

Briley, M.S., Raisman, R., Arbilla, S., Casadamont, M. and Langer, S.Z. (1982). Concomitant decrease in ^{3}H-imipramine binding in cat brain and platelets after chronic treatment with imipramine. Eur. J. Pharmacol., 81, 309-14

Briley, M.S., Raisman, R. and Langer S.Z. (1979). Human platelets possess high-affinity binding sites for ^{3}H-imipramine. Eur. J. Pharmacol., 58, 347-8

Brunello, N., Chuang, D. and Costa, E. (1982). Different synaptic locations of mianserin and imipramine binding sites. Science, 215, 1112-13

Gross, G., Göthert, M., Ender, H.-P. and Schümann, H.-J. (1981). ^{3}H-Imipramine binding sites in the rat brain: selective localization on serotoninergic neurons. Naunyn-Schmiedeberg's Arch. Pharmacol., 317, 310-14

Hrdina, P., Elson-Hartmann, K., Roberts, D. and Pappas, B. (1981). High affinity ^{3}H-desipramine binding in rat cerebral cortex decreases after selective lesion of noradrenergic neurons with 6-hydroxydopamine. Eur. J. Pharmacol., 73, 375-6

Laduron, P., Robbyns, M. and Schotte, A. (1982). [^{3}H]-Desipramine and [^{3}H]-imipramine binding are not associated with noradrenaline and serotonin uptake in the brain. Eur. J. Pharmacol., 78, 491-3

Langer, S.Z. (1980). Presynaptic regulation of the release of
    catecholamines. Pharmacol. Rev., 32, 337-62
Langer, S.Z. and Briley M.S. (1981). High-affinity ³H-imipramine
    binding : a new biological tool for studies in depression.
    Trends Neurosci., 4, 28-31
Langer, S.Z., Briley, M.S., Raisman, R., Henry, J.-F. and Morselli
    (1980a). Specific ³H-imipramine binding in human platelets:
    influence of age and sex. Naunyn-Schmiedeberg's Arch.
    Pharmacol., 313, 189-94
Langer, S.Z., Javoy-Agid, F., Raisman, R., Briley, M.S. and Agid,
    Y. (1981a). Distribution of specific high-affinity binding
    sites for imipramine in human brain. J. Neurochem., 37,
    267-71
Langer, S.Z., Moret, C., Raisman, R., Dubocovich, M.L. and Briley,
    M.S. (1980b). High affinity ³H-imipramine binding in rat
    hypothalamus is associated with the uptake of serotonin but
    not norepinephrine. Science, 210, 1133-5
Langer, S.Z., Raisman, R. and Briley, M.S. (1980c).   Stereo-
    selective inhibition of ³H-imipramine binding by antide-
    pressant drugs and their derivatives. Eur. J. Pharmacol.,
    64, 89-90
Langer, S.Z., Raisman, R. and Briley, M.S. (1981b). High affinity
    [³H]-DMI binding is associated with neuronal noradrenaline
    uptake in the periphery and the central nervous system. Eur.
    J. Pharmacol., 72, 423-4
Langer, S.Z., Raisman, R., Briley, M.S., Sechter, D. and Zarifian,
    E. (1980d). Platelets from depressed patients have a de-
    creased number of ³H-imipramine binding sites. Fed. Proc.,
    39, 1097
Langer, S.Z., Zarifian, E., Briley, M.S., Raisman, R. and Sechter,
    D. (1981c). High affinity binding of ³H-imipramine in brain
    and platelets and its relevance to the biochemistry of
    affective disorders. Life Sci., 29, 211-20
Langer, S.Z., Zarifian, E., Briley M.S., Raisman, R. and Sechter,
    D. (1982). High affinity ³H-imipramine binding : a new
    biological marker in depression. Pharmacopsychiatria, 15,
    4-10
Möhler, H. and Okada, T. (1977). Properties of ³H-diazepam
    binding to benzodiazepine receptors in the rat cerebral
    cortex. Life Sci., 20, 2101-10
Palkovits, M., Raisman, R., Briley, M.S. and Langer, S.Z. (1981).
    Regional distribution of ³H-imipramine binding in rat brain.
    Brain Res., 210, 493-8
Paul, S.M., Rehavi, M., Skolnick, P., Ballenger, J.C., and
    Goodwin, F.K. (1981). Depressed patients have decreased
    binding of ³H-imipramine to the platelet serotonin 'trans-
    porter'. Arch. Gen. Psychiatry, 38, 1315-20
Raisman, R., Briley, M.S., Bouchami, F., Sechter, D., Zarifian, E.

and Langer, S.Z. (1982a). ³H-Imipramine binding and serotonin uptake in platelets from untreated depressed patients
and control volunteers. Psychopharmacology, 77, 332-5

Raisman, R., Briley, M.S. and Langer S.Z. (1979a). High-affinity
³H-imipramine binding in rat cerebral cortex. Eur. J. Pharmacol., 54, 307-8

Raisman, R., Briley, M.S. and Langer, S.Z. (1979b). Specific
tricyclic antidepressant binding sites in rat brain. Nature,
281, 148-50

Raisman, R., Briley, M.S. and Langer, S.Z. (1980). Specific
tricyclic antidepressant binding sites in rat brain charac-
terised by high affinity ³H-imipramine binding. Eur. J.
Pharmacol., 61, 373-80

Raisman, R., Sechter, D., Briley, M.S., Zarifian, E. and Langer,
S.Z. (1981). High-affinity ³H-imipramine binding in platelets from untreated and treated depressed patients compared
to healthy volunteers. Psychopharmacology, 75, 368-71

Raisman, R., Sette, M., Pimoule, C., Briley, M.S. and Langer, S.Z.
(1982b). High-affinity [³H]-desipramine binding in the
peripheral and central nervous systems : a specific site
associated with the neuronal uptake of noradrenaline. Eur.
J. Pharmacol., 78, 345-51

Sette, M., Briley, M.S. and Langer, S.Z. (1983). Complex inhibition of ³H-imipramine binding by serotonin and non-tricyclic serotonin uptake blockers. J. Neurochem., in press

Sette, M., Raisman, R., Briley, M.S. and Langer, S.Z. (1981).
Localization of tricyclic antidepressant binding sites on
serotonin nerve terminals in rat hypothalamus. J. Neurochem., 37, 40-2

Squires, R.F. and Braestrup, C. (1977). Benzodiazepine receptors
in rat brain. Nature, 266, 732-4

Stanley, M., Virgilio, J. and Gershon, S. (1982). Tritiated
imipramine binding sites are decreased in the frontal cortex
of suicides. Science, 216, 1337-9

Tuomisto, J., Tukiainen, J. and Ahlfors, U.G. (1979). Decreased
uptake of 5-hydroxytryptamine in blood platelets from
patients with endogenous depression. Psychopharmacology, 65,
141-7

Characterization of high-affinity antidepressant binding to rat and human brain

Moshe Rehavi[1], Phil Skolnick[2] and Steven M. Paul[1]

INTRODUCTION

Studies examining the interaction of various radiolabeled psychotropic agents with neuronal membranes have played an important
role in elucidating the central sites of action of many of these
compounds. The benzodiazepines and opiate alkaloids, for example,
have been demonstrated to interact with a high degree of specificity at recognition sites on neuronal membranes following pharmacologically relevant doses. In contrast, antidepressants interact with many membrane sites with varying degrees of specificity
and affinity, including both pre- (Koe, 1976) and postsynaptic
(Snyder and Yamamura, 1977) re-uptake and/or receptor sites, and
perhaps other, as yet unidentified, binding or recognition sites
(Biegon and Samuel, 1979). Therefore, the *in vitro* conditions employed in studying the binding of radiolabeled antidepressants
should be clearly defined and optimized for selective and specific
'labeling' of a given membrane site. In this report, we will
review studies from our laboratories on the binding of [³H]-imi-
pramine and [³H]-desipramine to membrane preparations from rat and
human brain as well as platelets, emphasizing the conditions under
which these ligands will selectively label the serotonin and
norepinephrine transport sites, respectively. The clinical implications of these findings will also be discussed.

[³H]-IMIPRAMINE AND [³H]-DESIPRAMINE BINDING: METHODOLOGIC ISSUES

Langer and coworkers (Raisman *et al.*, 1979) demonstrated the
presence of high-affinity and saturable binding sites for [³H]-
imipramine to membrane preparations of rat brain. These authors

---
[1]Clinical Neuroscience Branch, NIMH, National Institutes of Health, Bethesda, MD
20205, USA
[2]Laboratory of Bioorganic Chemistry, NIADDK, National Institutes of Health,
Bethesda, MD 20205, USA.

speculated that this binding site might be a specific 'receptor' which mediates the antidepressant actions of tricyclic and other 'atypical' antidepressants (Langer *et al.*, 1980b). This con- clusion was based on the correlation between the potencies of a series of antidepressants in displacing [³H]-imipramine binding *in vitro* and their corresponding behavioral and/or clinical potencies in treating depression. In contrast, we observed a pharmaco- logical profile for [³H]-imipramine binding that differed from that initially reported by Langer *et al.* (1980a) which led us to conclude that the [³H]-imipramine binding site was associated with a serotonin uptake or transport site (Paul *et al.*, 1980). This hypothesis has been confirmed by more extensive studies in our laboratory (Paul *et al.*, 1981a) as well others (Langer *et al.*, 1980a) using a variety of different techniques. However, neither the exact structural nor functional relationship between the [³H]-imipramine binding site and the serotonin transport complex is completely understood.

In their initial report on [³H]-imipramine binding, Langer and coworkers employed a prefiltration-dilution method in which an aliquot of the incubation reaction was quickly diluted more than 100-fold in ice-cold buffer immediately prior to filtration through glass fiber filters (Raisman *et al.*, 1979). In attempting to circumvent this somewhat cumbersome prefiltration procedure, we observed that elimination of this predilution step resulted in a significant amount of [³H]-imipramine bound to filters in the absence of tissue (figure 1; cf. Paul *et al.*, 1981a). Further- more, a significant amount of the binding of [³H]-imipramine to filters was displaceable by an excess of non-radioactive anti- depressant, resulting in spurious 'specific' binding of [³H]- imipramine to filters. Further characterization of this 'filter binding' indicated that it was of low affinity, and the potencies of various tricyclic antidepressants in displacing this 'binding' were in the μM range. In contrast, rapid dilution of an aliquot of the incubation mixture resulted in almost totally eliminating the low-affinity 'binding' of [³H]-imipramine to glass fiber filters. 'Low-affinity' binding of [³H]-imipramine was also observed in denatured brain and peripheral tissues as well as in purified myelin and nuclear fractions of brain. Table 1 illus- trates a temperature-inactivation curve for [³H]-imipramine bind- ing to brain membranes. Specific binding was totally inhibited when membranes were pre-incubated at 56°C for 15 min prior to assay. However, higher pre-incubation temperatures resulted in an increase in 'specific' [³H]-imipramine binding to values approxi- mately fourfold higher than observed in unheated tissue. However, characterization of [³H]-imipramine binding in heat-treated mem- branes revealed that it was of low affinity and pharmacologically distinct from that observed in unheated membranes (table 1). Therefore, it appears that utilization of a prefiltration-dilution step is critical for the study of 'high-affinity' binding of tricyclic antidepressants to defined presynaptic sites.

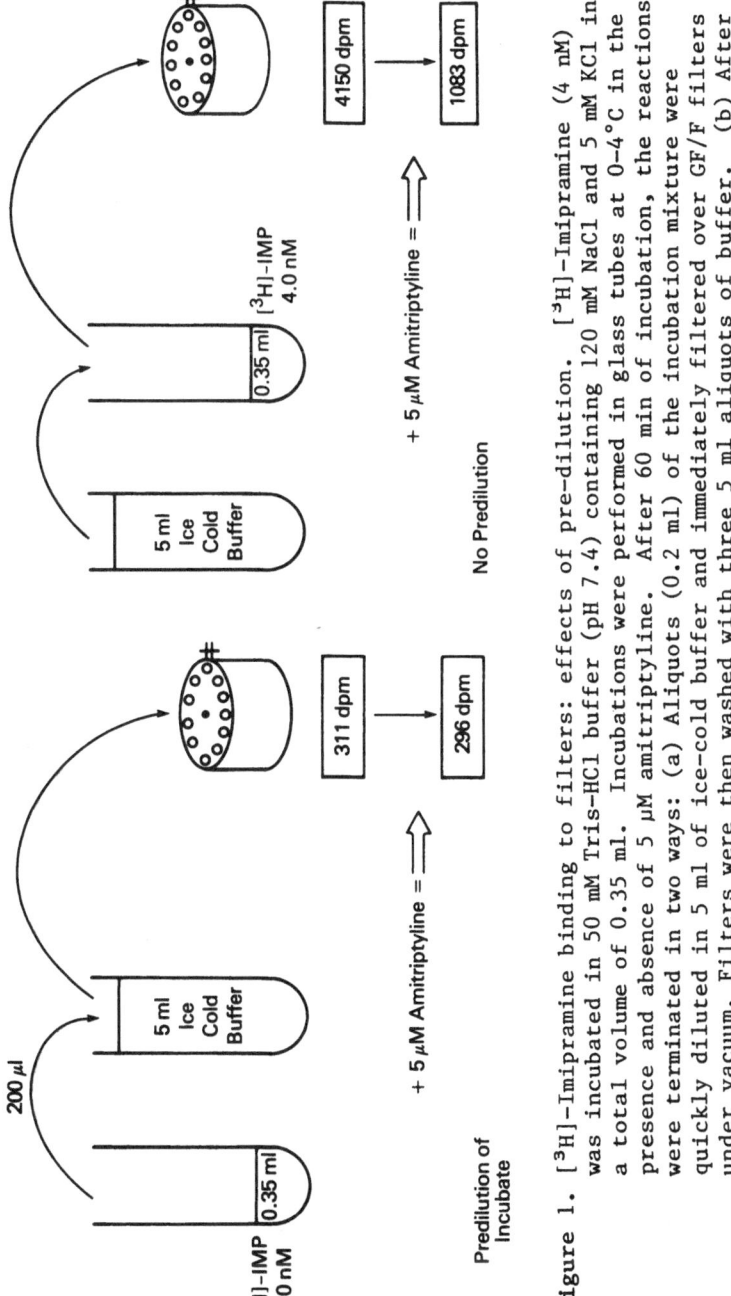

Figure 1. [³H]-Imipramine binding to filters: effects of pre-dilution. [³H]-Imipramine (4 nM) was incubated in 50 mM Tris-HCl buffer (pH 7.4) containing 120 mM NaCl and 5 mM KCl in a total volume of 0.35 ml. Incubations were performed in glass tubes at 0-4°C in the presence and absence of 5 µM amitriptyline. After 60 min of incubation, the reactions were terminated in two ways: (a) Aliquots (0.2 ml) of the incubation mixture were quickly diluted in 5 ml of ice-cold buffer and immediately filtered over GF/F filters under vacuum. Filters were then washed with three 5 ml aliquots of buffer. (b) After 60 min the entire incubation mixture was quickly diluted with 5 ml ice-cold buffer and filtered immediately. The tube was washed once more with 5 ml buffer and the filter washed twice with 5 ml aliquots of buffer.

Yet another important characteristic of the high-affinity binding of [³H]-imipramine to brain and platelet membranes is the absolute requirement for sodium ions. The use of sodium-free and sodium-enriched buffers permitted the differentiation of specific 'high-affinity' binding of either [³H]-imipramine or [³H]-desipramine to brain and/or platelet membranes and the binding to 'low affinity' sites in these same tissues (Rehavi *et al.*, 1983). Figure 2 illustrates the effects of sodium ions on the binding of [³H]-imipramine to the synaptosomal, myelin and nuclear fractions of rat brain. Only the binding to synaptosomal fractions was enhanced by sodium ions. The sodium ion dependency of both [³H]-imipramine and [³H]-desipramine binding is an important 'marker' for the high-affinity binding of tricyclic antidepressants to presynaptic neurotransmitter uptake sites.

RELATIONSHIP OF [³H]-IMIPRAMINE AND [³H]-DESIPRAMINE BINDING TO BIOGENIC AMINE UPTAKE PROCESSES

Our initial report describing [³H]-imipramine binding (Paul *et al.*, 1980) demonstrated the presence of high-affinity and saturable binding sites on human platelet membranes. Preliminary

Table 1. Effects of temperature on 'specific' [³H]-imipramine binding to rat brain membranes

Temperature (°C)	'Specific' binding (DPM)	$\dfrac{\text{Specific binding } (T)}{\text{Specific binding } (0°C)}$
0	470	1.0
56	0	0
65	404	0.9
76	940	2.0
90	1836	3.9
100	1843	3.9

Temperature of pre-incubation (°C)	IC_{50} for chlorimipramine (nM)
0	3
90	>100

Brain membranes were prepared as previously described (Raisman et al., 1979). Membranes were pre-incubated at various temperatures for 15 min, and then cooled on ice (0-4°C) prior to assay. A concentration of [³H]-imipramine of approximately 1.0 nM was used and the assay was carried out as described previously (Rehavi et al., 1980). Membranes pre-incubated at 90°C for 15 min were examined for the displacement of 'specific' [³H]-imipramine binding by chlorimipramine. The 'specific' binding of [³H]-imipramine in the denatured membranes was of low affinity and only weakly inhibited by chlorimipramine.

studies in our laboratory suggested that tertiary amine anti-depressants such as chlorimipramine, imipramine and amitryptyline were more potent in displacing [³H]-imipramine binding from rat and human brain membranes than the corresponding secondary amine derivatives (i.e. desmethylchlorimipramine, desipramine and nor-tryptyline) (Paul *et al.*, unpublished data; Rehavi *et al.*, 1980). This pharmacologic profile was identical to that reported for the inhibition of serotonin uptake into synaptosomes (Koe, 1976), and prompted an examination of the binding of [³H]-imipramine to platelets, since the latter has a well characterized uptake mech-anism for serotonin. More extensive structure-activity studies demonstrated an excellent correlation between the affinities of a

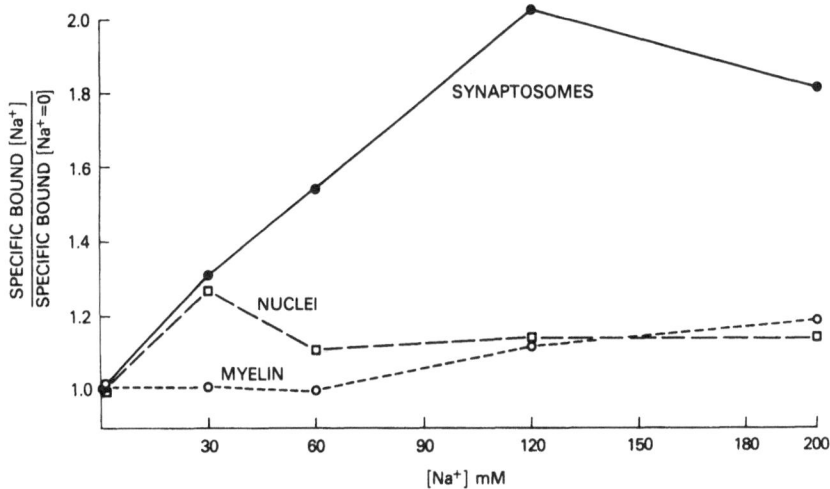

Figure 2. [Na$^+$] dependence of [³H]-imipramine binding to subcel-lular fractions of rat brain. Rat forebrain was hom-ogenized in 10 volumes of 0.32 M sucrose and the nuclei, synaptosomal and myelin fractions isolated according to the method of Whittaker and Barker (1972). The fractions were then disrupted with a Polytron (Brinkmann Instruments, setting 7, 20 s) in 50 mM Tris-HCl buffer (pH 7.4) containing 5 mM KCl and centrifuged at 30000g for 15 min. The disruption/centrifugation procedure was repeated three times. Binding of [³H]-imipramine (4 nM) to membranes was performed as pre-viously described (Raisman *et al.*, 1979). For each concentration of [Na$^+$], the binding in the presence or absence of 10 µM desipramine was measured. This is a representative experiment repeated twice with similar results.

large series of drugs for the imipramine binding site in platelets and their potencies as inhibitors of serotonin uptake (Paul *et al.*, 1980, 1981a). Moreover, if both the uptake and binding studies were performed under identical conditions (including a protein-free physiological medium), the concentrations of the various drugs as inhibitors of [^{3}H]-imipramine binding and serotonin uptake were almost identical (Paul *et al.*, 1981a). The correlation coefficients obtained between the potencies of various drugs as inhibitors of [^{3}H]-imipramine binding and serotonin uptake have now been reported by several laboratories to be between 0.89 and 0.98, similar to values reported for many drug receptor-effector interactions. The absence of a significant correlation between the potencies of various drugs at displacing [^{3}H]-imipramine binding and their potencies at other neurotransmitter uptake or receptor sites supports the selectivity of [^{3}H]-imipramine for the serotonin uptake site. The findings that there is a similar pharmacologic profile between the brain and platelet binding site (Rehavi *et al.*, 1980), and the lack of [^{3}H]-imipramine binding sites in peripheral tissue other than in platelets, further support this hypothesis.

More direct evidence for a structural relationship between the [^{3}H]-imipramine binding site and the presynaptic uptake mechanism for serotonin derives from two sources. Electrolytic or chemical lesions of the ascending serotonergic pathways from the raphe nuclei to various forebrain regions have been reported by several groups to destroy selectively high-affinity [^{3}H]-imipramine binding sites (cf. Paul *et al.*, 1981a; Langer *et al.*, 1980). We have also observed that the decrease in [^{3}H]-imipramine binding in individual animals is directly proportional to the decrease in serotonin uptake produced by these lesions (Paul *et al.*, 1981a). Since lesions to the midbrain raphe nuclei have been shown to be highly specific for denervating serotonin-containing presynaptic terminals, these results support the structural localization of [^{3}H]-imipramine binding sites to such terminals. Second, incubation of synaptosomal or platelet membranes with 2-nitroimipramine, a specific, slowly dissociating, essentially irreversible ligand of the [^{3}H]-imipramine binding site, results in a dose- and time-dependent decrease in both serotonin uptake and [^{3}H]-imipramine binding (Rehavi *et al.*, 1981a). Furthermore, 2-nitroimipramine was without effect on norepinephrine or dopamine uptake in synaptosomes, as well as a number of neurotransmitter-receptor systems (e.g. muscarinic, cholinergic, benzodiazepine), suggesting that the inhibition was specific for serotonin uptake.

Since the secondary amine tricyclic antidepressants such as desipramine and nortriptyline are more potent as inhibitors of norepinephrine uptake, we explored the possibility that high-affinity binding sites for [^{3}H]-desipramine were also present in rat brain. Incubation of brain membranes with low (i.e. nM) concentrations of [^{3}H]-desipramine followed by a prefiltration-dilution step as described for [³H]-imipramine binding revealed the presence of high-affinity and saturable binding sites for [³H]-desipramine (Rehavi *et al.*, 1981b, 1982a). In contrast to [³H]-imipramine binding, the secondary amine tricyclic antidepressants were more potent than their tertiary amine derivatives as inhibitors of [³H]-desipramine binding. Furthermore, there was no correlation between the potencies of a series of drugs in inhibiting [³H]-desipramine and [³H]-imipramine binding in cerebral cortical membranes, suggesting that each ligand labeled a different population of binding sites. Predictably, there was an excellent correlation between the potencies of a series of drugs in inhibiting [³H]-desipramine binding and the inhibition of norepinephrine uptake into synaptosomes. Like [³H]- imipramine binding, the binding of [³H]-desipramine displayed heat sensitivity, dependency on sodium ions, and a regional distribution throughout the CNS. High concentrations of [³H]-desipramine binding sites were found in the septum, cerebral cortex and hypothalamus (areas rich in norepinephrine-containing terminals), whereas lower densities of binding sites were observed in the medulla, cerebellum and corpus striatum. Direct evidence for a structural association between [³H]-desipramine binding sites and presynaptic norepinephrine uptake was revealed by studying the effects of intraventricular 6-hydroxydopamine on both the binding of [³H]-desipramine and norepinephrine uptake. A marked decrease in both norepinephrine uptake and [³H]-desipramine binding was observed in cerebral cortical membranes prepared from 6-hydroxydopamine lesioned animals compared to vehicle-treated animals, while no significant alterations were observed in either serotonin uptake or [³H]-imipramine binding (Rehavi *et al.*, 1982a). Similar results have now been reported by several groups (Lee and Snyder, 1981; Langer *et al.*, 1981) using a variety of techniques. Taken together with the characteristics of [³H]-imipramine binding outlined in the preceding section, these studies strongly support the hypothesis that radiolabeled imipramine and desipramine can be used to label (and perhaps quantitate) the uptake or transport sites for serotonin and norepinephrine, respectively.

DISCUSSION

High-affinity, sodium-dependent binding sites for [³H]-imipramine and [³H]-desipramine appear to be recognition sites which mediate the inhibition of serotonin and norepinephrine uptake elicited by tricyclic antidepressants and perhaps other chemically unrelated agents. The pharmacological significance of inhibiting biogenic amine uptake is unclear, particularly as it relates to antidepressant activity. Therefore, it is premature to refer to these binding sites as receptors for antidepressants. However, since these sites are functionally, and perhaps structurally, associated with uptake sites for biogenic amines, the use of radiolabeled antidepressants for further characterization of these uptake mechanisms seems possible. Recent studies in our laboratory on the solubilization and purification of the $[^3H]$-imipramine binding site from platelet membranes suggest that this site is part of a larger, supramolecular transport complex (Rehavi *et al.*, 1982b). It should not be surprising, therefore, if a number of drugs (e.g. digitalis glycosides) will be found to inhibit biogenic amine uptake by affecting other sites on this transport complex (e.g. a Na^+-K^+ ATPase) rather than interacting directly with $[^3H]$-imipramine binding sites.

Although there is both direct and indirect evidence that $[^3H]$-imipramine and $[^3H]$-desipramine binding sites are structurally associated with serotonin- and norepinephrine-containing presynaptic terminals, not all investigators concur with these findings. Laduron *et al.* (1982) have recently reported that $[^3H]$-imipramine and $[^3H]$-desipramine binding sites are not associated with biogenic amine uptake because of the differential subcellular distribution of the binding and uptake mechanisms. In their report 'specific' $[^3H]$-imipramine and $[^3H]$-desipramine binding was associated with the nuclear fraction of rat brain while serotonin and norepinephrine uptake were associated with the mitochondrial fraction (which presumably contained synaptosomes). These investigators, however, failed to characterize fully the binding of radiolabeled antidepressants in the individual subcellular fractions. In similar experiments performed in our laboratory (Rehavi *et al.*, 1983) we have characterized the binding of $[^3H]$-imipramine and $[^3H]$-desipramine (as well as the uptake of serotonin and norepinephrine) in the various subcellular fractions. In contrast to the results of Laduron *et al.* (1982), we observed that high-affinity, sodium-ion-dependent binding of radiolabeled imipramine and desipramine was predominantly localized in the synaptosomal fraction, with virtually no 'specific' binding in the nuclear fraction. In our experiments, a very significant quantity of 'displaceable' binding was observed in the myelin, but this binding was of very low affinity and *not* affected by sodium ions. Such 'low affinity' binding sites for tricyclic antidepressants have been reported for a variety of tissue proteins (as well as glass fiber filters and denatured tissue). Thus, the methodologic caveats described in this chapter must be considered when interpreting the results of binding studies which employ only a large excess of unlabeled drug to define 'specific' binding.

Despite the lack of a behavioral correlation between the clinical efficacy of various tricyclic antidepressants and their potencies in displacing radiolabeled imipramine and desipramine binding *in vitro*, several lines of evidence suggest that these 'binding sites' may still prove to be clinically relevant. We have emphasized the biochemical and pharmacological similarities between the high-affinity binding sites for [³H]-imipramine in human brain and platelet membranes (cf. Rehavi *et al*., 1980) and subsequently clinical studies have demonstrated that platelets from severely depressed patients possess fewer [³H]-imipramine binding sites than platelets from age- and sex-matched controls Briley *et al*., 1980; Paul *et al*., 1981). Furthermore, we have recently examined the binding of both [³H]-imipramine and [³H]-desipramine in suicide victims and compared them to values obtained from specimens of matched controls who succumbed to accidents or trauma (Paul *et al*., in preparation). A significant reduction in the number of [³H]-imipramine, but not [³H]-desipramine, binding sites was observed in the suicide brain specimens, and the magnitude of this reduction (∿30-40%) was similar to that observed in platelets from severely depressed patients. It is tempting to speculate that a decrease in the density of [³H]-imipramine binding sites (and perhaps an alteration in presynaptic serotonin uptake) in brain may be involved in the pathogenesis or pathophysiology of severe affective disorders characterized by suicidal behavior.

REFERENCES

Biegon, A. and Samuel, D. (1979). Binding of labeled anti-depressants to rat brain tissue. Biochem. Pharmacol., 28, 3361-6

Briley, M.S., Langer, S.Z., Raisman, R., Sechter, D. and Zarifian, E. (1980). Tritiated imipramine binding sites are decreased in platelets of untreated depressed patients. Science, 209, 303-5

Koe, B.K. (1976). Molecular geometry of inhibitors of the uptake of catecholamines and serotonin in synaptosomal preparations of rat cortex. J. Pharmacol. Exp. Ther., 199, 649-61

Laduron, P.M., Robbyns, M. and Schotte, A. (1982). [³H]Desipramine and [³H]imipramine binding are not associated with noradrenaline and serotonin uptake in brain. Eur. J. Pharmacol., 78, 491-3

Langer, S.Z., Moret, C., Raisman, R., Dubocovich, M.L. and Briley, M. (1980a). High affinity [³H]imipramine binding in rat hypothalamus: association with uptake of serotonin but not of norepinephrine. Science, 210, 1133-5

Langer, S.Z., Raisman, R. and Briley, M. (1980b). Stereoselective inhibition of [³H] imipramine binding by antidepressant drugs and their derivatives. Eur. J. Pharmacol., 64, 89-90

Langer, S.Z., Raisman, R. and Briley, M. (1981). High affinity [³H]DMI binding is associated with neuronal noradrenaline uptake in the periphery and central nervous system. Eur. J. Pharmacol., 72, 423-4

Lee, C.H. and Snyder, S.H. (1981). Norepinephrine neuronal uptake sites in rat brain membranes labeled with [^{3}H]desipramine. Proc. Natl. Acad. Sci., 78, 4250-6

Paul, S.M., Rehavi, M., Rice, K.C., Ittah, Y. and Skolnick, P. (1981a). Does high affinity [^{3}H]imipramine binding label serotonin reuptake sites in brain and platelet? Life Sci., 28, 2753-60

Paul, S.M., Rehavi, M., Skolnick, P., Ballenger, J.C. and Goodwin, F.K. (1981b). Depressed patients have decreased binding of tritiated imipramine to platelet serotonin 'transporter'. Arch. Gen. Psychiatry, 38, 1315-17

Paul, S.M., Rehavi, M., Skolnick, P. and Goodwin, F.K. (1980). Demonstration of specific high affinity binding sites for [^{3}H]imipramine on human platelets. Life Sci., 26, 953-9

Raisman, R., Briley, M. and Langer, S.Z. (1979). Specific tricyclic antidepressant binding sites in rat brain. Nature, 281, 148-50

Rehavi, M., Ittah, Y., Rice, K.C., Skolnick, P., Goodwin, F.K. and Paul, S.M. (1981a). 2-Nitroimipramine: a selective irreversible inhibitor of [^{3}H]serotonin uptake and [^{3}H]imipramine binding in platelets. Biochem. Biophys. Res. Comm., 99, 954-9

Rehavi, M., Paul, S.M., Skolnick, P. and Goodwin, F.K. (1980). Demonstration of specific high affinity binding sites for [^{3}H]imipramine in human brain. Life Sci., 26, 2273-9

Rehavi, M., Skolnick, P., Brownstein, M.J. and Paul, S.M. (1982a). High affinity binding of [^{3}H] desipramine to rat brain: a presynaptic marker for noradrenergic uptake sites. J. Neurochem., 38, 889-95

Rehavi, M., Skolnick, P., Hulihan, B. and Paul, S.M. (1981b). High affinity binding of [^{3}H]desipramine to rat cerebral cortex: relationship to tricyclic antidepressant-induced inhibition of norepinephrine uptake. Eur. J. Pharmacol., 70, 597-9

Rehavi, M., Skolnick, P. and Paul, S.M. (1982b). Solubilization and partial purification of the high affinity [^{3}H] imipramine binding site from human platelets. FEBS Lett., 150(2), 514-18

Rehavi, M., Skolnick, P. and Paul, S.M. (1983). Subcellular distribution of high affinity [^{3}H] imipramine binding and [^{3}H] serotonin uptake in rat brain. Eur. J. Pharmacol., in press

Snyder, S.H. and Yamamura, H.I. (1977). Antidepressants and the muscarinic acetylcholine receptor. Arch. Gen. Psychiatry, 34, 236-9

Whittaker, V. and Barker, L. (1972). The subcellular fractionation of brain tissue with special reference to the preparation of synaptosomes and their component organelles. In Methods of Neurochemistry, vol. 2 (ed. R. Fried), Marcel Dekker, New York, pp. 1-52

Section Six

Clinical Psychopharmacology of Peptides, Amino Acids and Related Compounds

The human psychopharmacology of peptides related to ACTH and $\propto$-MSH

R.M.Pigache[1]

INTRODUCTION

There is considerable interest in the diverse actions of ACTH (adrenocorticotrophin) -like peptides on the central nervous system (CNS), and in their application to man. Much of the experimental literature has been reviewed quite recently, e.g. in relation to structure–activity relationships (Van Nispen and Greven, 1982), animal pharmacology (Beckwith and Sandman, 1978; Bohus and De Kloet, 1979; Rigter and Crabbe, 1979; De Kloet and De Wied, 1980; Rigter, 1982), biochemical mechanisms (Wiegant *et al.*, 1981) and basic and human studies (Pigache and Rigter, 1981; Pigache, 1982a, b; Rigter *et al.*, 1982)

    The review that follows is meant to update those cited above, and in so doing will try to avoid repetition. The peptides to be dealt with comprise $ACTH_{1-39}$, $ACTH_{1-24}$, $ACTH_{11-24}$ and $ACTH_{1-10}$ and also fragments with sequences shared by ACTH and α-MSH: $ACTH_{4-10}$ and $ACTH_{4-7}$, and the orally active synthetic peptide $[Met(O_2)^4, D\text{-}Lys^8, Phe^9] ACTH_{4-9}$ (Org 2766). In rat, the sequence $ACTH_{4-7}$ is the shortest fragment possessing the full behavioral potency of $ACTH_{1-39}$ (or equally $ACTH_{1-24}$) in the pole–jump test (Greven and De Wied, 1973). The most extensively studied of these peptides in man, however, is Org 2766. Evidence that Org 2766 crosses the blood–brain barrier remains circumstantial (Pigache, 1982b), apart from data reported for rat (Verhoef and Witter, 1976; Verhoef *et al.*, 1977) which need replication with new high–performance liquid chromatography methods. Nonetheless, effects on the human electroencephalogram (EEG) following oral Org 2766 (Rockstroh *et al.*, 1981, 1982; Fehm–Wolfsdorf *et al.*, 1981), strongly support the assumption of central activity.

    The origin of interest in the central effects of ACTH lies more than 30 years ago and is documented by the reviews of Lidz *et*

---

[1]Organon Scientific Development Group, Oss, The Netherlands.

al. (1952) and Quarton *et al.* (1955) who referred to 'euphor-igenic' effects of the hormone, but could not dissociate these from the cortisol response or from the favorable therapeutic outcomes. During the next decade, however, De Wied (1969) was able to study the effects in rats of various ACTH fragments, e.g. $ACTH_{4-10}$, which had reduced corticotrophic activity. This led to the first study in man (Endroczi *et al.*, 1970) with such frag-ments, which are dealt with next.

EFFECTS OF $ACTH_{1-24}$, $ACTH_{11-24}$ AND $ACTH_{1-10}$

Endroczi *et al.* (1970) gave acute doses (0.5 mg) intravenously (i.v.) of $ACTH_{1-24}$ (a peptide which possesses full corticotrophic activity) to volunteers practiced in making a handgrip response to a stimulus of 12 cycles per second (c.p.s.) (tone or flicker) and no response to a 4 c.p.s. stimulus. The stimuli were presented alternately, i.e. a 'go, no-go' alternation task. After 50 to 100 practice trials, the spontaneous EEG following either type of stimulus became synchronized, i.e. exhibited alpha activity. The synchronization represented a habituation of earlier orienting responses. The action of $ACTH_{1-24}$ (compared with placebo) was to desynchronize the EEG following the 12 c.p.s. stimulation, i.e. dishabituation. Curiously, however, this desynchronization was not apparent during the first 1–2 h after peptide administration, but only 24 h later. The effects of $ACTH_{1-10}$ (1 and 2 mg i.v.) were the same as $ACTH_{1-24}$, whereas $ACTH_{11-24}$ (1 and 2 mg i.v.) had no effect at all. Thus the dishabituating property of $ACTH_{1-24}$, appeared to reside in its 1–10 amino acid sequence. However, the study was only single-blind and no statistical analysis was re-ported. The findings require replication.

Miller *et al.* (1974) studied the effects of a single dose of $ACTH_{1-24}$ (0.5 mg i.v.) on spontaneous EEG, contingent negative variation, and other psychophysiological variables, in a double-blind comparison with placebo. Measurements were made 1 h after treatment during the acquisition of a 'go, no-go' task (fixed fore-period reaction-time paradigm). There were no EEG effects and none on the Benton Visual Retention Test or the Rod and Frame Test. This discrepancy with the Endroczi *et al.* (1970) result might be explained by procedural differences. A discrepancy with the results of Rockstroh *et al.* (1981) for Org 2766 (see later) should also be noted.

Any interpretation of the foregoing results is complicated by the possibility that the peptides would have stimulated cortisol release. Many behavioral effects of corticosterone in rat, e.g. facilitation of active-avoidance extinction and impairment of passive-avoidance, are contrary to those of ACTH fragments lacking corticotrophic activity (see review by Bohus and De Wied, 1980). Equivalent opposing effects of cortisol and certain ACTH-like fragments might occur also in man.

EFFECTS OF ACTH$_{4-7}$

In contrast to the absence of effects at 1 h after ACTH$_{1-24}$ treatment described by Endroczi *et al.* (1970), a recent Russian report (Medvedev *et al.*, 1980) notes marked behavioral effects with the short ACTH$_{4-7}$ core fragment (devoid of adrenocorticotrophic activity) as soon as 45 min after intranasal (i.n.) administration (40-60 mg). [N.B. When given intranasally, much larger doses of peptide may be needed to elicit effects equivalent to an injected dose, as with synthetic $α^{1-18}$-corticotropin (Geyer and Templ, 1976).] Medvedev *et al.* report five statistically significant effects of ACTH$_{4-7}$, in a double-blind comparison with placebo:

   (i)   decreased omission and commission errors, increased rate
         of information processing and decreased time to complete a
         proof-reading task;
  (ii)   increased immediate (but not delayed) recall of nonsense
         syllables;
 (iii)   increased digit span;
  (iv)   improved running addition of sequential digit pairings;
   (v)   improved immediate recall of geometric shapes.

These results for ACTH$_{4-7}$ contrast with the largely non-significant findings of numerous studies using similar cognitive tests (for reviews see Pigache and Rigter, 1981; Pigache 1982a, b) with ACTH$_{4-10}$ and Org 2766. They are reminiscent, however, of some of the earlier claims made for the peptides and certainly need replication. It is possible, of course, that the ACTH$_{4-7}$ results may be attributable to bias (not immediately apparent in the condensed and translated report) or to a property peculiar to the ACTH$_{4-7}$ sequence. The next section deals with examples of how ACTH peptides differ.

DIFFERENCES BETWEEN ACTH-LIKE PEPTIDES

Differing structure-activity relationships between various ACTH-like peptides were first reported by Greven and De Wied (1973) and have been the subject of a recent review (Van Nispen and Greven, 1982). The present comments are restricted to the peptides under consideration.

Although ACTH$_{4-7}$ and ACTH$_{4-10}$ are similar (and similar to ACTH$_{1-24}$) in terms of delaying pole-jump extinction and facilitating passive-avoidance in rats (Greven and De Wied, 1973), they do differ in terms of certain opiate-like properties (table 1). While these differences might not be directly relevant to their possibly different activities in man, they allow the possibility that other differences might exist. Similarly, there are qualitative differences (table 2) between ACTH$_{4-10}$ (which resembles ACTH$_{1-24}$) and Org 2766.

Table 1. Differences between $ACTH_{4-7}$ and $ACTH_{4-10}$

Test	Effects		References
	$ACTH_{4-7}$	$ACTH_{4-10}$	
Inhibition of mouse vas deferens contraction	inactive	active	Plomp and Van Ree (1978)
Displacement of ^{125}I-morphine from morphine antiserum	inactive	active	Plomp and Van Ree (1978)
Affinity for opiate binding sites	virtually inactive	active (weak)	Terenius *et al.* (1975)
Induction of excessive grooming	active	virtually inactive	Wiegant *et al.* (1977)

Table 2. Differences between $ACTH_{4-10}$ and Org 2766

Test	Effects		References
	$ACTH_{4-10}$	Org 2766	
Social interaction (familiar environment)	decreased*	–	File and Vellucci (1978)
	decreased*	–	File (1979)
	–	increased*†	File (1981)
	decreased	increased §	Clarke and File (1981)
Social interaction (unfamiliar environment)	decreased*	increased*	Niesink and Van Ree (1982)
Affinity for opiate binding sites	active (weak)	inactive	Pigache (1982b)

*Intraperitoneal
†Dose-related effect
 Intraseptal route
§Also increased in a comparison with α-MSH (File, 1981).

Finally, it appears that in some situations Org 2766 has both agonist and antagonist activities in rats, depending on the dose given. In active-avoidance tests the dose-response relationship for Org 2766 is linear (Greven and De Wied, 1980), but in other tests (listed in table 3) the relationship is more like an inverted 'U'. To explain the downturn of effects with 'high' doses of the peptide ('high' and 'low' are relative terms, with absolute doses varying according to the task), Fekete and De Wied (1982a) have suggested that the major metabolite of Org 2766, i.e. the COOH-terminal tripeptide (Phe-D-Lys-Phe, otherwise PDLP), could be responsible. When PDLP was given intracerebroventricularly (i.c.v.) it acted just like 'high'-dose Org 2766 (table 3), leading the authors to suggest that 'high' doses of Org 2766 possibly generate enough PDLP to reverse the effects produced by lower doses of the parent peptide. We do not know if such reversals of response would occur in man, nor which doses should be considered 'high'.

The predictive value for man of experimental models in rat remains uncertain. However, differing properties of short peptides

Table 3.   Effects of 'low-' and 'high'-dose Org 2766 and of 'PDLP' in rats

Test	Effects Org 2766		PDLP (COOH-terminal tripeptide Org 2766)	References
	'Low' dose	'High' dose		
Active avoidance (extinction)	delayed	-	delayed*	Van Nispen and Greven (1982)
	-	delayed †	-	Greven and De Wied (1980)
Passive avoidance	facilitation ‡ (not blocked by naltrexone)	inhibition (blocked by naltrexone)	inhibition (blocked by naltrexone)	Fekete and De Wied (1982a)
Intracranial§ self-stimulation	facilitation	inhibition	unknown	Fekete et al. (1982)
Exploratory** behavior	increased	decreased	unknown	File (1981)

*Potency one-tenth $ACTH_{4-10}$ (on weight basis)
†Dose-related effects
‡Potency x 1000 $ACTH_{4-10}$ (Fekete and De Wied, 1982b)
§Medial septal area
**Time spent head-dipping

related to ACTH and α-MSH justify caution in generalizing from one peptide to another. From another standpoint, behavioral differences between Org 2766 and its metabolites (mainly PDLP) must also complicate any question of whether a given clinical effect would represent 'substitution therapy' or 'direct pharmacological action' by the peptide.

VIGILANCE AND EEG EFFECTS OF ACTH$_{4-10}$ AND ORG 2766

Both ACTH$_{4-10}$ and Org 2766 improve vigilance performance in man. This has been a constant effect following acute dosing with the peptides (for review see Pigache, 1982b). Thus a significant decrease in long reaction times during a 30 min serial reaction-time task was reported following subcutaneous (s.c.) ACTH$_{4-10}$ (30 mg) (Gaillard and Sanders, 1975), following each of three dose levels (5, 10 and 20 mg) of Org 2766 given per os (p.o.) (Gaillard and Varey, 1979), and almost significantly so ($p < 0.06$) following Org 2766 (10 mg p.o.) in hypophysectomized patients (Gaillard and Zwaan, 1978). A subsequent study by O'Hanlon (cited in Pigache, 1982b) showed that Org 2766 (40 mg p.o.) and dexamphetamine (10 mg p.o.) equally and significantly prevented a time-related decrement in performance during a long (105 min) vigilance task. These results were obtained in healthy young subjects tested 90 min after dosing. In a later study (cited in Pigache, 1982b), using somewhat different procedures, O'Hanlon failed to find a comparable effect of Org 2766 (40 mg p.o.) in healthy elderly subjects. Results in vigilance studies are highly sensitive to variations in the task parameters. In an attempt to reconcile the above discrepant findings, O'Hanlon *et al.* (1982) recently adopted a different procedure to permit analysis according to 'signal detection theory'. Twenty college students performed a TV monitoring task that involved a difficult discrimination. In successive trials (spaced every 2.5 s) they were shown either video noise or the noise plus a 'hidden' signal and were asked each time to indicate, at one of four levels of confidence, whether or not a signal had occurred. In comparison with the earlier task the new paradigm depended less on memory and more on the processes of perception, decision-making and response selection. It was also shorter (60 min) and was given just 15 min after Org 2766 (40 mg p.o.), or placebo, administration. A preliminary analysis indicates that the subjects performed better after Org 2766. Gross performance measures (e.g. percent signals detected) indicated a trend ($p < 0.1$, two-tail).

Interesting and sometimes stronger differences were seen with finer measures (e.g. a significant, $p < 0.02$, reduction under Org 2766, compared with placebo, of the signal distribution, but no change of the noise distribution). For these comparisons the necessary data were not forthcoming from every subject. The results suggest that the peptide facilitated perceptual discrimination between the stimuli.

The above conclusion would seem to agree with an earlier statement of Rockstroh *et al.* (1981) that Org 2766 (40 mg p.o.) 'facilitates the fixation of a single and simple set of stimuli'. This referred to EEG evoked responses showing shorter N 100 latencies ($p < 0.05$), a tendency toward greater N 100 amplitudes and increased P 300 amplitudes ($p < 0.10$) in a fixed fore-period (6 s) reaction-time task, where Org 2766 (40 mg p.o.) was compared with placebo. These results have been replicated in a second, similar, study (Rockstroh *et al.*, 1982), performed and analyzed double-blind. Fehm-Wolfsdorf *et al.* (1981), in an almost identical experiment, except that subjects had to respond to each of two different stimuli presented in separate trials, found that Org 2766 (40 mg p.o.) impaired the switching of attention, as measured by the same EEG variables.

The foregoing effects of Org 2766 on various tests and measures related to attention are summarized in table 4. They require, however, some interpretation. The N 100 changes in the EEG evoked response are said to relate to 'detection/selection of simple cue characteristics' (Hillyard *et al.*, 1978; Parasuraman and Beatty, 1980) and the P 300 to better 'stimulus evaluation/ categorization in relation to a neural template' (Hillyard *et al.*, 1978; Parasuraman and Beatty, 1980; McCarthy and Donchin, 1981). Both processes appeared to be improved by Org 2766 treatment.

The decrements in performance, as seen under placebo, in the vigilance tasks may be attributable to sensory adaptation, habituation or a loss of incentive-motivation. It is not easy to distinguish between these possibilities, empirically. Habituation (or 'reactive inhibition') occurs to both the non-specific (irrelevant) aspects of a task, with a resultant progressive loss of arousal, and to the 'critical' stimuli whenever these are not perceived as being different from the background (i.e. as salient). The ensuing decrease in arousal during a monotonous task decreases further any likelihood of detecting critical stimuli. Since acute doses of Org 2766 do not increase general arousal (Pigache, 1982b), or alter any sleep parameter (Nicholson and Stone, 1980), it would seem that Org 2766 attenuates a vigilance decrement by attenuating sensory adaptation, or impairing habituation (i.e. interference with the encoding of irrelevant stimulus characteristics), or increasing incentive-motivation. The first proposition is possible, the second seems fairly unlikely for a peptide which, so far, has failed to modify human memory. However, increased incentive-motivation, i.e. an increase in the subjective 'value' of a stimulus, has already been proposed as a mechanism underlying ACTH and Org 2766 effects (De Kloet and De Wied, 1980; Bohus, 1981; Pigache and Rigter, 1981). Increased incentive-motivation could also account for the Org 2766 improvement of stimulus detection and of evaluation/categorization. These pro-

Table 4. Profile of Org 2766 effects in man

Subjects (*n*)	Daily dose (mg)	Treatment duration (days)	Effects	References
Acute dosing				
Healthy students (26)	5,10,20	1	↓ habituation*	Gaillard and Varey (1979)
(18)	40	1	↓ habituation	O'Hanlon (cited in Pigache,(1982b)
(20)	40	1	↑ discrimination	O'Hanlon et al. (1982)
(30)	40	1	↑ stimulus detection/ selection† ↑ evaluation/ categorization†	Rockstroh et al. (1981)
(32)	40	1	↓ switching of attention	Fehm-Wolfsdorf et al. (1981)
Subchronic dosing 'Symptomatic'				
elderly (50)	10,20	14	↓ anxiety ↓ depression ↑ competence ↑ attention ↑ energy	Ferris and Reisberg (1981)
⟩43⟨	10-20	7	↓ anxiety	Willner (1981)
Mild-moderate dementia (mixed)(35)	40	28	↓ withdrawal/apathy ↑ sociability	Braverman et al. (1981)

↑ increase, ↓ decrease

* Or ↑ motivation

† Replicated in subsequent study (Rockstroh et al., 1982)

cesses make for the salience of relevant stimuli and belong to selective attention. The impairment which followed Org 2766, i.e. in switching attention between two relevant stimuli (Fehm-Wolfsdorf *et al.*, 1981), would not ordinarily be considered a counterpart to enhanced selective attention, but the stimuli concerned had different motivational loadings (one was always followed by an aversively loud tone). Perhaps the peptide caused attention to 'lock on' more firmly to both stimuli, though possibly unequally, and an impairment in switching attention was the consequence.

A number of theoretical and possibly semantic issues have been raised in this section. It is evident that further work must be done with Org 2766 to clarify the results. Moreover, this work should develop from a model of attention that, potentially, would be able to integrate all the data. It may also be hoped that beneficial effects following acute Org 2766 administration will persist with chronic treatment.

EFFECTS OF ORG 2766 IN THE ELDERLY

Effects of subchronic treatment with Org 2766 in elderly 'symptomatic' volunteers and in mildly demented patients are summarized in table 4. These findings, and others, have been extensively reviewed quite recently (Pigache and Rigter, 1981; Pigache 1982a, b). In addition, a study in 39 patients with moderate to severe primary degenerative dementia has just been completed by Martin *et al*. (1982). These researchers found no convincing effects of Org 2766 (40 mg p.o. for 1 month), but they suggested, however, that the patients might have been at the end-stage of the disease, with little capacity for improvement.

As Raskin (1981) remarked recently, the long-standing difficulty of translating geriatric rating scale scores into clinically meaningful measures of change persists. In the Braverman *et al*. (1981) study of Org 2766, changes with the Plutchik Geriatric Rating Scale in mildly demented patients (of mixed etiology) amounted to about 15% (more of course for the patients who responded) and was considered to be clinically significant. It may be hoped that the effects of Org 2766 will be especially useful in demented outpatients, perhaps enabling them to maintain their lives longer in the community.

A qualitative appraisal of the effects produced, so far, in aged and demented subjects, with subchronic Org 2766 treatment indicates that the peptide improved rated: competence, attention, energy, mood and sociability. These effects may be compared to the 'behavioral qualities' identified and grouped under two general classes of behavior (table 5) by Wittenborn (1981), representing 'loss of awareness' and 'distractibility'. Wittenborn (1981) adds, that, in some subjects, the two classes might be 'mutually dependent and parts of the same behavioural complex'. Before arriving at his classification Wittenborn (1981) analyzed the item content of 40 observer rating scales for geriatric subjects and grouped together semantically or behaviorally equivalent qualities, which appeared to change after treatment with various 'geriatric drugs' (cyclandelate, Hydergine®, meclofenoxate, naftidrofuryl, papaverine and piracetam). The behavioral qualities referred to in table 5 appeared to respond much more to these 'geriatric drugs' than to other psychotropic drugs, e.g. major or minor tranquilizers and antidepressants. However, the 'geriatric drugs' might have had some antidepressant actions which, by improving affective tone, could have increased alertness and awareness, too. Wittenborn (1981) proposes that 'some behavioural qual-

Table 5. Behavioral qualities common to geriatric rating
scales (Wittenborn, 1981)

'Loss of awareness' (items)	'Distractibility' (items)
disorientation	restlessness
loss of memory	emotional lability
loss of alertness	
incontinence	

ities may be more susceptible to amelioration in elderly people
than other qualities'. It would be interesting to know if there
might be intrinsic limits to how much such qualities could change,
but this might depend on the advent of drugs with sufficient
impact.

Single doses of Org 2766 given to healthy young subjects
produced effects (table 4) that have been ascribed to increased
motivation (Gaillard and Varey, 1979). For the sake of parsimony,
it was argued elsewhere (Pigache and Rigter, 1981; Pigache,
1982a,b) that increased motivation might underly the improved mood
seen after subchronic dosing in the elderly (table 4). However,
it is also possible that Org 2766 acted otherwise, on pharmacologically sensitive behaviors such as those identified by
Wittenborn (1981) (table 5).

ACUTE VERSUS CHRONIC ADMINISTRATION OF ORG 2766

Perhaps the acute dose effects of Org 2766 in young adults do not
connect with those of subchronic dosing in the elderly. An example
of acute and subchronic treatments having different effects was
seen in rats, where acute doses of Org 2766 had no effect on
glucose metabolism (Delanoy and Dunn, 1978) whereas subchronic
treatment (10 days) significantly increased glucose utilization in
limbic areas (McCulloch *et al.*, 1982). The same tests and treatment regimens will need to be applied at both ends of the human
lifespan in order to clarify whether the duration of dosing would
account for the different responses noted, or rather that the
peptide should be considered to have multiple actions (Rigter *et
al.*, 1982).

In the same vein, it is extremely interesting that very
prolonged administration (8.5 months) of Org 2766 to rats, from 16
months of age, reduced neuronal loss and astrocyte reactivity in
the hippocampus, which occurred in controls as a function of age
(Landfield *et al.*, 1981). A behavioral concomitant of this apparent protection against brain aging was seen in the better acqui-

sition of reversal learning by Org 2766 treated rats. Reversal learning is a paradigm used to evaluate selective attention in rats (e.g. Mackintosh, 1969). It is impaired both by aging (Elias and Elias, 1976) and by hippocampal lesions (Niki, 1966). An effect of chronic Org 2766 treatment on attentional processes would also mirror the effects ascribed to acute treatments in rat (De Wied, 1974; Sandman and Kastin, 1977) and man (see earlier section). Further neurotropic action of Org 2766 (and other ACTH peptides) was seen following treatments lasting no more than 18 days, which facilitated the recovery of sensorimotor function in rats with sciatic nerve injuries (Bijlsma *et al.*, 1981). If the neurotropic actions of ACTH peptides in rat can be extrapolated to man, we may hope that prolonged treatment with Org 2766 will attenuate the gradual cerebral degeneration in dementia. Such an action would not have to relate to any of the effects reviewed earlier, for treatments given for one month or less.

OTHER POSSIBLE INDICATIONS FOR ACTH-LIKE PEPTIDES

Although much of this paper has concentrated on the treatment of dementia, it may be that ACTH-like peptides would produce more favorable results in other patient groups. There are good reasons for extending Org 2766 treatment to younger patients (perhaps to Down's syndrome, but probably not to infantile epilepsy currently treated with ACTH (Willig and Lagenstein, 1980)), to degenerative nervous system diseases other than primary degenerative dementia, and to demyelinating diseases. It is not possible to do everything at once, however, and for the time being it seems wise to follow existing leads and to establish whether or not the peptide will be beneficial to the growing population of demented patients. This work is in progress.

REFERENCES

Beckwith, B.E. and Sandman, C.A. (1978). Behavioural influences of the neuropeptides ACTH and MSH: a methodological review. Neurosci. Behav. Rev., 2, 311-38

Bijlsma, W.A., Jennekens, F.G.I., Schotman, P. and Gispen, W.H. (1981). Effects of corticotrophin (ACTH) on peripheral nerve regeneration: structure-activity study. Eur. J. Pharmacol., 70, 73-9

Bohus, B. (1981). Neuropeptides in brain functions and dysfunctions. Int. J. Ment. Health, 9, 6-44

Bohus, B. and De Kloet, E.R. (1979). Behavioural effects of neuropeptides (endorphins, enkephalins, ACTH fragments) and corticosteroids. In Interaction within the Brain-Pituitary-Adrenocortical System, (ed. M.T. Jones, B. Gillham, M.F.

Dallman and S. Chattopadhyay), Academic Press, London, pp. 7-16

Bohus, B. and De Wied, D. (1980). Pituitary-adrenal system hormones and adaptive behaviour. In General, Comparative and Clinical Endocrinology of the Adrenal Cortex, vol. 3, (ed. I.C. Jones and I.W. Henderson), Academic Press, London, pp. 265-347

Braverman, A., Hamdy, R., Meisner, P. and Perera, N. (1981). Clinical trial of Org 2766 ($ACTH_{4-9}$ analogue) in the treatment of elderly people with impaired function. Paper presented at III World Congress of Biological Psychiatry, Stockholm, June 28 - July 3

Clarke, A. and File, S.E. (1981). Social interaction in male rats after septal administration of ACTH [4-10] and Org 2766. Br. J. Pharmacol., 74, 277P

De Kloet, E.R. and De Wied, D. (1980). The brain as target tissue for hormones of pituitary origin: behavioral and biochemical studies. Front. Neuroend., 6, 157-201

Delanoy, R.L. and Dunn, A.J. (1978). Mouse brain deoxyglucose uptake after footshock, ACTH analogs, α-MSH, corticosterone or lysine vasopressin. Pharmacol. Biochem. Behav., 9, 21-6

De Wied, D. (1969). Effects of peptide hormones on behaviour. Front. Neuroend., 1, 97-140

De Wied, D. (1974). Pituitary-adrenal system hormones and behavior. In The Neurosciences, Third Study Program, (ed. F.O. Schmitt and F.G. Worden), MIT Press, Cambridge MA, pp. 653-66

Elias, P.K. and Elias, M.F. (1976). Effects of age on learning ability: contributions from the animal literature. Exp. Ageing Res., 2, 164-86

Endroczi, E., Lissak, K., Fekete, T. and De Wied, D. (1970). Effects of ACTH on EEG habituation in human subjects. Prog. Brain Res., 32, 254-62

Fehm-Wolfsdorf, G., Elbert, T., Lutzenberger, W., Rockstroh, B., Birbaumer, N. and Fehm, H.L. (1981). Effects of $ACTH_{4-9}$ analog on human cortical evoked potentials in a two-stimulus reaction time paradigm. Psychoneuroendocrinology, 6, 311-19

Fekete, M., Bohus, B., Van Wolfswinkel, L., Van Ree, J.M. and De Wied, D. (1982). Comparative effects of $ACTH_{4-9}$ analog (Org 2766), $ACTH_{4-10}$ and [D-Phe^7] $ACTH_{4-10}$ on medial septal self-stimulation behaviour in rats. Neuropharmacology, in press

Fekete, M. and De Wied, D. (1982a). Naltrexone sensitive facilitation and naltrexone sensitive inhibition of passive avoidance behavior by the $ACTH_{4-9}$ analog (Org 2766). Eur. J. Pharmacol., 81, 441-8

Fekete, M. and De Wied, D. (1982b). Potency and duration of

action of the ACTH$_{4-9}$ analog (Org 2766) as compared to ACTH$_{4-10}$ and [D-Phe^7] ACTH$_{4-10}$ on active and passive avoidance behaviour of rats. Pharmacol. Biochem. Behav., 16, 387-92

Ferris, S.H. and Reisberg, B. (1981). Clinical studies of neuropeptide treatment in impaired elderly. Paper presented at III World Congress of Biological Psychiatry, Stockholm, June 28 - July 3

File, S.E. (1979). Effects of ACTH$_{4-10}$ in the social interaction test of anxiety. Brain Res, 171, 157-60

File, S.E. (1981). Contrasting effects of Org 2766 and α-MSH on social and exploratory behavior in the rat. Peptides, 2, 255-60

File, S.E. and Vellucci, S.V. (1978). Studies on the role of ACTH and of 5 HT in anxiety, using an animal model. J. Pharm. Pharmacol., 30, 105-10

Gaillard, A.W.K. and Sanders, A.F. (1975). Some effects of ACTH$_{4-10}$ on performance during a serial reaction task. Psychopharmacol. (Berl.) 42, 201-8

Gaillard, A.W.K. and Varey, C.A. (1979). Some effects of an ACTH$_{4-9}$ analog (Org 2766) on human performance. Physiol. Behav., 23, 78-84

Gaillard, A.W.K. and Zwaan, E.J. (1978). Some effects of Org 2766 on serial reaction time in hypophysectomized patients. (Report to Organon)

Geyer, G. and Templ, H. (1976). Nasale Applikation eines synthetischen α$^{1-18}$-corticotropins. Deutsche Medizinische Wochenschrift, 49, 1806-8

Greven, H.M. and De Wied, D. (1973). The influence of peptides derived from corticotrophin (ACTH) on performance. Structure activity studies. Prog. Brain Res., 39, 429-42

Greven, H.M. and De Wied, D. (1980). Structure and behavioral activity of peptides related to corticotrophin and lipotrophin. In Hormones and the Brain (ed. D. De Wied and P.A. Van Keep), MTP Press, Lancaster, pp. 115-27

Hillyard, S.A., Picton, T.W. and Regan, D. (1978). Sensation, perception and attention: analysis using ERP's. In Event-Related Brain Potentials in Man (ed. E. Callaway, P. Tueting and S. Koslow), Academic Press, New York, pp. 223-322

Landfield. P.W., Baskin, R.K. and Pitler, T.A. (1981). Brain aging correlates: retardation by hormonal-pharmacological treatments. Science, 214, 581-4

Lidz, T., Carter, J.D., Lewis, B.I. and Surratt, C. (1952). Effects of ACTH and cortisone on mood and mentation. Psychosom. Med., 14, 363-77

McCarthy, G. and Donchin, E. (1981). A metric for thought: a comparison of P 300 latency and reaction time. Science, 211, 77-80

McCulloch, J., Kelly, P.A.T. and Van Delft, A.M.L. (1982). Alterations in local cerebral glucose utilisation during chronic treatment with an ACTH$_{4-9}$ analog. Eur. J. Pharmacol., 78, 151-8

Mackintosh, N.J. (1969). A further analysis of the overtraining reversal effect. J. Comp. Physiol. Psychol., 67, Suppl. 1-18

Martin, J.C., Cockram, L.C., Ballinger, B.R., Pigache, R.M. and McPherson, F.M. (1982). Evaluation of the clinical efficacy of Org 2766 in patients suffering from severe senile dementia. Paper presented at 13th Collegium International Neuro-psychopharmacologicum, Jerusalem, June 20-25

Medvedev, V.I., Bakharev, V.D., Grechko, A.T. and Nezovibat'Ko, V.N. (1980). Effect of vasopressin and adrenocorticotrophic hormone fragment ACTH$_{4-7}$ on human memory. Human Physiol., 6, 307-10

Miller, L.H., Kastin, A.J., Sandman, C.A., Fink, M. and Van Veen, W. (1974). Polypeptide influences on attention, memory and anxiety in man. Pharmacol. Biochem. Behav., 2, 663-8

Nicholson, A.N. and Stone, B.M. (1980). A synthetic ACTH$_{4-9}$ analogue (Organon 2766) and sleep in healthy man. Neuropharmacology, 15, 1245-6

Niesink, R.J.M. and Van Ree, J.M. (1982). Analysis of the facilitatory effect of the ACTH$_{4-9}$ analogue Org 2766 on active social contact in rats. Life Sci., in press

Niki, H. (1966). Response perseveration following the hippocampal ablation in the rat. Jap. Psychol. Res., 1, 1-9

O'Hanlon, J.F., Van Arkel, A., De Vries, G. and Volkerts, E. (1982). Effects of ACTH$_{4-9}$ analog upon psychological factors underlying human performance in a vigilance task. Paper presented at 13th Collegium International Neuropsychopharmacologicum, Jerusalem, June 20-25

Parasuraman, R. and Beatty, J. (1980). Brain events underlying detection and recognition of weak sensory signals. Sciene, 210, 80-3

Pigache, R.M. (1982a). Effects of ACTH-like peptides on cognition and affect in the elderly. In Neuropeptides and Hormone Modulation of Brain Function and Homeostasis, (ed. J.M. Ordy, J.R. Sladek and B. Reisberg), Raven Press, New York, in press

Pigache, R.M. (1982b). A peptide for the aged? Basic and clinical studies. In Psychopharmacology of Old Age, (ed. D. Wheatley), Oxford University Press, Oxford, pp. 67-96

Pigache, R.M. and Rigter, H. (1981). Effects of peptides related to ACTH on mood and vigilance in man. Front. Hormone Res., 8, 193-207

Plomp, G.J. and Van Ree, J.M. (1978). Adrenocorticotrophic

hormone fragments mimic the effect of morphine *in vitro*.
Br. J. Pharmacol., 64, 223-7

Quarton, G.C., Clark, L.K., Cobb, S. and Bauer, W. (1955). Mental
disturbance associated with ACTH and cortisone: a review of
explanatory hypotheses. Medicine, 34, 13-50

Raskin, A. (1981). Special considerations in the assessment of
psychopathology in the elderly. Psychopharm. Bull., 17,
104-7

Rigter, H. (1982). A peptide for the aged? Animal studies. In
Psychopharmacology of Old Age, (ed. D. Wheatley), Oxford
University Press, Oxford, pp. 97-112

Rigter, H. and Crabbe, J.C. (1979). Modulation of memory by
pituitary hormones and related peptides. Vitamins and
Hormones, 37, 153-241

Rigter, H., Van Delft, A.M. and Pigache, R.M. (1982). ACTH-like
neuropeptides and ageing. In Integrative Neurohormonal
Mechanisms, (ed. E. Endroczi), in press

Rockstroh, B., Elbert, T., Lutzenberger, W., Birbaumer, N., Fehm,
H.L. and Voigt, K.-H. (1981). Effects of an $ACTH_{4-9}$ analog
on human cortical evoked potentials in a constant fore-
period reaction time paradigm. Psychoneuroendocrinology,
6, 301-10

Rockstroh, B., Elbert, T., Lutzenberger, W., Birbaumer, N., Voigt,
K.-H. and Fehm, H.L. (1982). Distractibility under the
influence of an $ACTH_{4-9}$ derivative. (Report to Organon),
to be published

Sandman, C.A. and Kastin, A.J. (1977). Pituitary peptide influ-
ences on attention and memory. In Neurobiology of Sleep and
Memory, (ed. R.R. Drucker-Colin and J.L. McGaugh), Academic
Press, New York, pp. 347-60

Terenius, L., Gispen, W.H. and De Wied, D. (1975). ACTH-like
peptides and opiate receptors in the rat brain: structure-
activity studies. Eur. J. Pharmacol., 33, 395-9

Van Nispen, J.W. and Greven, H.M. (1982). Structure-activity
relationships of peptides derived from ACTH, β-LPH and MSH
with regard to avoidance behavior in rats. Pharmacol.
Ther., 16, 67-102

Verhoef, J. and Witter, A. (1976). *In vivo* fate of a behaviourally
active $ACTH_{4-9}$ analog in rats after systemic administration. Pharmacol. Biochem. Behav., 4, 583-90

Verhoef, J., Witter, A. and De Wied, D. (1977). Specific uptake
of a behaviourally potent [^{3}H] $ACTH_{4-9}$ analog in the septal
area after intraventricular injection in rats. Brain Res.,
131, 117-28

Weigant, V.M., Gispen, W.H., Terenius, L. and De Wied, D. (1977).
ACTH-like peptides and morphine: interaction at the level
of the CNS. Psychoneuroendocrinology, 2, 63-9

Weigant, V.M., Zwiers, H. and Gispen, W.H. (1981). Neuropeptides and brain cAMP and phosphoproteins. <u>Pharmacol. Ther.</u>, 12, 463-90

Willig, R.P. and Lagenstein, I. (1980). Therapieversuch mit einem ACTH-Fragment ($ACTH_{4-10}$) bei frühkindlichen Anfällen. <u>Monatsschr. Kinderheilkd.</u>, 128, 100-3

Willner, A.E. (1981). Influence of an analog of $ACTH_{4-9}$ (Org 2766) on mood in elderly symptomatic volunteers. Paper presented at <u>III World Congress of Biological Psychiatry</u>, Stockholm, June 28-July 3

Wittenborn, J.R. (1981). The assessment of behavioral changes in geriatric patients. <u>Psychopharm. Bull.</u>, 17, 96-103

Clinical psychopharmacology of endorphins

H.M.Emrich[1] and C.Gramsch[1]

INTRODUCTION

One of the most active topics in current psychopharmacology is the investigation of CNS-active endogenous ligands of pharmacological agents, e.g. studies as to the possible existence of an endogenous diazepam-like material, endogenous neuroleptics, etc. Such developments result not only from the discovery of the endorphins (i.e. endogenous morphine-like substances) which opened a novel field of research, but were also associated with novel concepts of the operation of the CNS and the introduction of advanced pharmacological technology.

Historically, endorphins were discovered when specific opiate receptors were studied not only indirectly by pharmacological characterization but also directly by use of receptor binding studies (Pert and Snyder, 1973). These findings raised questions as to the possible biological significance of these receptors and as to the chemical identity of the natural ligands; as a consequence, Hughes *et al.* (1975) were able to isolate and characterize an opiate-active material in the brain containing the pentapeptides met-enkephalin and leu-enkephalin. Further biochemical research revealed a whole family of opiate-active peptides which may be classified as the transmitter-like pentapeptides (enkephalins) and larger molecules (e.g. β-endorphin, α-neo-endorphin, β-casomorphin, dynorphin; for review, see Emrich, 1981; Höllt *et al.*, 1981).

From the mode of action of endorphins, a spectrum of activity similar to that of morphine might be anticipated. Generally, it has been shown that this is indeed the case. In particular, it has been established that chronic administration of endorphins, in a fashion similar to opiates, results in the induction of tolerance and physical dependence; thus, a physiological analgesic and/

[1]Max-Planck-Institut für Psychiatrie, Kraepelinstrasse 10, D-8000 München 40, FRG.

or tranquilizing drug of therapeutic potential cannot be derived simply from an endorphin-like chemical structure. Differences between the actions of endorphins and of opiates depend mainly on pharmacokinetic and physicochemical differences. However, recent investigations (Childers *et al.*, 1979; Lord *et al.*, 1977; Robson and Kosterlitz, 1979; Wüster *et al.*, 1980) have demonstrated the specificity of certain opioid agonists and antagonists on different subtypes of opiate receptors (μ, δ, ϵ). The possible clinical implications of these findings cannot as yet be evaluated, since clinical experience in humans up to now is confined to the application of β-endorphin, the enkephalin analog FK 33-824 and the opiates. The primary effects of these substances are mediated by μ-receptors and, in the case of the psychotomimetic partial agonists, such as cyclazocine and nalorphine, their psychotogenic properties are apparently independent of their opiate-receptor affinity (Shearman and Herz, 1982). More specific agonists for e.g. δ-receptors, such as [D-Ala^2,D-Leu^5]-enkephalin, have not yet been examined clinically; therefore, the possible psychotropic action of these subtypes of opioids, e.g. psychic effects initiated by the activation of different subtypes of opiate receptors, is up to now completely a '*terra incognita*'.

From the analgesic and tranquilizing effects of opioid-peptides, a central functional role in psychic responses to stress may be predicted. In fact, a plethora of animal studies have shown that opioid peptides act as modulators of nociception, temperature control and motor behavior under conditions of stress (for review see Millan and Emrich, 1981). On the contrary, in human studies comparatively few investigations have as yet positively demonstrated an involvement of endorphinergic systems in stress phenomena, whereas a great number of studies showed negative results (for review see Emrich, 1981). The main reason underlying this discrepancy may be the fact that for ethical reasons in human studies the intensity of enforceable stress may, in many cases, be insufficient to activate an endorphinergic response.

The clinical psychopharmacology of opioids is confronted with problems concerning (a) possible beneficial effects of opiate-like substances in various types of psychiatric disorders, and (b) a possible mediation of the psychotropic effects of other classes of substances via an activation of endorphinergic systems. Furthermore, (c) the possible therapeutic and/or antitherapeutic actions of specific opioid antagonists (naloxone, naltrexone) demand consideration.

PSYCHOTROPIC ACTIONS OF OPIOIDS

In response to the question as to the psychopharmacological profile of action of opioids, their euphorogenic and anxiolytic properties are of pertinence; this prompts the hypothesis of a possible antidepressant property of opioids. Interestingly, endorphin research in the past has been undertaken in completely the opposite direction: based on the endorphin hypothesis of schizophrenia (Terenius *et al.*, 1976), schizophrenic patients were treated with the specific opiate antagonist naloxone. This approach evolved partially from the concept (Terenius) that some types of partial agonists (e.g. cyclazocine and nalorphine) exert their psychotogenic effects via a specific action on opiate receptors. This concept was derived from the contention that the psychotogenic effects of cyclazocine and nalorphine are naloxone-reversible (Jasinski *et al.*, 1967) which is apparently not the case (see also Shearman and Herz, 1982). The strategy to try to counteract schizophrenic symptoms by application of naloxone was furthermore based on experiments which detected elevated levels of endorphins (radioreceptor assay) in the CSF of schizophrenic patients (Terenius *et al.*, 1976). However, attempts to replicate these findings (radioimmunoassay: Emrich *et al.*, 1979a; radio-receptor assay: Naber *et al.*, 1981) have proven unsuccessful. Therefore, the essential theoretical basis for the naloxone treatment of schizophrenic patients is conspicuously weak, and an alternative explanation for certain interesting results acquired with this drug must possibly be constructed (see below).

Investigations as to a possible beneficial effect of β-endorphin in psychotic patients were initiated by Kline and coworkers in 1977. In a series of open studies, Kline *et al.* (1977) investigated possible effects of β-endorphin in different types of psychoses and neuroses. The profile of action of β-endorphin was described as tranquilizing and mood-elevating. In some cases hallucinatory effects were also observed. Subsequently, the clinical efficacy of β-endorphin was investigated under double-blind conditions by Catlin's group (Gerner *et al.*, 1980), by the NIMH group (Pickar *et al.*, 1981), and by Berger's group in Stanford (Berger *et al.*, 1980). From the present state of knowledge, an antidepressant effect of β-endorphin may be recognized as clear (Gerner *et al.*, 1980; Gorelick *et al.*, 1981), whereas its anti-schizophrenic properties are highly questionable

Investigations using the enkephalin-derivative FK 33-824 (Jørgensen *et al.*, 1979; Nedopil and Rüther, 1979) point to a weak antischizophrenic effect; its possible antidepressant efficacy has not as yet been evaluated satisfactorily.

The finding that endogenous opioids apparently exert anti-depressant effects in patients suffering from primary depression renders inconceivable the idea that there may be a constitutional defect of endorphinergic systems in endogenous depression. This question has recently been discussed extensively, and in a synthesis of the body of information concerning biochemical and pharmacological data no substantial evidence pointing to such a hypothesis could be derived (Emrich, 1982). Nevertheless, although there may not be a deficiency in endorphin function in depression, exogenous application of opiate-like material is possibly of therapeutic use (e.g. the application of buprenorphine; Emrich *et al.*, 1982).

ACTIVATION OF ENDOGENOUS OPIOIDS BY ELECTROCONVULSIVE THERAPY

Although the interesting findings of Grahame-Smith's group (1978) demonstrated a mobilization of central monoamines by an exposure to electroconvulsive therapy (ECT), the neurochemical basis of the therapeutic action of this manipulation remains an open question. Holaday's group (Belenky and Holaday, 1979; Holaday *et al.*, 1981) recently obtained compelling evidence for an activation of central endorphinergic systems by ECT. In line with these results are the findings of Emrich *et al.* (1979a) in which an increase in plasma levels of β-endorphin immunoreactivity was evaluated 10 min following ECT in depressed patients, a result which has recently been reproduced by Inturrisi *et al.* (1982).

From these findings a possible endorphinergic component of the mode of action of ECT may be hypothesized.

ACTIVATION OF ENDORPHINS BY NEUROLEPTIC DRUGS

According to the findings of Costa's group (Hong *et al.*, 1979) and of Höllt and Bergmann (1982), chronic treatment with haloperidol or other neuroleptic drugs results in an elevation in levels of endorphins in the striatum, pituitary and plasma. From these findings and, in particular, the observation (Höllt and Bergmann, 1982) that chronic haloperidol treatment exerts a specific facilitation of β-endorphin biosynthesis (via an activation of messenger RNA; cf. Höllt, 1981), the hypothesis may be raised that therapeutic actions of neuroleptic drugs may be mediated via a potentiation of the functional activity of endorphins.

Clinical investigations in this regard have focused on two types of variables: On the one hand, the activating effect of chronic neuroleptic treatment upon endorphinergic systems was studied at the level of determination of β-endorphin immunoreactivity in plasma; on the other hand, the question was raised whether the therapeutic effects of neuroleptics might be counteracted by naloxone treatment. Investigation of β-endorphin immunoreactivity in plasma of schizophrenic patients prior to and during long-term neuroleptic therapy showed a small but highly significant increase during the course of medication (Gramsch and Emrich, unpublished data). Interestingly, the opposite is true in treatment of schizophrenic patients with high-dosage diazepam (this study was performed in cooperation with Haas and Beckmann, at Mannheim; Haas *et al.*, 1982). This reduction of β-endorphin immunoreactivity in plasma may be due to the antistress effect of diazepam (Millan and Duka, 1981). The naloxone trial, employing 2 x 20 mg per day for 2 days in schizophrenic patients revealing productive psychotic symptoms, was designed to counteract the beneficial effects of neuroleptic drugs. In comparison to a placebo control, no blockade by naloxone of the antipsychotic effect of neuroleptic drugs could be demonstrated. However, the interpretation of these observations is difficult since, probably owing to the short half-life of naloxone, endorphin-activating effects may develop during the course of this treatment (cf. Reker *et al.*, 1983).

ACTION OF THE OPIATE-ANTAGONIST NALOXONE IN DIFFERENT TYPES OF PSYCHOSES

The rationale for the therapeutic administration of naloxone in schizophrenic patients, as discussed above, was that competitive inhibition of a hypothetical opioid hyperactivity in schizophrenia may thus be attained. From the sum of naloxone studies performed in recent years (see Emrich, 1981) it has to be concluded that the (low) doses sufficient to precipitate withdrawal symptoms in opiate addicts are ineffective in schizophrenic patients, whereas higher dosages (4.0-25.0 mg, i.v.) induce a relatively small but statistically significant antipsychotic effect (Emrich *et al.*, 1977, 1979b; Pickar *et al.*, 1982; Watson *et al.*, 1978). In several studies, this therapeutic effect exhibited a time lag of 2-3 h and it is presently and open question whether this therapeutic effect may be interpreted as reflecting opiate receptor blockade or possibly an endorphin-activating activity of naloxone as demonstrated by Reker *et al.* (1983).

SIGNIFICANCE OF ENDORPHINS IN HEROIN ADDICTION

The neurochemical bases of heroin addiction is attributable to a modulation of processes at a hierarchy of organizational levels:

(a) adaptive processes at the receptor/second messenger level;

(b) adaptive processes concerning endorphins (for a summary see Herz, 1981).

According to a hypothesis formulated by Goldstein (1976) there might exist a constitutional basis for the development of heroin addiction, i.e. the existence of an endorphin deficiency in this (sub-) population. To address a part of this hypothesis, β-endorphin immunoreactivity in the plasma of seven heroin addicts was evaluated before and during heroin withdrawal. No abnormality of β-endorphin immunoreactivity in plasma could be observed. During heroin withdrawal a relatively small but highly significant increase of β-endorphin immunoreactivity could be demonstrated. From these data, no convincing support for the endorphin deficit hypothesis of heroin addiction can be deduced.

SUMMARY

Endorphins undoubtedly play a major role in physiological re-sponses to stress, although in humans these effects cannot be demonstrated easily. The pharmacological profile of opioids resembles that of opiates, although at present specific actions on subtypes of opiate receptors differing from the μ-receptor cannot be evaluated. An antidepressant effect of opioid peptides in humans has clearly been demonstrated, whereas its effects in schizophrenic patients are questionable. Neuroleptic drugs exert an activating effect upon endorphinergic systems. However, it cannot as yet be demonstrated that their antipsychotic effects are mediated via an endorphinergic mode of action. A similar action of ECT has been found, and it has been hypothesized that the antidepressant effect of ECT reflects, at least partially, this endorphinergic mode of action. Furthermore, the role of endor-phins in heroin addiction is discussed.

Acknowledgement

One of us (H.M.E.) was supported by a grant (Heisenberg-Programm) from the Deutsche Forschungsgemeinschaft.

REFERENCES

Belenky, G.L. and Holaday, J.W. (1979). The opiate antagonist naloxone modifies the effects of electroconvulsive shock (ECS) on respiration, blood pressure and heart rate. Brain Res., 177, 414–17

Berger, P.A., Watson, S.J., Akil, H., Elliott, G.R., Rubin, R.T., Pfefferbaum, A., Davis, K.L., Barchas, J.D. and Li, C.H. (1980). β-Endorphin and schizophrenia. Arch. Gen. Psychiatry, 37, 635–40

Childers, S.R., Creese, I., Snowman, A.M. and Snyder, S.H. (1979). Opiate receptor binding affected differentially by opiates and opioid peptides. Eur. J. Pharmacol., 55, 11–18

Emrich, H.M. (ed.) (1981). The Role of Endorphins in Neuro-psychiatry (Modern Problems in Pharmacopsychiatry, vol. 17), Karger, Basel

Emrich, H.M. (1982). A possible role of opioid substances in depression. In Typical and Atypical Antidepressants: Clin-ical Practice (ed. E. Costa and G. Racagni), Raven Press, New York, pp. 77–84

Emrich, H.M., Cording, C., Pirée, S. Kölling, A., von Zerssen, D. and Herz, A. (1977). Indication of an antipsychotic action of the opiate antagonist naloxone. Pharmakopsychiatrie, 10, 265-70

Emrich, H.M., Höllt, V., Kissling, W., Fischler, M., Laspe, H., Heinemann, H., von Zerssen, D. and Herz, A. (1979a). β-Endorphin-like immunoreactivity in cerebrospinal fluid and plasma of patients with schizophrenia and other neuropsychiatric disorders. Pharmakopsychiatrie, 12, 269-76

Emrich, H.M., Möller, H.-J., Laspe, H., Meisel-Kosik, I., Dwinger, H., Oechsner, R., Kissling, W. and von Zerssen, D. (1979b). On a possible role of endorphins in psychiatric disorders. Actions of naloxone in psychiatric patients. In Biological Psychiatry Today, (ed. J. Obiols, C. Ballús, E. González Monclús and J. Pujol), Elsevier/North-Holland Biomedical Press, Amsterdam, pp. 789-805

Emrich, H.M., Vogt, P. and Herz, A. (1982). Possible antidepressive effects of opioids. Action of buprenorphine. Ann. NY Acad. Sci., 398, 108-12

Gerner, R.H., Catlin, D.H., Gorelick, D.A., Hui, K.K. and Li, C.H. (1980). β-Endorphin: intravenous infusion causes behavioral change in psychiatric inpatients. Arch. Gen. Psychiatry, 37, 642-7

Goldstein, A. (1976). Opioid peptides (endorphins) in pituitary and brain. Science, 193, 1081-6

Gorelick, D.A., Catlin, D.H. and Gerner, R.H. (1981). β-Endorphin studies in psychiatric patients. In The Role of Endorphins in Neuropsychiatry (Modern Problems in Pharmacopsychiatry, vol. 17) (ed. H.M. Emrich), Karger, Basel, pp. 236-45

Grahame-Smith, D.G., Green, A.R. and Costain, D.W. (1978). Mechanism of the antidepressant action of electroconvulsive therapy. Lancet, i, 254-7

Haas, S., Emrich, H.M. and Beckmann, H. (1982). Analgesic and euphoric effects of high dose diazepam in schizophrenia. Neuropsychobiology, 8, 123-8

Herz, A. (1981). Role of endorphins in addiction. In The Role of Endorphins in Neuropsychiatry (Modern Problems in Pharmacopsychiatry, vol. 17) (ed. H. M. Emrich), Karger, Basel, pp. 175-80

Höllt, V. (1981). Effects of neuroleptic drugs on endogenous opioid peptides in the rat. In The Role of Endorphins in Neuropsychiatry (Modern Problems in Pharmacopsychiatry, vol 17), (ed. H. M. Emrich), Karger, Basel, pp. 1-18

Höllt, V. and Bergmann, M. (1982). Effect of acute and chronic haloperidol treatment on the concentrations of immunoreactive β-endorphin in plasma, pituitary and brain of rats. Neuropharmacology, 21, 147-54

Höllt, V., Haarmann, I., Seizinger, B.R. and Herz, A. (1981). Levels of dynorphin-(1-13) immunoreactivity in rat neurointermediate pituitaries are concomitantly altered with those of leucine enkephalin and vasopression in response to various endocrine manipulations. Neuroendocrinology, 264, 39–45

Holaday, J.W., Tortella, F.C. and Belenky, G.L. (1981). Electroconvulsive shock results in a functional activation of endorphin systems. In The Role of Endorphins in Neuropsychiatry (Modern Problems in Pharmacopsychiatry, vol. 17) (ed. H.M. Emrich), Karger, Basel, pp. 142–57

Hong, J.S., Yang, H.-Y.T., Gillin, J.C., di Giulio, A.M., Fratta, W. and Costa, E. (1979). Chronic treatment with haloperidol accelerates the biosynthesis of enkephalins in rat brain. Brain Res., 160, 192–5

Hughes, J., Smith, T.W., Kosterlitz, H.W., Fothergill, L.A., Morgan, B. A. and Morris, H. R. (1975). Identification of two related pentapeptides from the brain with potent opiate agonist activity. Nature, 258, 577–9

Inturrisi, C.E., Alexopoulos, G., Lipman, R., Foley, K. and Rossier, J. (1982). β-Endorphin immunoreactivity in the plasma of psychiatric patients receiving electroconvulsive treatment. Ann. NY Acad. Sci., 398, 413–22

Jasinski, D.R., Martin, W.R. and Haertzen, C.A. (1967). The human pharmacology and abuse potential of *N*-allyl-noroxymorphone (naloxone). J. Pharmacol. Exp. Ther. 157, 420–6

Jørgensen, A., Fog, R. and Veilis, B. (1979). Synthetic enkephalin analogue in treatment of schizophrenia. Lancet, 1, 935

Kline, N.S., Li, C.H., Lehmann, H.E., Lajtha, A., Laski, E. and Cooper, T. (1977). β-Endorphin-induced changes in schizophrenic and depressed patients. Arch. Gen. Psychiatry, 34, 1111–13

Lord, J.A.H., Waterfield, A.A., Hughes, J. and Kosterlitz, H.W. (1977). Endogenous opioid peptides: multiple agonists and receptors. Nature, 267, 495–9

Millan, M.J. and Duka, Th. (1981). Anxiolytic properties of opiates and endogenous opioid peptides and their relationship to the actions of benzodiazepines. In The Role of Endorphins in Neuropsychiatry (Modern Problems in Pharmacopsychiatry, vol. 17) (ed. H. M. Emrich), Karger, Basel, pp. 123–41

Millan, M.J. and Emrich, H.M. (1981). Endorphinergic systems and the response to stress. Psychother. Psychosom., 36, 43–56

Naber, D., Pickar, D., Post, R.M., van Kammen, D.P., Waters, R.N., Ballenger, J.C., Goodwin, F.K. and Bunney, W.E. Jr (1981). Endogenous opiate activity and β-endorphin immunoreactivity in CSF of psychiatric patients and normal volunteers. Am. J. Psychiatry, 138, 1457–62

Nedopil, N. and Rüther, E. (1979). Effects of the synthetic analogue of methionine enkephalin FK 33-824 on psychotic symptoms. Pharmakopsychiatrie, 12, 277–80

Pert, C.B. and Snyder, S.H. (1973). Opiate receptors: demonstration in nervous tissue. Science, 179, 1011-14

Pickar, D., Davis, G.C., Schulz, S.C., Extein, I., Wagner, R., Naber, D., Gold, P.W., van Kammen, D.P., Goodwin, F.K., Wyatt, R. J., Li, C. H. and Bunney, W. E. Jr (1981). Behavioral and biological effects of acute β-endorphin injection in schizophrenic and depressed patients. Am. J. Psychiatry, 138, 160-6

Pickar, D., Vartanian, F., Bunney, W.E. Jr, Maier, H.P., Gastpar, M.T., Prakash, R., Sethi, B.B., Lidman, R., Belyaev, B.S., Tsutsulkovskaja, M.V.A., Jungkunz, G., Nedopil, N., Verhoeven, W. and van Praag, H. (1982). Short-term naloxone administration in schizophrenic and manic patients. Arch. Gen. Psychiatry, 39, 313-19

Reker, D., Anderson, B., Yackulic, C., Cooper, T.B., Banay-Schwartz, M., Leon, C. and Volavka, J. (1983). Naloxone, tardive dyskinesia and endogenous beta-endorphin. Psychiatry Res., in press

Robson, L.E. and Kosterlitz, H.W. (1979). Specific protection of the binding sites of D-Ala^2-D-Leu^5-enkephalin (δ-receptors) and dihydromorphine (μ-receptors). Proc. R. Soc. Lond., 205, 425-32

Shearman, G.T. and Herz, A. (1982). Non-opioid psychotomimetic-like discriminative stimulus properties of *N*-allylnormethazocine (SKF 10,047) in the rat. Eur. J. Pharmacol., 82, 167-72

Terenius, L., Wahlström, A., Lindström, L. and Widerlöv, E. (1976). Increased CSF levels of endorphins in chronic psychosis. Neurosci. Lett., 3, 157-62

Watson, S.J., Berger, P.A., Akil, H., Mills, M.J. and Barchas, J.D. (1978). Effects of naloxone on schizophrenia: reduction in hallucinations in a subpopulation of subjects. Science, 201, 73-6

Wüster, M., Schulz, R. and Herz, A. (1980). The direction of opioid agonists towards μ-, δ- and ε-receptors in the vas deferens of the mouse and the rat. Life Sci., 27, 163-70

GABA receptor agonists: pharmacological spectrum and clinical actions

G.Bartholini[1] and P.L.Morselli[1]

INTRODUCTION

Stimulation of GABA receptors has been reported to modify the activity of a variety of cerebral neurotransmitter systems (see below). As these systems are affected in various neuropsychiatric disorders, GABA receptor agonists represent a potential class of new drugs with a wide therapeutic spectrum.

This review focuses briefly on the pharmacological spectrum and the clinical action of progabide (SL 76 002; (4-{[(4-chloro-phenyl) (5-fluoro-2-hydroxyphenyl)-methylene]amino} butanamide) (Kaplan *et al.*, 1980), the first apparently non-toxic, specific GABA receptor agonist available for clinical studies. Thus, the action of this compound on norepinephrine (NE), 5-hydroxytrypta-mine (5-HT, serotonin) and dopamine (DA) neurons will be empha-sized in the light of the therapeutic results in affective dis-orders, dyskinesia and epilepsy.

(For details on the pharmacological actions of progabide, see Worms *et al.*, 1982; Lloyd *et al.*, 1982; Scatton *et al.*, 1982; Scatton and Bartholini, 1982.)

NE AND 5-HT NEURONS - DEPRESSION

Progabide on acute administration increases dose-dependently the concentrations of 3,4-dihydroxyphenylethyleneglycol sulfate - the major cerebral metabolite of NE - in limbic forebrain areas of the rat without alteration of the NE levels (Scatton *et al.*, 1982). Also, the α-methyl-*p*-tyrosine-induced disappearance of the amine is accelerated by progabide (Scatton *et al.*, 1982). These effects indicate an enhancement of NE turnover and, as they are blocked by picrotoxin, result from a GABA-mediated mechanism (Scatton *et al.*,

---

[1]L.E.R.S. Synthélabo, 58 rue de la Glacière, 75013 Paris, France.

1982). As iontophoretic administration of progabide or other GABAergic agents on locus coeruleus cells reduces their firing rate (Guyenet and Aghajanian, 1979), the acceleration of NE turnover by GABA receptor stimulation probably occurs via an indirect mechanism, i.e. via changes of neuronal inputs on noradrenergic neurons. Whatever the mechanism, the increased NE turnover by progabide should lead to an enhanced noradrenergic transmission. Similarly, tricyclic antidepressants, by inhibition of the NE re-uptake, increase the availability of the amine at the receptor sites and therefore noradrenergic transmission (Schildkraut, 1965). Indeed, both progabide and antidepressants antagonize the reserpine-induced ptosis which results from a reduced availability of NE in the synaptic cleft.

Progabide administered to rats daily for 14 days leads to a reduction of the enhanced NE turnover observed after a single injection; this occurs in the absence of changes of postsynaptic β-antagonist binding or of NE-sensitive adenylate cyclase and is probably the result of a tolerance of the noradrenergic system which develops to GABA receptor agonists; it is likely that the absence of receptor changes is a consequence of this tolerance (Zivkovic *et al.*, 1982). Tricyclic antidepressants on repeated treatment lead, in contrast, to a down-sensitization of β- binding and of the NE-sensitive adenylate cyclase activity (Sulser *et al.*, 1978).

Serotonergic neurons are also affected by GABA receptor stimulants but in the opposite manner than noradrenergic cells. Thus, progabide on acute administration reduces the 5-HT turnover in the rat striatum as indicated by (a) the diminution of 5-HT disappearance after α-propyl-dopacetamide; (b) the decreased accumulation of 5-HTP after inhibition of aromatic L-amino acid decarboxylase by NSD 1015; (c) the accumulation of 5-HT after pargyline (Scatton *et al.*, 1982). This effect probably occurs by direct stimulation of GABA receptors localized on raphe cells which are inhibited by iontophoretically administered GABA (Gallager and Aghajanian, 1976). Repeated treatment with progabide accentuates the reduction in 5-HT turnover (Zivkovic *et al.*, 1982). This further reduction in 5-HT turnover is accompanied by the development of a supersensitivity of postsynaptic target cells as indicated by the increase in spiroperidol binding sites (Briley, personal communication). Under these conditions, as progabide antagonizes the 5-HTP-induced head twitches (Worms, personal communication), serotonergic transmission should be reduced - even if this reduction may be partially compensated by receptor up-regulation.

In contrast, tricyclic antidepressants on acute administration increase 5-HT transmission as a consequence of the 5-HT re-uptake inhibition (Schildkraut, 1965); however, this leads under repeated treatment to a down-regulation of postsynaptic receptors (Peroutka and Snyder, 1980). According to these data,

5-HT uptake blockers, 5-HT receptor antagonists (e.g. mianserin) and GABA receptor agonists (e.g. progabide) decrease 5-HT transmission under chronic treatment.

Support for this view is provided by the fact that amitryptyline or mianserin antagonize 5-HT-mediated effects (Maj *et al.*, 1979; Ogren *et al.*, 1979) and progabide reduces the 5-HTP-induced head twitches. The three classes of compounds are effective in behavioral animal models predictive of antidepressant activity such as olfactory bulbectomy and learned helplessness (Broekkamp *et al.*, in preparation). In the case of progabide, this effect is blocked by bicuculline, indicating a GABA receptor-mediated event (Broekkamp *et al.*, in preparation).

In conclusion, progabide and probably other GABA receptor agonists represent a new class of antidepressant drugs; similarly to tricyclic compounds, progabide affects NE- and 5-HT-mediated transmission. However, the effects of progabide on monoamines differ from those of tricyclics (see above) and it is still unknown which common denominator is relevant to the antidepressant action. Also, the mechanism of progabide likely involves a primary change in NE and 5-HT cell firing rate whereas tricyclic antidepressants affect primarily synaptic events, i.e. monoamine re-uptake.

Clinical Results in Depression

Data in man support the hypothesis that GABA-agonists have a therapeutic action in depressive syndromes.

In a preliminary open study on 15 depressive (11 endogenous and four reactive) patients, progabide administered at doses of 20-30 mg kg^{-1} per day led within 8-15 days to a significant improvement in seven (six endogenous and one reactive) cases with mobilization of defenses, disappearance of death thoughts and culpability, reappearance of critical judgement and frank elevation of mood (Morselli *et al.*, 1980).

A second, more recent, 28-day double-blind controlled study was run against imipramine (1.6-3.3 mg kg^{-1} per day) in patients suffering from major depressive episodes (DSM III) or depressive reactions. The antidepressant action of progabide (20-30 mg kg^{-1} per day) was found to be similar to that of the tricyclic for the global clinical rating and the Hamilton rating scale for depression. The disappearance or significant reduction of depressive symptoms with resumption of daily activity was observed in eight out of 11 cases with progabide and nine out of 11 cases with imipramine.

In both studies, progabide was very well tolerated with a minimal incidence of minor and short-lasting side-effects such as light drowsiness, dry mouth, nausea (Morselli *et al.*, 1981, 1982).

These data confirm that GABA receptor agonists have a therapeutic action in major depression and support the hypothesis that changes in GABA-mediated regulation of monoaminergic neurons play a role in the pathophysiology of the disease.

DA NEURONS - DYSKINESIA/MANIA

Progabide, as well as other GABA receptor agonists such as muscimol, inhibits the activity of striatal and mesolimbic DA neurons in various animal species (rat, cat, etc.) (Scatton *et al.*, 1982). Thus, the synthesis of the neurotransmitter is diminished by progabide as indicated by the decreased tyrosine hydroxylase activity and the accumulation of dopa following inhibition of aromatic L-amino acid decarboxylase in the rat. Similarly, the release of DA is decreased as progabide reduces both the disappearance of the amine following α-methyl-*p*-tyrosine and the DA liberation from the cat caudate nucleus (perfused by means of the push-pull cannula). These effects of progabide are blocked by bicuculline, indicating mediation by GABA receptors. Finally, they are likely the consequence of the inhibition of firing rate of DA neurons and become more pronounced after their activation (e.g. after neuroleptic drugs, Scatton *et al.*, 1982).

The progabide-induced decrease in dopaminergic transmission, as well as in its enhancement by neuroleptics, is confirmed by behavioral results. Thus, progabide, although *per se* it does not induce catalepsy, potentiates the cataleptogenic action of neuroleptics (Lloyd *et al.*, 1979). This effect is explained by the diminution in DA neuron activity, DA release and the availability of the amine at the receptor sites for competing with neuroleptics.

Not only are the dopaminergic neurons affected by GABAergic stimulation but also their postsynaptic cells (Bartholini *et al.*, 1980). Thus, repeated co-administration of progabide and neuroleptics reduces (1) the tolerance which develops to the cataleptogenic action of the latter; (2) the supersensitivity to dopaminergic agents; and (3) the increase in DA receptors as indicated by the enhanced B_{max} of ^{3}H-spirone binding (Briley, personal communication); these are all events which occur following sustained neuroleptic treatment.

DA neurons are inhibited by GABA receptor agonists also in the limbic system. However, the doses of these drugs which decrease limbic DA turnover are higher than those effective in the extrapyramidal systems. This indicates that mesolimbic DA neurons are less sensitive to GABAergic inhibition than nigro-striatal cells (Bartholini *et al.*, 1979).

The inhibition of DA neuron activity by progabide and the prevention of the up-regulation of DA receptors following neuroleptics represent the biochemical basis for the therapeutic action of GABA receptor agonists in disorders which involve an absolute or relative increase in dopaminergic transmission. These disorders include neuroleptic-induced dyskinesia, L-dopa-induced dyskinesia and mania. Results in monkeys with a ventrotegmental lesion show that small doses of progabide block the dyskinetic syndrome in-duced by dopamine receptor agonists such as piribidil or by L-dopa (Lloyd *et al.*, 1981a).

Clinical Results in Dyskinesia

Clinical evidence has been provided for the effectiveness of progabide in various forms of dyskinesia. Thus, in a preliminary open study on eight patients suffering from neuroleptic-induced dyskinetic syndrome (as confirmed by electromyography), progabide was administered at doses of 10-30 mg kg^{-1} per day for at least 6-8 weeks. An evident improvement was observed in six cases after two weeks whereas disappearance of abnormal movements took place in four cases after six weeks of treatment (Sevestre *et al.*, 1982).

A more recent double-blind controlled study on a larger number of subjects suffering from neuroleptic-induced dyskinesia confirmed these findings (Sevestre *et al.*, in preparation).

Similar results have been obtained in L-dopa-induced involun-tary movements (Constantinidis, personal communication).

Mania

The potential therapeutic action of GABA receptor agonists in mania is supported by the fact that valproate has been shown to be effective in preventing manic episodes in bipolar patients (Emrich *et al.*, 1981). No clinical data are available as yet with pro-gabide in mania. Should the compound be effective, a single medication would thus be available for preventing and curing psychotic depression and mania.

CELLULAR EXCITABILITY - EPILEPSY

GABA receptor agonists decrease cellular excitability and antagon-ize its enhancement induced by various mechanisms (Lloyd *et al.*, 1979; Worms *et al.*, 1982). In contrast to classical anticonvulsant agents such as ethosuccimide and diphenylidantoin - which are active in only some animal models of epilepsy - progabide and muscimol are effective in seizures which (1) involve changes in GABAergic transmission (bicuculline-, picrotoxin- or cortical penicilline-induced seizures) or (2) are apparently independent of GABA-related parameters (seizures induced by strychnine or ECS; audiogenic seizures). This wide spectrum of GABA receptor agonists in animal models parallels the efficacy of these compounds in various forms of human epilepsy (see below). It is interesting to note that even in humans two populations of epileptic patients have been identified, one in which the focal and perifocal zones of the brain exhibit alterations of GABA-related parameters (GABA binding, GAD activity, GABA-T activity) and another in which no such changes are detectable (Lloyd *et al.*, 1981b). This points to different etiopathogenetic mechanisms involving or not involving GABAergic transmission.

Another advantage of GABA receptor agonists is the low incidence of side-effects. Thus, progabide exerts its anticonvulsant action at doses far lower than those inducing sedation and muscle relaxation. This differentiates GABA receptor agonists from other anticonvulsants including benzodiazepines which cause the above-mentioned side-effects at doses close to those effective in seizures (Lloyd *et al.*, 1979; Worms *et al.*, 1982).

Clinical Results in Epilepsy

The anti-epileptic activity of progabide has been demonstrated in a series of clinical studies conducted mostly on severe epileptic patients poorly responding to the available anti-epileptic medication.

In a first preliminary open study on 36 epileptic patients suffering from partial and/or generalized seizures, administration of progabide (20–30 mg kg^{-1} per day) for 4–8 weeks led to a significant reduction of seizure frequency in 47% of the cases (Baruzzi *et al.*, 1980). These preliminary observations have been successively confirmed by two controlled double-blind trials vs placebo. In both studies, progabide significantly reduced the incidence of complex partial seizures, showing in addition a therapeutic action on generalized seizures (Loiseau *et al.*, 1981; Van der Linden *et al.*, 1981); an evident clinical improvement was manifest in 59% and 45% of the patients, respectively.

Long-term studies (12–18 months) have given additional evidence for the anti-epileptic action of progabide; they have also shown that no tolerance develops to the therapeutic action of the compound administered as monotherapy or associated with other drugs (Martinez-Lage *et al.*, in preparation; Loiseau *et al.*, in preparation).

These studies have demonstrated that progabide, on long-term administration, is well tolerated, causing a minimal incidence of minor and transient side-effects such as drowsiness, nausea and hypotonia.

On the whole, it appears that progabide exerts a therapeutic action in 45–50% of the patients who respond poorly to 'classical' anti-epileptic drugs. This is in good agreement with the finding that 50–60% of patients undergoing neurosurgery because of poor responsiveness to pharmacological treatment have an alteration of GABA-mediated transmission (see above; Lloyd *et al.*, 1981b).

SUMMARY

Stimulation of GABA receptors (e.g. by progabide, a new GABA receptor agonist), affects noradrenergic and serotonergic transmission in animals and, on chronic administration, causes changes in 5-HT$_2$ receptors similar to those caused by ECS. Based on double-blind trials versus imipramine, it has been shown that progabide is effective in psychotic depression.

Progabide reduces DA turnover in animals and prevents supersensitivity caused by neuroleptic agents. This double mechanism on dopaminergic transmission appears to be the basis for the clinical action of the compound in various forms of dyskinesia (L-dopa- and neuroleptic-induced dyskinesia). It also suggests that progabide will be effective in mania.

Progabide decreases cellular excitability in animal brain and antagonizes seizures whatever their origin (GABA-mediated or GABA-unrelated mechanisms). Clinically, the compound is effective in various forms of epilepsy resistant to 'classical' medication in the absence of major side-effects such as sedation or muscle relaxation. The wide spectrum in animals seems to parallel the effects in humans. In this respect, it is interesting to note that, in epileptic patients, two populations have been distinguished, one with cerebral alteration of, and one with normal, GABA-related parameters in focal and perifocal brain areas.

REFERENCES

Bartholini, G., Scatton, B. and Zivkovic, B. (1980). Effect of the new GABA agonist SL 76 002 on striatal acetylcholine: relation to neuroleptic-induced extrapyramidal alterations. In Long-term Effects of Neuroleptics (ed. F. Cattabeni, G. Racagni, P. F. Spano and E. Costa), Raven Press, New York, pp. 207-13

Bartholini, G., Scatton, B., Zivkovic, B. and Lloyd, K.G. (1979). On the mode of action of SL 76 002, a new GABA receptor agonist. In GABA-Neurotransmitters (ed. P. Krogsgaard-Larsen, J. Scheel-Kruger and H. Kofod), Munksgaard, Copenhagen, pp. 326-39

Baruzzi, A., Pazzaglia, P., Loiseau, P., Cenraud, B., Zarifian, E., Mitchard, M. and Morselli, P.L. (1980). Preliminary observations on the effects of SL 76 002, a new GABA agonist in the epileptic patient. In Advances in Epileptology. The Xth Epilepsy International Symposium (ed. J.A. Wada and J.K. Penry), Raven Press, New York, p. 356

Emrich, H.M., von Zerssen, D., Kissling, W. and Möller, H.-J. (1981). Therapeutic effect of valproate in mania. Am. J. Psychiatry, 138, 256

Gallager, D. W. and Aghajanian, G.K. (1976). Effect of antipsychotic drugs on the firing of dorsal raphe cells. II. Reversal by picrotoxin. Eur. J. Pharmacol., 39, 357–64

Guyenet, P. and Aghajanian, G.K. (1979). ACh, substance P and met-enkephalin in the locus coeruleus. Pharmacological evidence for independent sites of action. Eur. J. Pharmacol., 53, 319–28

Kaplan, J.P., Raizon, B.M., Desarmenien, M., Feltz, P., Headley, P.M., Worms, P., Lloyd, K.G. and Bartholini, G. (1980). New anticonvulsants: Schiff bases of γ-aminobutyric acid and γ-aminobutyramide. J. Med. Chem., 23, 702–4

Lloyd, K.G., Arbilla S., Beaumont, K., Briley, M., De Montis, G., Scatton, B., Langer, S.Z. and Bartholini, G. (1982). GABA receptor stimulation. II. Specificity of progabide (SL 76 002) and SL 75 102 for the GABA receptor. J. Pharmacol. Exp. Ther., 220, 672–7

Lloyd, K.G., Broekkamp, C.L.E., Cathala, F., Worms, P., Goldstein, M. and Aseno, T. (1981a). Animal models for the prediction and prevention of dyskinesia induced by dopaminergic drugs. In Apomorphine and Other Dopaminomimetics, vol. II, Clinical Pharmacology (ed. U. Corsini and G. L. Gessa), Raven Press, New York, pp. 123–33

Lloyd, K.G., Munari, C., Bossi, L., Stoeffels, C., Talairach, J. and Morselli, P.L. (1981b). Biochemical evidence for the alterations of GABA-mediated synaptic transmission in patho-logical brain tissue (stereo EEG or morphological definition) from epileptic patients. In Neurotransmitters, Seizures and Epilepsy (ed. P.L. Morselli, K.G. Lloyd, W. Löscher, B. Meldrum and E. Reynolds), Raven Press, New York, pp. 325–37

Lloyd, K.G., Worms, P., Depoortere, H. and Bartholini, G. (1979). Pharmacological profile of SL 76 002, a new GABA receptor agonist. In GABA-Neurotransmitters (ed. P. Krogsgaard-Larsen, J. Scheel-Kruger and H. Kofod) Munksgaard, Copenhagen, pp. 308–25

Loiseau, P., Cenraud, B., Bossi, L. and Morselli, P.L. (1981). Double-blind cross-over trial with progabide versus placebo in severe epilepsy. In Advances in Epileptology. The XIIth Epilepsy International Symposium (ed. M. Dam, L. Gram and J. K. Penry), Raven Press, New York, pp. 135–9

Maj, J., Lewandowska, A. and Rawtow, A. (1979). Central antisero-tonin action of amitryptyline. Pharmakopsychiatrie, 12, 281–3

Morselli, P.L., Bossi, L., Henry, J.F., Zarifian, E. and Bartholini, G. (1980). On the therapeutic action of SL 76 002, a new GABA-mimetic agent: preliminary observations in neuropsychiatric disorders. Brain Res. Bull., 5, Suppl. 2, 411–14

Morselli, P.L., Fournier, V., Macher, J.P., Bottin, D., Huber, J.P. and Orofiamma, B.(1982). GABA agonists in depressive syndromes. In Frontiers in Neuropsychiatric Research (ed. E. Usdin, et al.), (Macmillan, London, in press

Morselli, P.L., Henry, J.F., Macher, J.P., Bottin, P., Huber, J.P. and Van Landeghem, V.H. (1981). Progabide and mood. In Biological Psychiatry (ed. C. Perris, G. Struwe and B. Jansson), Elsevier/North-Holland Biomedical Press, Amsterdam, pp. 440-3

Ogren, S.A., Fuxe, K., Agnati, L.F., Gustafson, A., Jonsson, G. and Holm, A.C. (1979). Reevaluation of the indoleamine hypothesis of depression. Evidence for a reduction of functional activity of central 5HT systems by antidepressant drugs. J. Neural Transm., 46, 85-103

Peroutka, S.J. and Snyder, S.H. (1980). Long-term antidepressant treatment lowers spiroperidol labelled serotonin receptors. Science, 210, 88-90

Scatton, B. and Bartholini, G. (1982). γ-Aminobutyric acid (GABA) receptor stimulation. IV. Effect of progabide (SL 76 002) and other GABAergic agents on acetylcholine turnover in rat brain areas. J. Pharmacol. Exp. Ther., 220, 689-95

Scatton, B., Zivkovic, B., Dedek, J., Lloyd, K.G., Constantinidis, J., Tissot, R. and Bartholini, G. (1982). γ-Aminobutyric acid (GABA) receptor stimulation. III. Effect of progabide (SL 76 002) on norepinephrine, dopamine and 5-hydroxytryptamine turnover in rat brain areas. J. Pharmacol. Exp. Ther., 220, 678-88

Schildkraut, J.J. (1965). The catecholamine hypothesis of affective disorders: a review of supporting evidence. Am. J. Psychiatry, 122, 509-22

Sevestre, P., Rondot, P., Bathien, N., Morselli, P.L. and Van Landeghem, V.H. (1982). The effect of progabide, a specific GABA-agonist, on neuroleptic-induced tardive dyskinesia. Results of a pilot study. Presented at 13th Collegium International Neuro-psychopharmacologicum, Jerusalem, June 20-25, Abstracts, vol. 2, p. 663

Sulser, F., Vetulani, J. and Mobley, P.L. (1978). Mode of action of antidepressant drugs. Biochem. Pharmacol., 27, 257-61

Van der Linden, G.J., Meinardi, H., Meijer, J.W.A., Bossi, L. and Gomeni, C. (1981). A double blind cross-over trial with progabide (SL 76 002) against placebo in patients with secondary generalized epilepsy. In Advances in Epileptology. The XIIth Epilepsy International Symposium (ed. M. Dam, L. Gram and J.K. Penry), Raven Press, New York, pp. 141-4

Worms, P., Depoortere, H., Durand, A., Morselli, P.L., Lloyd, K.G. and Bartholini, G. (1982). γ-Aminobutyric acid (GABA) receptor stimulation. I. Neuropharmacological profiles of progabide (SL 76 002) and SL 75 102, with emphasis on their anticonvulsant spectra. J. Pharmacol. Exp. Ther., 220, 660-71

Zivkovic, B., Scatton, B., Dedek, J. and Bartholini, G. (1982). GABA influence on noradrenergic and serotoninergic transmissions: possible implications in mood regulation. In New Vistas on Depression (ed. S.Z. Langer, R. Takahashi and M. Briley), Pergamon Press, New York, in press

Benzodiazepine receptor-mediated experimental 'anxiety' in rhesus monkeys after infusion of 3-carboethoxy-ß-carboline (ß-CCE)

Steven M. Paul[1], Philip Ninan[1], Thomas Insel[2] and Phil Skolnick[3]

INTRODUCTION

The presence of specific recognition (viz. receptor) sites for benzodiazepines in brain that are functionally (and perhaps structurally) coupled to both recognition sites for γ-aminobutyric acid (GABA) and a chloride ionophore has been firmly established (cf. Tallman *et al.*, 1980; Paul *et al.*, 1981; Skolnick and Paul, 1982). Both direct and indirect evidence suggest that this 'supramolecular complex' mediates the pharmacological actions of benzodiazepines as well as other structurally unrelated compounds which share common properties with the benzodiazepines (Paul *et al.*, 1981; Skolnick and Paul, 1982). Whether this supramolecular complex has a physiological role in the absence of an exogenous ligand (drug) has been a source of considerable speculation, particularly regarding its function in the pathophysiology of anxiety and related disorders (cf. Paul and Skolnick, 1981).

The report by Braestrup *et al.* (1980) that certain C-3 substituted β-carbolines possess very high affinities for the benzodiazepine receptor stimulated investigation of the pharmacologic actions of these compounds. In general, β-carbolines such as 3-carboethoxy-β-carboline (β-CCE) have been reported to antagonize the actions of benzodiazepines (Tenen and Hirsch, 1980; Cowen *et al.*, 1981; and others). However, more recent work suggests that subtle modification of the C-3 position of this compound results in dramatic changes in pharmacological activity with a spectrum from convulsant (Braestrup *et al.*, 1982; Schweri *et al.*, 1982) to benzodiazepine-like (Skolnick *et al.*, in prep-

[1]Clinical Neuroscience Branch, NIMH, National Institutes of Health, Bethesda, MD 20205, USA.
[2]Clinical Neuropharmacology Branch, NIMH, National Institutes of Health, Bethesda, MD 20205, USA.
[3]Laboratory of Bioorganic Chemistry, NIADDK, National Institutes of Health, Bethesda, MD 20205, USA.

aration). These observations, supported by more detailed neurochemical findings (Skolnick *et al.*, 1982), suggest that the benzodiazepine receptor has several functional 'domains' (or subsites), and that binding of a ligand to a given domain on the receptor can result in opposite pharmacologic and behavioral effects.

Recently, we have examined this hypothesis by studying the behavioral and physiological actions of β-CCE in the rhesus monkey (Ninan *et al.*, submitted). Although most reports in rodents suggest that β-CCE antagonizes the pharmacologic actions of diazepam and related benzodiazepines with no marked behavioral actions by itself (however, see File, 1982), our data suggest that in primates β-CCE elicits a behavioral and physiological state of anxiety manifested by dramatic elevations in plasma cortisol and epinephrine, blood pressure and heart rate. Furthermore, both the behavioral and physiological effects of β-CCE are blocked by pretreatment with the benzodiazepine receptor antagonist, Ro 15-1788 (Hunkeler *et al.*, 1981). These results suggest that the benzodiazepine receptor may not only be involved in the anxiolytic actions of benzodiazepines and related compounds, but may also play a pivotal role in both the pathogenesis of 'anxiety' and its pathophysiologic sequelae in man.

MATERIALS AND METHODS

Adult male rhesus monkeys (7-10 kg) were administered β-CCE i.v. (2.5 mg kg^{-1}) in 10 ml of 20% diluted Emulphor® - 80% 0.9% NaCl (cf. Skolnick *et al.*, 1980) during a 2 min interval. All animals were previously fitted with femoral venous catheters under ketamine anesthesia and placed in chairs at least 24 h prior to administration of drug or vehicle. The i.v. catheters were kept patent by administering a slow i.v. infusion of sterile 0.9% NaCl over the course of the experiment. The dose of β-CCE used (2.5 mg kg^{-1}) was empirically chosen based on the reported affinity of this compound for the benzodiazepine receptor (∿1 nM) and previous studies demonstrating its very rapid metabolism when incubated with rodent plasma at 37°C (Mendelson *et al.*, 1982).

In this experimental protocol, animals were administered β-CCE or vehicle on the morning of day 1. On day 2, the same animals were administered Ro 15-1788 (5 mg kg^{-1}) 10 min prior to receiving an identical dose of β-CCE. In all studies, blood samples (1 ml) were collected at 20 min intervals beginning 40 min prior to the drug or vehicle infusion, and continuing for up to 4 h. Blood pressure and pulse rate were monitored automatically at 5 min intervals using a Dinamap Research Monitor (Model 1245) (Applied Medical Research). Plasma cortisol levels were measured by radioimmunoassay (New England Nuclear, Boston, MA). Behavior of the animals was videotaped during both vehicle and drug administration for subsequent rating by 'blind' investigators.

RESULTS

Administration of β-CCE (2.5 mg kg^{-1}) elicited significant behavioral changes in all of the monkeys examined. Although both the time course and intensity of these changes varied among individual animals, they were easily distinguished from vehicle-treated animals. The behavioral effects of β-CCE included: increased rotation of the head and neck; hyperexcitability to external stimuli (e.g. hand clap); increased vocalizations; defecation and urination; hand clasping and hand wringing; intense scratching (sufficient to cause bleeding in some animals); and a heightened responsiveness to threatening stimuli. Many of these actions were apparent within 10 min after injection, and lasted for up to 2 h. In a number of animals, this increase in excitability was followed by a period of sedation, and in some cases sleep. Concomitant with the behavioral effects of β-CCE, there was a dramatic increase in heart rate (pulse) and mean arterial blood pressure. Figure 1 depicts the β-CCE-induced elevation of heart rate and blood pressure in a typical experiment. These changes are most likely caused by an increase in circulating plasma catecholamines observed following β-CCE administration (Ninan *et al.*, submitted). Since elevations of plasma cortisol can occur under stressful or anxiety-provoking situations in both laboratory animals and man, we examined the effects of β-CCE administration on plasma cortisol. A dramatic and highly significant elevation of plasma cortisol was observed following β-CCE administration (Figure 2). The elevations in plasma cortisol peaked at about 80 min and lasted for as long as 5-6 h (figure 2 and unpublished observations).

   If the behavioral and physiological effects of β-CCE were mediated by a specific interaction with the benzodiazepine receptor, then pre-treatment with a benzodiazepine antagonist should prevent or blunt the response to β-CCE. Pre-treatment of monkeys with Ro 15-1788 (5 mg kg^{-1}) 10 min prior to injection of β-CCE completely reversed the elevation of plasma cortisol (figure 2) and greatly attenuated the elevation of both blood pressure and heart rate (data not shown). Ro 15-1788 had no significant behavioral or physiological actions when administered alone, although there was a slight trend toward decreased heart rate and blood pressure (unpublished observations).

DISCUSSION

β-CCE binds to benzodiazepine receptors with high affinity and has been previously shown to antagonize some of the pharmacological actions of benzodiazepines in rodents (Tenen and Hirsch, 1980; Cowen *et al.*, 1981; and others), while eliciting no obvious behavioral changes when administered alone. However, a very recent

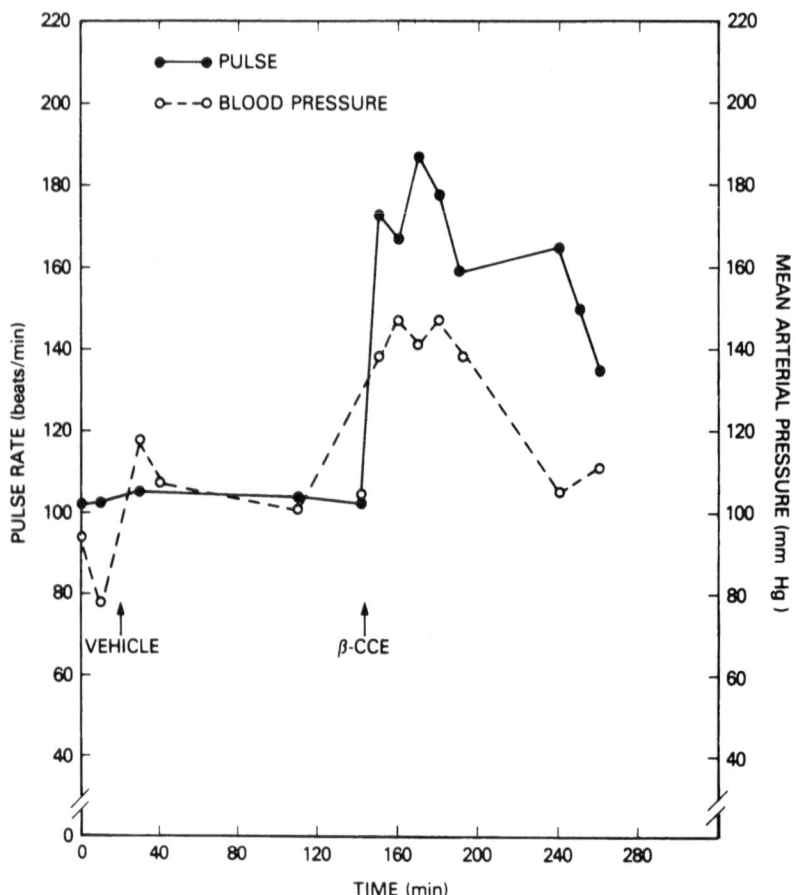

Figure 1. Effects of β-CCE on pulse rate and mean arterial blood
pressure. In this representative experiment, a male
rhesus monkey was injected with vehicle, and the pulse
rate and mean arterial blood pressure monitored for 2 h.
Following administration of β-CCE (2.5 mg kg^{-1} i.v.), a
marked rise in both blood pressure and pulse rate was
observed.

report (File, 1982) suggests that, in a test of social interaction, this compound exerted an action 'opposite' to that of the
benzodiazepines, which could be interpreted as 'anxiety'. However,
to our knowledge, the physiological and behavioral actions of
β-CCE have not been examined in primates.

In the rhesus monkey, β-CCE elicited a profound elevation in
the circulating levels of stress-related hormones such as cortisol

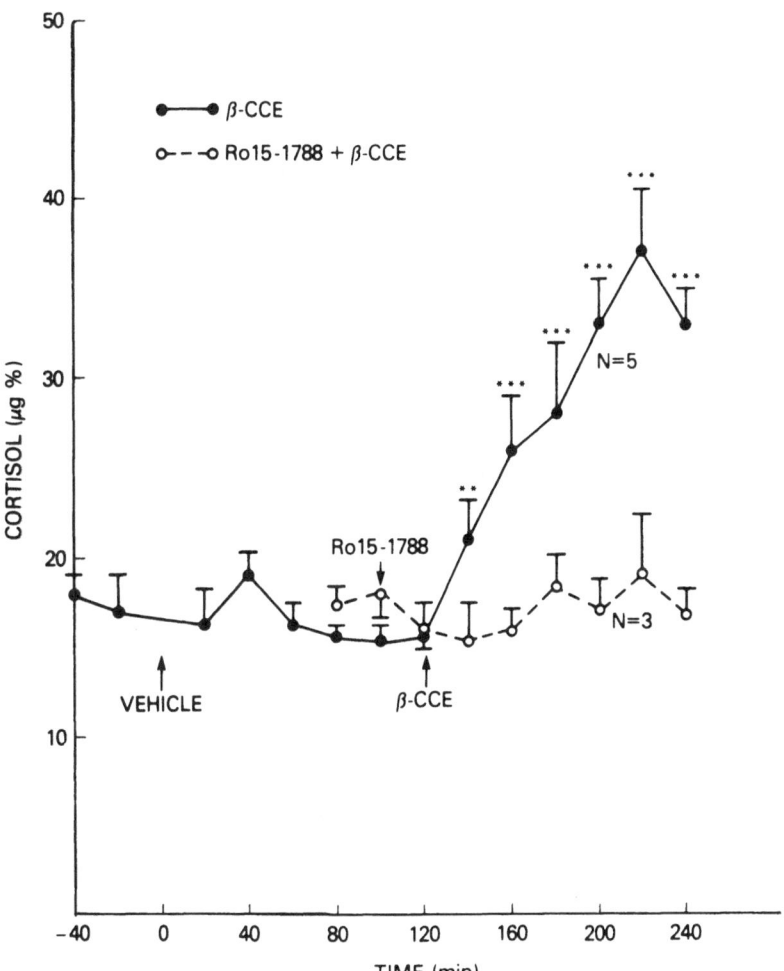

Figure 2. Effects of β-CCE and Ro 15-1788 on plasma cortisol
levels.   Rhesus monkeys were injected with vehicle, and
the plasma cortisol levels were monitored by
radioimmunoassay as described in the text.   At the times
indicated by arrows, β-CCE (2.5 mg kg^{-1} i.v.) was
administered alone (filled circles) or 10 min after
treatment with Ro 15-1788 (5 mg kg^{-1} i.v.) (open
circles). Symbols: ** $p < 0.01$, *** $p < 0.001$ compared
to a combination of Ro 15-1788 + β-CCE at the corresponding time point.   These data were evaluated using
Student's t-test.

and epinephrine. Concomitant with these endocrine changes, a dramatic increase in the somatic manifestation of 'anxious' behavior was also observed, reflected as an elevated heart rate and blood pressure. Furthermore, a wide range of behaviors were elicited by β–CCE which were not observed in vehicle-treated animals, many of which could be interpreted as 'anxious'.

The effects of β–CCE on the endocrine, somatic and behavioral parameters used in these studies are reminiscent of those typically observed in anxious patients and/or animals and humans exposed to anxiety-provoking or stressful situations. That these effects are mediated through the benzodiazepine receptor is supported by the blockade or muting of these effects by pre-treatment with the specific benzodiazepine receptor antagonist, Ro 15–1788. Taken together, these results suggest that the benzodiazepine–GABA receptor-chloride ionophore complex not only mediates the pharmacological actions of the benzodiazepines but may also subserve the affective and physiological expression of anxiety.

REFERENCES

Braestrup, C., Nielsen, M. and Olsen, C. (1980). Urinary and brain β-carboline-3-carboxylates as potent inhibitors of brain benzodiazepine receptors. Proc. Natl Acad. Sci. USA, 77, 2288–92

Braestrup, C., Schmiechen, R., Neef, G., Nielsen, M. and Petersen, E. (1982). Interaction of convulsive ligands with benzodiazepine receptors. Science, 216, 1241–3

Cowen, P., Green, A., Nutt, D. and Martin, I. (1981). Ethyl-β-carboline-3-carboxylate lowers seizure threshold and antagonizes flurazepam-induced sedation in rats. Nature, 290, 54–5

File, S. (1982). Animal anxiety and the effects of benzodiazepines. In Pharmacology of Benzodiazepines (ed. S. Paul, P. Skolnick, J. Tallman and E. Usdin), Macmillan, London, in press

Hunkeler, W., Mohler, H., Pieri, L., Polc, P., Bonetti, E., Cumin, R., Schaffner, R. and Haefely, W. (1981). Selective antagonists of benzodiazepines. Nature, 290, 514–16

Mendelson, W., Cain, M., Cook, J., Paul, S. and Skolnick, P. (1982). Do benzodiazepine receptors plays a role in sleep regulation: studies with the benzodiazepine antagonist, 3-hydroxymethyl-β-carboline (3-HMC). In Beta-Carbolines and Tetra-isoquinolines (ed. E. Usdin), Alan R. Liss, New York, in press

Paul, S., Marangos, P. and Skolnick, P. (1981). The benzodiazepine-GABA receptor chloride ionophore complex: common site of minor tranquilizer action. Biol. Psychiat., 16, 213–29

Paul, S. and Skolnick, P. (1981). Benzodiazepine receptors and psychopathological states: towards a neurobiology of anxiety.

In Anxiety: New Research and Changing Concepts (ed. D. Klein
    and J. Rabkin), Raven Press, New York, pp. 215-33
Schweri, M., Cain, M., Cook, J., Paul, S. and Skolnick, P. (1982).
    Blockade of 3-carbomethoxy-β-carboline induced seizures by
    diazepam and the benzodiazepine antagonists Ro 15-1788 and
    CGS 8216. Pharmacol., Biochem. Behav., in press
Skolnick, P., Lock, K.-L., Paugh, B., Marangos, P., Windsor, R.
    and Paul, S. (1980). Pharmacologic and behavioral effects of
    EMD 28422: a novel purine which enhances [^{3}H]diazepam binding
    to brain benzodiazepine receptors. Pharmacol., Biochem. Be-
    hav., 12, 685-9
Skolnick, P. and Paul, S. (1982). Molecular pharmacology of the
    benzodiazepines. Int. Rev. Neurobiol., 23, 103-40
Skolnick, P., Schweri, M., Kutter, E., Williams, E. and Paul, E.
    (1982). Inhibition of [^{3}H]diazepam and 3-carboethoxy-β-
    carboline binding by irazepine: evidence for binding to
    different 'domains' of the benzodiazepine receptor. J. Neuro-
    chem., in press
Tallman, J., Paul, S., Skolnick, P. and Gallager, D. (1980).
    Receptors for the age of anxiety: molecular pharmacology of
    the benzodiazepines. Science, 207, 274-81
Tenen, S. and Hirsch, J. (1980). β-Carboline-3-carboxylic acid
    ethyl ester antagonizes diazepam activity. Nature, 288,
    609-10

Contributors' index*

---

* Numbers indicate starting pages of chapters

Subject index*

---

*Numbers indicate starting pages of chapters.